REAL FOOD, FAKE FOOD

FAKE FOOD

and Everything in Between

Also by Geri Harrington

Health and Life-style

The Health Insurance Fact and Answer Book
The Medicare Answer Book
Never Too Old: A Complete Guide for the Over-Fifty Adult

Energy

Total Warmth: The Complete Guide to Winter Well-Being
Fireplace Stoves, Hearths and Inserts
The Wood-Burning Stove Book

Gardening and Cookery

Cash Crops for Thrifty Gardeners
The New College Cookbook
Grow Your Own Chinese Vegetables
The Salad Book
Summer Garden, Winter Kitchen
The College Cookbook

REAL FOOD, FAKE FOOD

and Everything in Between

The Only Consumer's Guide to Modern Food

Geri Harrington

Macmillan Publishing Company, Inc.
New York

Macmillan Publishing Company
866 Third Avenue, New York, N.Y. 10022
Collier Macmillan Canada, Inc.

Library of Congress Cataloging-in-Publication Data
Harrington, Geri.
    Real food, fake food, and everything in between.
    Bibliography: p.
    Includes index.
    1. Food additives. 2. Food—Composition.
3. Nutrition. I. Title.
TX553.A3H37   1987   613.2   86–31327
ISBN 0–02–548420–6

Macmillan books are available at special discounts for bulk purchases
for sales promotions, premiums, fund-raising, or educational use.
For details, contact:

    Special Sales Director
    Macmillan Publishing Company
    866 Third Avenue
    New York, N.Y. 10022

Designed by Nancy Sugihara

10 9 8 7 6 5 4 3 2 1

Printed in the United States of America

to Hillel Black

*because over the years he's always been there with support and
encouragement when it was needed*

Contents

PART THREE

Real Food

PART FOUR

Real Food at Risk

PART FIVE

When the Government Lends a Helping Hand

PART SIX

Getting the Facts

PART SEVEN

Taking Charge of Your Life and Your Health

Acknowledgments

There is not enough room to list the names of all the many great people who helped make this book possible by furnishing me with data, materials, help, encouragement, and advice. But I do want to thank especially Dr. Denham Harman, whose lucid explanation of his free radical theory clarified much I had not understood about the aging process of the body. Also, special thanks to Dr. Edward R. Pinckney who always responded by phone and by mail with a wealth of information and published and unpublished materials, which have given me a firm grounding in the role of fats in human nutrition. I would like to thank also the many staffers at the Food and Drug Administration who patiently answered my questions even when it meant time-consuming research on their part, especially Rees B. Davis, assistant director for packaging technology, Dennis M. Dignan, food technologist, and Emil Corwin of the press office. And at the U.S. Department of Agriculture, especially Hettie Ohringer and Frank Hepburn of the Nutrient Data Research Branch, and Ruth Matthew, Carol Davis, and Diane Odlin of Human Nutrition Information Services, as well as Nancy Raper for making food supply data available, and especially a nutrient analysis of the national food supply. In addition, I owe an ongoing debt for all the help I have received here and over many years from Dr. Lester Hankin of the Connecticut Agricultural Experiment Station, and from Michael Jacobson and Bonnie Liebman of the Center for Science in the Public Interest.

Last but not least I want to express my appreciation to the entire staff of the Wilton Library, especially those indefatigable reference librarians, David Ostergren and Beth Mason, as well as Marion Simplicio, all of whom always found out what I needed to know even when I wasn't entirely sure myself how to describe it.

INTRODUCTION

What This Book Can Do for You

Man, alone among the animals, will eat almost anything. Of course, tastes differ: some South American Indians relish white grubs, while the Chinese eat sea cucumbers. Most Americans will eat whatever is either sweet enough or salty enough, no matter what it is made of or how much processing it has undergone. The only problem is that while we are pleasing our palates, we are shortchanging our health.

Since the primary function of food is to nourish, any food that does not nourish as it was meant to is not real. If it is presented as real food, it is fake. If we are fooled into eating it instead of real food, we are unwittingly doing ourselves harm.

Theoretically all the "foods" in the market are edible; that is, more or less safe to eat (how safe we will see later on). But it is getting harder and harder to distinguish real foods—foods that are inherently nourishing— from products that are less nourishing or nourishing only by reason of added supplements. But there are more new, fabricated foods invented every day.

Fortunately, consumers are beginning to realize that what they eat has a lot to do with how well they feel, how successfully they resist disease, how they cope with pollution and stress, and even how long they live. Because they care, they have already led food manufacturers to make low-salt soup, canned fruits in lighter syrup, and ice cream with real flavorings. Baby food no longer contains monosodium glutamate (MSG), and meat is leaner. More and more consumers want to know which food is real and which, for instance, contains more salt, sugar, and even artificial ingredients than real food would require. How to tell the difference so you can make an informed choice is what this book is all about.

PART ONE

Understanding Modern Food

CHAPTER 1

How to Know What You're Eating

It's not easy to know what you're eating—some food today may be perfectly edible and good-tasting but not nourishing in the way you expect—and that's important. If you understand what you are eating, you may still choose a particular food; on the other hand, you may prefer to do without it. A food may contain nutrient supplements to replace those lost in processing. If you are avoiding supplements or keeping track of them, you need to know. Or a food may merely contain more fat or more salt than you would ordinarily expect, upsetting your low-fat or low-salt diet. Fortunately, it is often possible to identify this kind of food.

The first place to look for clues is right on the package. And over 60 percent of consumers do read the labels on foods. However, many don't realize that the information to be found there is often misleading. Despite government attempts to assure accuracy, most manufacturers use packages and labels as billboards to promote the product rather than to help the consumer.

Take, for example, some low-calorie TV dinners that brag about "all natural ingredients," no sugar, and only 60% as much sodium as comparable products. Unfortunately the package is liable to feature these pluses but not the fact that over 70 percent of the calories come from fat. If you are looking for a low-fat—as well as a low-calorie—product, you might have a problem with this. Most nutrition-conscious consumers are looking not only to reduce their caloric but also their fat intake, and this high a fat content might make a diet product no less fatty than the standard no-diet ones.

3

This type of omission illustrates a common problem for the consumer. It is completely truthful, but the consumer may come away with a false impression of the contents of the package.

Another way a package may be misleading without actually being untruthful is by stipulating a smaller-than-usual serving size. Reading the package may make you think the product is low-calorie. This practice is widespread, so the consumer should always compare serving sizes before comparing calories or nutrient information.

Food packages may exaggerate benefits by oversimplifying. Bran cereals that advertise that "fiber prevents cancer" don't go out of their way to tell you only oat bran is thought to have potential for preventing cancer. A corn oil that claimed using it would lower high blood pressure impressively cited five studies to support its claims. The National Council of Better Business Bureaus, in reviewing the advertising for fairness and accuracy, said the studies cited weren't conclusive.

Translating advertising claims can be difficult. One chicken noodle soup claimed it contained more protein than a peanut butter sandwich, "calorie for calorie." It does. You may not realize, however, that since a peanut butter sandwich contains ten times as many calories as a bowl of the soup, it also contains ten times as much actual protein.

The consumer's first real insight into whether a food is real is provided by a careful look at the label's nutrition information and ingredients list. Remember, the list of ingredients contains not only the chemical additives that are required to be listed but also *added* vitamin and mineral nutrients. And this kind of nutrition information may be a smoke screen to disguise what you are really buying. Fake foods, such as some cold breakfast cereals, have little food value in themselves; most of their nutrition comes from the few added vitamin and mineral supplements. If you discover the only food value in the product is in the added vitamin and mineral supplements, you may decide it would be cheaper and simpler to take your own supplements instead of paying premium prices for them as additives.

Crude fiber information is nutritionally meaningless. Do not make the mistake of comparing it to dietary fiber. (For a fuller discussion, see Chapter 22, Fiber—Why Bran Is Not Enough.) The source of fiber is important; cellulose is often wood or lint fiber—not necessarily what you want to eat or the kind that will produce the desired result; for example, some kinds of fiber are constipating.

Often reading ingredients requires translating them. For instance, wheat flour is not the same as whole wheat flour. Enriched wheat flour is bleached white flour with a few nutrients put back in to replace the many that have been processed out of the whole wheat. "Vegetable oils" doesn't mean the oil is unsaturated; coconut oil and palm oil are more highly saturated than beef fat.

It is also important to bear in mind that not all additives are listed. If the government has established permissible ingredients for a given product, called "standards of identity," the package need not list any of those ingredients. But "permissible ingredients" may include many additives, artificial colors, and other undesirable items.

In many cases it may not be possible to determine whether a product is real solely by looking at well-designed labels. But there are other telltale signs, such as the following.

` Basic Checklist

Many of the foods you may want to avoid or at least eat less of have the following characteristics:

A fancy name. The manufacturer may not want to use the word *imitation* in the name of the product. He avoids this by using a made-up name. Miracle Whip, for a mayonnaise-type product; "coffee whitener" to describe a nondairy product; "King Krab," for noncrab fish.

"Flavored." Vanilla-flavored ice cream is not made with real vanilla; vanilla ice cream is. The less forthright the name or description, the less likely the product is to be the real thing.

New. There aren't any truly new foods. Some foods from other parts of the world may not be familiar to us but they have been around a long time in their native lands. If a food is promoted as being new, examine it carefully. Unless it is a whole fresh fruit or vegetable that you've never seen before, be suspicious. It is probably merely another fabricated item. While a few new products, such as unsweetened sorbets, are improvements, many are not. Most "new" foods are highly processed laboratory concoctions that may be less desirable than the originals. Many new yogurt products, for example, are less desirable than plain yogurt, to which you can add your own fresh fruits and vegetables or unsweetened preserves. Many are high in fat and sugar and not as healthful. You can usually recognize this type of "new" product because it will contain unfamiliar chemical additives not found in the original.

Unnecessary ingredients. Real food shouldn't need added flavor. No product *needs* artificial anything. Peanut butter, cottage cheese, and many other products need not contain anything but basic ingredients (such as peanuts and, maybe, peanut oil). There is no reason peanut butter should contain any sugar whatsoever. (In fact, sugar is one of the most overused additives because it is often used to cover lack of real flavor.)

Highly promoted. When is the last time you saw a cents-off coupon for pearl tapioca, fresh pineapple, bananas, olive oil, or honey? Although all are well-advertised products with brand names, they are seldom promoted by coupons because the profit margin is low compared to cat and dog food, highly sugared cereals, vegetable oils, and instant pudding mixes. Newspapers feature cents-off coupons, but sometimes you can go through an entire eight-page four-color supplement and not find one "food" you'd want to buy at any price.

Gussied-up. Real food is plain food. A butter-basted turkey can't compare with a high-quality turkey that has not been injected with fat. Frozen vegetables in butter or seasoned sauces are less desirable than plain frozen vegetables you dress up yourself. Ten varieties of cream or cottage cheese don't make as much sense as one package of plain with which you can do whatever you like.

Price. Real food is usually cheaper. If it is more expensive, it's because the manufacturer has had to use better ingredients because the additives that disguise inferior quality have been left out. It may also be more expensive because the manufacturer thinks the consumer wants real food enough to pay more for it. Nutrient for nutrient, real food is always a better buy. Real rice and real potatoes, for example, are a real bargain compared to seasoned rice and instant potatoes.

In addition to being able to identify the nature of individual products by studying the products themselves, it is important to recognize industry trends in fabricated foods. The following classic examples of fabricated foods are an indication of the type of products that are being made today.

Fabricated Food Trends

Food from Outer Space

Space exploration has accelerated the creation of new types of food because it has special requirements. Among the many problems the astronauts have had to contend with are limited storage space, eating under conditions of weightlessness, and the problem of food preparation, with weight and space limitations controlling the availability of cooking and refrigeration equipment. The first space food was dehydrated food in pouches. The astronauts added water and reconstituted the food by kneading it and squeezing it from a tube, like toothpaste, so that food particles would not get loose and float around the tiny cabin. Many ingenious variations on this method were devised, from highly compressed foods to a spacecraft, parts of which were edible.

On more recent voyages an effort has been made to create food that looks and tastes more like what the astronauts are used to on Earth. This is difficult because the result in space is not always what earthbound food scientists think it will be; food even tastes different in space. Also a certain amount of hype has crept into the picture; for example, Pepsi and Coke angled to be first in space (the compromise was both of them going). The element of hype that surrounds certain areas of the space program is unfortunate when it affects the consumer's food. Certainly the requirements for food designed for those conditions should not be glossed over when the same food is promoted to the public as being suitable for an on-Earth diet. Yet some products create initial consumer acceptance by capitalizing on their association with the space program; if an entire astronaut meal were included in a taste test, it might put the product in better perspective.

Hard-boiled "Eggs"

It used to be that you could trust a hard-boiled egg. If you found yourself eating at a questionable "greasy-spoon" counter joint, you ordered a hard-boiled-egg sandwich and the sandwich maker shelled an egg then and there or, at worst, took a whole egg from a dish full of them. He sliced the egg, slathered mayonnaise on the bread, and you had a genuine hard-boiled-egg sandwich. But not anymore. Hard-boiled "eggs" can now be created by a process called extrusion, in which various oils, stabilizers, binders, artificial food colors, and other ingredients are made into a paste, then forced through a machine called an extruder into whatever shape is desired by the manufacturer.

If you happen to see your sandwich being made, the counterman may work from a dish of sliced eggs, along with sliced tomatoes and other fixings. What you don't know is whether these eggs came from a chicken or from an extruded sausagelike roll cut up into "hard-boiled-egg" slices. These "egg" rolls are really ingenious. The eggless "yolk" can be made from vegetable oil, milk solids, emulsifiers, and other additives, appropriately colored and flavored and surrounded by equally unreal "egg white." Another "egg" manufacturer makes the yolk in a similar fashion, adding vitamins and various other ingredients and pasteurizing it before freezing it. Not only is this available to restaurants, it is also used by hospitals, where the nutrition needs of the ill should be given higher priority. Given time, you may even be able to buy this product in the supermarket and make party canapes with it, adding dollops of synthetic caviar (a suspension the Russians developed about fifteen years ago, composed of casein and gelatin fabricated into a water-immiscible liquid to form jellylike beadlets, firmed with a tanning agent and colored according to whether the caviar is imitation sturgeon, salmon, or other fish eggs). If you have eaten caviar lately, did you think it tasted a bit "unusual" ?

These eggs, incidentally, are sometimes described as being beneficial to the consumer because they are "low in cholesterol," without any mention of all the good egg nutrients they totally lack and all the chemical additives they contain. And if you're keeping track of your cholesterol and nutrient intake, not knowing whether an egg is real may result in a nutrient-deficient diet.

Enriched White Bread

Enriched bread is so called because, while much of the good has been taken out of it, a few nutrients have been put back, thus enriching it. The nutrients put back are usually the synthetic vitamins and minerals: niacin, riboflavin, thiamine, vitamin D, calcium, and iron. Real whole grain breads, on the other hand, contain all the above plus biotin, pantothenic acid, pyridoxine, copper, manganese, phosphorus, potassium, and two amino acids, lysine and tryptophan—and these are natural, not synthetic.

"Pimiento-stuffed" Olives

Pimiento-stuffed olives used to be stuffed only with strips of real pimiento. Now they may contain a gum instead that only incidentally contains a bit of minced pimiento.

Restaurants That Smell Enticing

All those good smells you associate with home cooking—Mom's apple pie, baked ham, fresh-baked bread—can now be bought in a spray can. Precooked food from a central commissary, reheated in a microwave oven and kept hot under lights, doesn't generate those mouth-watering odors, so many restaurants spray their dining rooms to create the illusion of the presence of real food. Don't be fooled by an appetizing smell—it, too, may be fake.

Fabricated Foods You May Not Recognize

Even taking all possible precautions, you may not be able to evaluate certain foods. Meat, for example, may be so heavily processed or have so many artificial ingredients that you might, at best, consider some of it to be "in between" real and fake. Milk, except for imitation milk, filled milk, and similar products, all of which are clearly labeled, is real; but its nutritional value may have been altered by processing, pasteurization, homogenization, blending, and other techniques. Cheese presents the same problem. Fish may be totally denatured and then formed to look like shrimp, crab, lobster, and other expensive shellfish, or perhaps treated with preservatives that may not agree with you. In the next chapter we will talk about products that fall into this category.

CHAPTER 2

Fabricated, Processed, and Altered Foods

Only a food chemist can really know what today's food is made of or what's been done to it. Artificial flavor may be added to cottage cheese; spaghetti may be made out of fish paste; caviar may be jelled vegetable oil. In addition, there's an increasingly large gray area between the real and the out-and-out fake. Fake "food" may contain a bit of the real thing—for example, butter is now frequently added to margarine. As time goes on, more and more processes and additives are entering into the manufacture of an increasing percentage of our foods, and the consumer who wishes to eat only real food must buy carefully and selectively. Here are some examples of the choices confronting the consumer who goes to the market.

Manufactured Meat—No Home on the Range

If you haven't had a good steak lately, don't blame the cook; blame today's methods of raising beef. The quality of beef has deteriorated to the point that a United States congressman actually stood up at a congressional hearing to complain about its lack of taste and flavor. Congressman Leo W. O'Brien (New York) hit the nail on the head when he said, "I have an idea that our mothers had a little better meat to work with in the beginning." He was speaking in 1965; in the twenty-two years since, it has all been downhill.

Beef used to come from animals that roamed free on the range, eating from the land. They grew at a natural pace, maturing in three or four years, and were slaughtered when they left the range. That was called raising beef.

10

Today beef is not raised, it is manufactured. From the day of its birth the average beef animal is treated like processed food. The range is a dim memory, replaced by unnatural "feedlots" where the animals are crowded together so that they are handy. Raising range-fed animals is considered inefficient, and modern meat manufacturing is nothing if not efficient.

If a man is what he eats, it's hard to know what to call beef animals. Their "feed" is liable to be almost anything that can be artificially flavored and scented to get the animal to eat it. In his devastating description of the meat industry, *Modern Meat,* Orville Schell describes his visit to a feed company that was using discarded waxed cardboard cartons as an ingredient. Ranchers in France and other European countries are experimenting with similar unnatural and nonnutritious materials; the nutrients are made up with some feed and supplements. Some experimental foods have been notably unsuccessful, including feathers and the animals' own waste, but scientists are still working to make them a viable alternative.

Since growing conditions are now so unhealthy, animals must be given all types of medicines to prevent the spread of disease. The meat growers reaped an unexpected bonus when they accidentally found that a side effect of administering antibiotics was to speed animal growth. They tried giving these potent drugs subtherapeutically (in other words, even when the animals weren't sick) and found the animals thus treated were ready for market in record time. On the heels of this discovery the use of antibiotics accelerated rapidly, and in 1984 it was reported in a publication by the Committee on the Scientific Basis of the Nation's Meat and Poultry Inspection Program that antibiotics were being added to the feed of farm animals in quantities of between nine and fifteen million pounds a year. (See Chapter 25, The Antibiotic Steak.)

In the meantime, scientific methods were developed to encourage the animals to gorge themselves on food to fatten them up faster. Just as with chickens, beef feedlots are lit around the clock, and the animals, totally confused by the lack of a natural night, eat twenty-four hours a day. Due possibly to these methods and possibly to lack of natural exercise, beef fat has changed materially so that today it is a much less healthful and desirable and a much more saturated product than formerly.

Much has been written about the stress all this inflicts on the animals; it is another factor that affects the quality and the nutrition value of the meat unfavorably. The meat industry has solved this problem with still another group of drugs: the animals are fed tranquilizers.

Unknown hazards to the consumer exist in all these practices, which permeate the flesh. For instance, the report referred to before described how chlorine in water used in processing the meat "has been recovered from animal lipids, depending on the concentration of chlorine to which the carcass has been exposed.'' The danger to the consumer has become so great that in 1985 the National Residue Program (NRP), the principal regulatory mechanism for determining the presence and level of chemicals in meat and poultry, targeted the following animals for continuous monitoring: horses, bulls, cows, heifers, steers, calves, sheep, lambs, goats, hogs, young and mature chickens, young and mature turkeys, ducks, geese, and rabbits.

The consumption of beef has dropped considerably in the last few years, due largely to the public's fear of cholesterol and saturated fat. To stop falling sales, the meat industry is presently raising leaner, but not tastier, beef. It doesn't seem to have occurred to them that improving the taste might also make a difference.

In addition to the processing of meat on the hoof, there are even further meat fabrications.

Soy ''Meat''

Soy products are useful because they create meatlike items, which vegetarians can use to make their diet more interesting and to provide needed protein. As long as these products are sold as soy made into meat, no objection can be made on the ground that they are not real meat; however, the processing it takes to make soy into a meatlike product may not be clear to the consumer.

To turn soy into meat, soybean proteins are dissolved into alkali. The resultant sticky liquid is then extruded through tiny holes, and the fibers are recoagulated in an acid bath. They are then spun into ropes with the appropriate texture, depending on whether chicken, ham, fish, or beef muscle tissue is wanted. At this point the product is more or less odorless, tasteless, and colorless, but that is soon remedied with fat, artificial flavorings, and artificial colors. (Real flavorings and colors are infrequently used because their flavor is not as stable, controllable, or cheap.) At this stage the product can be further processed by dehydration, compression, freezing, and the like. An example of the finished product is ''bacon'' chips, as well as some of the vegetable protein (soy) mixtures that many supermarkets featured for a time as an additive to hamburger (to produce a more inexpensive ground beef). Soy is a versatile product and can be disguised as any of a number of other foods.

Tenderized Beef

Pretenderized beef is another product you may unwittingly purchase. Beef manufactured by today's methods is already more tender than range-fed beef ever could be, but cattlemen have found a way to make it even more so: tenderizing enzymes are injected into the live animal just before slaughter, and the tenderizer is dispersed through the animal's tissue through the pumping of its heart. Without a label, the consumer has no way of knowing whether this has taken place.

Beef Flakes

Many consumers are not familiar with all the various cuts of beef and, once they have identified porterhouse, sirloin, and chuck steaks, must turn to the butcher for information as to how to cook the day's special. Among the possible beef "cuts" is one that has been made from flake-cut beef particles held together by processing that has released soluble myosin during mixing, thus allowing the flakes to be given "steak" shape and texture by controlled pressure. If this is not what you had in mind for your steak dinner, be sure you know what you are buying.

Mechanically Deboned Meat

Mechanically deboning meat (MDM) is another comparatively innovative process. Instead of—and in some instances, in addition to—hand deboning, this kind is done by grinding the bones (with whatever meat still adheres to them) and then forcing them against screens or perforated drums. The meat goes through the holes but, theoretically, the bones and sinews do not. Of course, this process utilizes meat that formerly was left on the bones by hand deboning; a certain percentage of ground bone, however, gets through the holes and is incorporated with the meat. In its April 1978 issue the *National Food Review* described the result as "a paste-like product."

Consumer groups have fought the use of MDM in processed meat products, but in 1978 a regulation allowing a 20 percent MDM content in processed meats was passed. This is represented as a "consumer benefit" in the form of cheaper meat. That the product is a cheaper product is apparently not relevant.

Consumer groups have not totally given up the fight. They have retreated to another position. Their new goal is to have meat thus processed labeled *mechanically deboned meat*. The meat processors not only are fighting this designation but are demanding the right to add extra "calcium" (the ground bone fragments) to the nutrient listing of these products.

Ham

It might seem strange to think of water as an additive, but if you have bought whole hams lately, you may have noticed that it is almost impossible to get one that is not labeled *water added*. A water-added ham is just that: ham that has had water injected into it. Instead of producing a delicious natural ham, this ham is made "moist and juicy" artificially—and you pay ham prices for the added water. You also pay a price in flavor; ham is another food that doesn't have the full rich flavor it used to.

The water-added process developed from a curing method that originally involved immersing the ham in brine, a form of pickling. This was "improved" by a process that pumped the brine directly into the meat through hollow needles. Fast as this process was, compared to the old method, it was speeded up even more when processors discovered they could inject the brine directly into arterial cavities. In addition to speed, this new method had another advantage: it made it possible to "overpump"the ham and led to what the United States Department of Agriculture (USDA) characterized as "dishonest ham."

Regulations were passed to try to curb the worst of these abuses, but in the 1950s processors discovered that adding phosphates to the brine had two salutary effects (from the processors' point of view). It speeded fluid absorption into ham tissues and increased the amount of total fluid absorbed. For some reason the USDA was not bothered by these "dishonest hams" and did not ban the use of phosphates for this purpose.

Theoretically, the consumer was still protected from overpumping by the original order that had required pumped hams to be brought back to their original weight. In spite of that, processors were able to get around this regulation and hams were marketed that contained as much as 30 percent water. In the following years the pressure on the USDA from the industry increased, and water was officially sanctioned as an additive in ham.

Aside from the detrimental effect on flavor, quality, and nutrient density, water-added hams—which may by law be 10 percent water—are a poor buy, with 10 percent of the price the consumer pays going for nonfood. If you can find ham that is not labeled *ham—water added*, it's worth 10 percent more to get all ham and true flavor. One more note of caution: if hams are cured within the state in which you buy them, the law allows up to 30 percent water added—in which case one-third of your ham money is buying water.

Poultry

Self-basting poultry, especially turkey, is popular with many cooks who doubt their own ability to produce a juicy, moist roast. The manufacturer generally injects a mixture of vegetable oils, water, salt, emulsifiers, and artificial flavor and color under the skin at several points. This mess melts during roasting, and the natural flavor, if any, of the turkey is overwhelmed by the far less desirable flavors.

Aside from the fact that nothing is easier to roast than a good turkey, and that it doesn't take a minute longer to do it yourself without its being artificially gussied up, this type of product encourages the manufacturer to cut corners and produce a less than excellent bird. A good turkey is naturally moist, flavorful, and practically foolproof to roast. But not all turkeys are good, and the cook must have confidence that a dry, tasteless bird is the manufacturer's fault, not hers. If it is treated with processed oils and flavors, how can you tell whether it was of good quality to start with? Ask yourself why a self-basting turkey pretends to baste itself with "butter" when it generally contains nothing of the sort.

A simple, foolproof way to roast a turkey is to butter or oil the underside of a piece of heavy-duty foil large enough to completely cover the turkey, with tucked-in sides. Then roast it in a 350-degree Fahrenheit oven according to size and whether or not it is stuffed, removing the foil for the last hour of cooking. (If you're not sure it's done when it's supposed to be, just jiggle a drumstick. If the turkey is done, it will move freely. Once you have made a few roasts, you'll know when it's done without checking.) No fuss, no basting; just a moist, juicy, beautifully brown roast turkey served with the knowledge that you did it all yourself—and didn't contribute to the family's intake of unneeded additives and oils. Don't encourage the production of inferior birds made salable by additives; if it hasn't occurred to poultry manufacturers to produce inferior birds, why give them the idea? If your turkey comes out dry and tasteless, don't hesitate to complain to the butcher; if he tells you to buy a butter-basted turkey next time, tell him you know how to roast a turkey if it is good to start with. You'll find he won't give you an argument; he knows you are right.

Fast-food "Chicken"

As beef has declined in popularity, the demand for chicken has increased, and nowhere has the increase been more spectacular than in the fast-food industry. First there was the colonel's fried chicken, a tasty, reasonably nutritious product. Today the newcomer on the scene is chicken nuggets.

Easy to eat, nuggets are a favorite of both children and adults who never seem to stop to think what they are eating. For some reason most people assume all nuggets are small chunks of chicken breast. They couldn't be more wrong. Some nuggets are minced chicken bits, formed with the help of binders and all sorts of other chemical additives, artificial chicken flavoring, and so on into their familiar shape. They are then cooked in whatever fat the company happens to be using; this could include beef tallow. All you can be sure of is that it isn't butter or chicken fat. Since most fast foods are high in fat and in sodium, nuggets may be, too; how else do you think they get to be so tasty?

Processed Meats

Although it's been shown time and again that bacon, salami, sausage, and other processed meats are a poor buy for your protein food dollar, their popularity persists even among those who need to get all the food value they can for their money. Expensive protein, however, isn't the only disadvantage to these foods.

Compared to other protein sources, such as chicken and fish, processed meats are much higher in fat and sodium. The manufacturers recognize this as a drawback and have responded to it by putting out "lean" versions, but not all of them are bargains.

The reason *lean* does not always mean low in fat is the government labeling regulation controlling appellations of *lean, extra lean, lite,* or *low-fat*. There are no guidelines that say how much fat a lean or any other less-fat product may contain. Any product that contains less fat than the leading brand or than its company's own regular product can call itself lean in comparison. In other words, salami can be called lean if it contains less fat than salami usually has. Inasmuch as many foods of this type get as much as 80 percent of their calories from fat, *lean* doesn't have much meaning. Even if it were half as fat, salami would still not compare favorably to chicken or fish. It can also qualify to be called lean if it contains less fat than its standard of identity, the FDA's profile of acceptable ingredients for a given product.

Average Values of Delicatessen Meats

Product	Fat %	Protein %	Nitrite ppm	Sodium mg/100g	Calories/ 100 g
frankfort and kielbasa	29.0	14.7	13.4	933	332
bologna	28.3	13.8	12.0	957	326
salami and wurst	27.8	17.4	10.2	1145	330
loafs and rolls	18.9	15.5	10.2	959	264

SOURCE: Connecticut Agricultural Experiment Station, September 1984. Report by Dr. Lester Hankin, "Quality of Delicatessen Meats."

Not all processed meats are this high in fat, but without a chart, the consumer has no way of knowing which are which. For instance, among those with under 30 percent of calories from fat are Klement's Jellied Beef Loaf, Armour Turkey Ham, and Eckrich Canadian Style Bacon.

When fat content is high, there isn't room for much nutrition—especially since what room there is must be shared with fillers, sugar, starch, seasonings, gelatin, sodium nitrite, artificial colors and flavors, and preservatives. No wonder it has been estimated that a hot dog roll contains about as much protein as the hot dog.

The saving grace is, of course, that this type of meat is usually consumed in small quantities, especially compared to half a chicken or a small steak, but it certainly isn't your best nutrition buy.

Milk

Milk that has been processed through homogenization and pasteurization and blended to create a bland, uniform product regardless of its origin (you used to be able to tell milk from a Jersey cow from milk from another breed), and that comes from an animal that has been scientifically manufactured to create that fluid, is still a comparatively real product. It's certainly the best we're going to get unless we live near a dairy farm and get to drink the milk reserved for the family. (And the beef raised especially for them). But milk and milk products lend themselves to imitation, and the consumer seems to have accepted this without question. The question should be, why not the real thing?

The answer is that manufacturing milk and milk products is a business, and a business's prime objective is to make a profit. The ideal milk, from a business point of view, would come from the laboratory, not from a dumb, often cantankerous critter with a mind and needs of its own. If the consumer would allow it, milk and milk products could probably be made entirely without the aid of the cow. Fortunately, at the present time that would not be acceptable; but some steps have already been taken in that direction.

Elsewhere in this book you will read about antibiotics, detergents, pesticides, and other modern milk ingredients; here let's look at how the industry's profits have grown through the public's acceptance of less-than-real milk products.

Whole milk is looked upon as undesirable by consumers who are trying to lower their cholesterol intake. Instead of simply drinking less milk and eliminating fast foods, junk foods, processed foods, and high-cholesterol snacks from their diet, they switch to skim milk. The industry, which used to consider skim milk practically a waste product—along with whey—of the production of cream and butter, now has a lucrative market for skim milk itself and myriad uses for it, such as ice milk, sherbet, low-fat cottage and other cheeses, and many processed foods. The creams and butter separated from whole milk are sold at much more than the cost of whole milk and used to make the more expensive cream cheese and ice cream. Unfortunately, separating the cream separates much of the fat-soluble vitamins (and, for all we know, other valuable nutrients), making the skim milk less than the complete food nature intended.

When we substitute totally artificial products for the real thing, we are shortchanging ourselves even more. Imitation milk, made from vegetable oil, corn syrup, artificial coloring and flavoring, and all the usual stabilizers, emulsifiers, and so on, is not widely available but seems to be a success wherever it is sold, because it's cheap. Similar to "filled milk" (see Glossary in Chapter 16, Dairy Products—A Gray Area), it contains no milk whatsoever. It is, however, a moneymaker, though, as you can see from the chart, a modest one compared to other fake milk products. Remember, it can't even call itself *imitation* something if it doesn't have the nutrient approximation of the real thing. If it calls itself imitation, it has been "fortified" with vitamin supplements—like the ones you are told you don't need because your balanced diet contains so many nutrients—to approximate what we know of the food value of the real thing.

As you can see from the chart, you are paying much more for imitation or fabricated food than for real food. If this were not the case, the manufacturer would have no incentive to go to the trouble of inventing foods.

Comparison of Profitability of Real, Imitation, and Fabricated Milk and Milk Products

Product	Percentage Increase in Retail Price over the Cost of Ingredients
whole milk	174.5
filled milk	184.2
coffee cream	220.9
coffee "whitener"	374.9
sour cream	312.1
imitation sour cream	660.8
whipping cream	169.7
nondairy topping	686.8
ice cream	268.8
imitation ice cream	311.3

SOURCE: Adapted from comparisons of dairy vs. nondairy substitutes made by Robert R. Holland, head of the Food-Science Department, Cornell University, 1968.

Whenever real food is replaced by substitute food, you can assume the latter is more profitable to the manufacturer and a poorer buy for the consumer, both in price and in food value. No matter how much "food" is fortified, we simply do not know as much as nature does about what natural foods contain that is needed for a healthy human system. The more we learn about the complexity of food and about how we handle it in the body, the more we find that interactions and subtle processes are critically important; tossing in a little vitamin D or some vitamin C won't make food real.

CHAPTER 3

More Fabricated, Processed, and Altered Foods

Any food that is a dietary staple is attractive to food fabricators. The profit levels on staple foods are difficult to enhance because there is very little that distinguishes one manufacturer's milk, Cheddar cheese, or potatoes from another. A way around this is to invent a unique product—like Cheez Whiz or Egg Beaters—that will appeal to the consumer who buys the staple (in this case, cheese or eggs) but will be different enough to stand out from the crowd. Happily for the manufacturer, the margin of profit for fabricated foods is much higher than for staples (see the chart called Comparison of Profitability of Real, Imitation, and Fabricated Milk and Milk Products on p. 19). Sometimes, as in the case of instant potatoes and processed cheese, the new products are available to many manufacturers, who must then use heavy brand-name advertising to distinguish among them. This is much easier to do than with staples, because fabricated foods can be changed more easily than real foods and the consumer told the change is a "benefit." Here are some more examples of this kind of fabricated foods.

Cheese

Real cheese is good food; but many products the consumer thinks of as cheese bear little resemblance to the real thing. Unfortunately, the more the product has been altered, the more liable it is to be nutrient-deficient and to contain additives you may prefer not to eat. The consumer's problem is how to tell the real cheese from the other kind.

Processed Cheese

Processed cheese is not natural. It didn't even pretend to be until just recently. As consumers have become more health conscious, *natural* has become a new advertising buzz word. Since there is no government ruling as to what may be called natural, the word appears on some unlikely food packages and cannot be counted on as a guide.

Processed cheese is, by definition, made by grinding various cheeses, melting them together, and combining them with additives, including emulsifiers, such as sodium citrate and disodium phosphate, to create a bland, uniform, pasty substance that even the government describes as "a homogenous plastic mass." This concoction is then poured into store-ready cartons, where it cools and hardens into "processed American cheese." The texture, color, and fat content are all controlled so as to produce an unnaturally uniform product with a "cheese" flavor, whatever that may be. It has been designed to be as versatile as possible, with a melting point (70 degrees Farenheit.) suitable for grilled cheese sandwiches, casseroles, pizzas, and cheese sauces. From a manufacturer's standpoint, this type of assembly-line "food" is infinitely more desirable than the unpredictable real cheeses— and, of course, much more profitable. The quality of the cheeses used may vary considerably from top to poor grades, with the consumer none the wiser, and the mass is aerated after heating to increase its volume (much as ice cream is pumped full of air so that a smaller quantity fills a larger carton). Beatrice Trum Hunter in *Consumer Beware* says of processed cheese, "The end products have undergone such modifications that they scarcely deserve classification as food."

Processed cheeses could probably be produced in more than one "flavor," but manufacturers have not found this necessary, so most of them taste something like Cheddar cheese, considered the most popular flavor for the consumer who would buy this kind of product. So uniform has this "flavor" become that the term "American" applied to cheese is almost a dead give-away that it is processed cheese. Instead of developing additional cheese flavors, processed cheeses are used to create the "variety" of foods that the food processors are so proud of. These include:

pasteurized process cheese
pasteurized process cheese with fruits, vegetables, or meats
pasteurized process pimiento cheese
pasteurized process cheese food
pasteurized process cheese food with fruits, vegetables, or meats
pasteurized process cheese spread
pasteurized process cheese spread with fruits, vegetables, or nuts

Any one of the combination cheese products on the list could be made at home in a few minutes with real cheese and real other ingredients, without additives or artificial flavors and colors. Since most fabricated products are more expensive than the real thing, the consumer could probably buy a blender or food processor with the savings and make the spreads at home quickly, inexpensively, and nutritiously.

The consumer who wants to eat real food is better off buying the plainest form it comes in. Most staple cheeses can easily be turned into all sorts of blends, spreads, and dips. Cottage cheese, mixed at home with raw vegetables, or pineapple, just prepared, will retain more nutrients than the same good foods prepared and combined in a factory days before you eat it.

The more cheese is processed and gussied up, the greater the temptation for the processor to increase profits by using cheaper ingredients. The Food and Drug Administration (FDA) files are full of instances of this kind of food. For example, in September 1985 the FDA's Atlanta district office, following up a tip from a USDA inspector, paid an unexpected visit to Mrs. Stratton's Salads, a Birmingham, Alabama, company manufacturing a product called Mrs. Stratton's Smooth Pimento Spread.

The label listed the ingredients as "pasteurized process cheese spread, American cheese substitute, salad dressing, sweet red peppers, non-fat milk powder, whey powder, and 0.1 percent potassium sorbate." All it claimed to be was a "spread," without the word cheese being mentioned in the name. But even those inexpensive ingredients apparently did not provide the margin of profit the manufacturer had in mind.

What the investigator found in comparing the actual ingredients with the label was that the so-called pasteurized process cheese spread ($1.65 a pound) was really imitation pasteurized process American cheese (63¢ a pound), that no nonfat milk powder had been used, and that the main ingredient by weight was the salad dressing—which, therefore, should have been listed first, not third. And as if all that were not enough, the red bits in this "pimento" spread, which supposedly contained $1.29-per-pound peeled pimientos, were really 63-cents-per-pound red peppers (correctly identified in the ingredients but called "pimentos" in the name of the product—possibly the assumption was that the consumer wouldn't know the difference between pimientos and red peppers).

Cheese Substitutes

An even more lucrative product is cheese substitutes, which is particularly popular for use on pizzas and is cheaper to manufacture and keeps longer than real cheese. Cheese substitute technology is used to imitate many types, including mozzarella, provolone, and even—the irony of it!—processed American cheese.

One food processor explains, "These products are based on combining casein with vegetable oils, flavors, minerals, and vitamins under suitable conditions to produce products that are functionally and nutritionally equivalent to natural cheese." The resulting product is designed to "successfully meet consumer needs." What needs substitute cheese meets that aren't better met by real cheese are difficult to imagine.

If you would like to know how to tell which cheese items are the most profitable for the company, note which are the most heavily advertised, especially on television. Note, also, which ones offer the most cents-off coupons (they are often the higher-profit items). Avoid cheeses that are "convenience" items, such as individually wrapped slices (where you pay a premium for the wrapping instead of the food), or cheese-and-food combinations. A box of cottage cheese and a can of pineapple, bought separately, will inevitably be a better buy than the two combined in one carton—and you will have pineapple left over to top ice cream or to add to roast ham or broiled pork chops.

Nonfoods—Out of the Frying Pan

There are a number of nonfoods that the consumer is buying deliberately. Not only is the consumer fully aware they are not the real thing; that is exactly why he or she is buying them.

The general hysteria over the dangers of cholesterol, generated in part by ignorance and partly by the heavy promotion of manufacturers who see it as a highly profitable opportunity, have led to the development of some products that, while they are not real food, may not be harmful, except that they replace good real food that consumers have been made afraid to eat. One of these is the butter replacement called Butter Buds.

Butter Buds

Butter Buds are distributed by Red Star, makers of a natural yeast that is preservative-free, a recommendation in itself. Butter Buds tastes something like butter. It is described by the manufacturer as "a highly concentrated flavor of butter extracted from whole cream, then spray-dried to a stable, water soluble powder." Its label description reads simply "natural butter flavor, butter flavor, or natural flavoring." It also contains malto-dextrose, corn syrup solids, guar gum, baking soda, salt, spray-dried butterfat to improve mouth feel, annatto, and turmeric. This makes it a more desirable product than margarine because it is a "natural" rather than a totally chemical product, although it would be even better without the malto-dextrin and corn syrup. The FDA has approved the use of the words "natural butter flavor" on the label.

Michael Jacobson, of the Center for Science in the Public Interest, in the organization's publication *Nutrition Action* gave it cautious approval. He says, "As far as health benefits, my hunch is that it is more healthful than butter in terms of heart disease." Not all scientists agree. Dr. Sami Hashim, director of the division of metabolism and nutrition at St. Luke's Hospital, New York, is dubious about the short-chain fatty acids that Butter Buds contains. The fatty acids are a type found in rancid fat and may not be desirable in their action in the human body. There has not been a great deal of comment to date on this product because it is still somewhat limited in its potential applications.

With a little adapting Butter Buds can be used in most of the foods where butter is called for; for instance, dissolved in any vegetable oil, it makes a buttery popcorn topping. It is not suitable for cooking, such as frying or sautéing, and doesn't work as a spread.

A big advantage of Butter Buds is that it is much lower in fat than butter; butter is 81 percent fat, Butter Buds, 13.5 plus or minus 1.0 percent, which makes it popular for low-fat, low-cholesterol diets. And it is even lower in actual use because the flavor of Butter Buds High Concentrate is eighty times the flavor strength of butter and a 4-ounce portion is supposedly equal to 2 pounds of butter (but with 99 percent less cholesterol and 94 percent fewer calories).

Another advantage that consumers will appreciate is that Butter Buds do not have to be refrigerated but can be stored in any cool dry area. From what is known so far, Butter Buds, even with its limitations, seems to be a better, less chemical product than margarine, but if cholesterol isn't a factor, real butter is best of all.

Egg Beaters

Egg Beaters is another product invented for the cholesterol wary; it allows one to continue to eat scrambled eggs and similar foods without worrying about the dangers that we are told lurk in whole eggs.

Egg Beaters is basically egg whites, without the yolks. Of course, the food value of an egg, which is considerable, is mostly in the yolk. In an effort to re-create the food value of the whole egg, the manufacturer has added the protein, vitamin, and mineral levels that, as far as we know, approximate those in a whole egg. This makes it all right with the FDA but, considering the present state of our nutritional knowledge, is no guarantee that it is the complete food that egg is. This is how egg yolk and egg white compare in nature:

Nutrient	Egg Yolk (mg. per 100 grams, edible portion)	Egg White (mg. per 100 grams, edible portion)
protein	16.00	10.9
fat	30.6	trace
calcium	141.0	9.0
phosphorus	569.0	15.0
sodium	52.0	146.0
potassium	98.0	139.0
vitamin A	3,400.0	0
thiamine	.22	trace
riboflavin	.44	.27
iron	5.5	.1

SOURCE: *USDA Composition of Foods.*

The sodium content of Egg Beaters (egg white is naturally high in sodium) has been reduced to only 20 milligrams, and, of course, the fat is naturally low. What Egg Beaters has that eggs don't is corn oil (though less than 1%), vegetable gums, calcium phosphate, artificial color, and mono- and diglycerides, as well as synthetic vitamins and minerals. None of these additives is thought to be harmful, except possibly the artificial color, which is to be supposed to be safe. (See also Chapter 12, How Safe Are Artificial Food Colors?)

As mentioned before, the added nutrients do not make Egg Beaters real eggs, and nowhere is that more obvious than in the taste. I would far rather reduce my egg intake, if necessary, and enjoy the ones I did eat. But the consumer who is tempted by them will be reassured to know that the Center for Science in the Public Interest (CSPI) considers them "a healthful substitute for eggs."

Egg whites eaten raw can cause a biotin deficiency; if you eat Egg Beaters, be sure to cook them thoroughly.

Fabricated Potatoes

Potatoes are another staple food that seem to have inspired the food fabricators to new creative heights. All the consumer has to do is compare the price of a sack of potatoes to a box of instant potatoes to see what the big attraction is.

Potato chips can be a fairly "natural" product, made entirely of potatoes, with only salt added. They still must be deep-fried, so the fat content will be considerable, but aside from that they aren't all that bad. They can't compete with potatoes in other forms (baked, boiled, or mashed) for nutritional content, and they are high in calories (because of the fat), but the best of them are free of salt, chemicals, and preservatives. On the other hand, if you don't read the label, you may buy a brand containing a lot more than potato slices and frying fat. Some chips can be almost totally fabricated, made from dehydrated potato that has been turned into a paste, extruded, and formed into a shape to stack neatly into a tennis ball can, complete with additives, salt, and, usually, a premium price.

After a snack of these chips, dinner may include instant mashed potatoes from dehydrated flakes, with artificial color and flavor and other additives, so completely denatured by processing that they have been fortified with vitamin C in imitation of the natural vitamin C that has been lost.

Fabrication can produce endless variations in the form of potato puffs, potato cakes, french fries, hash browns, scalloped potatoes, home fries, and anything else popular enough to be worth imitating. Obviously, anything that comes in a box is more liable to be fabricated than anything in the frozen food case, but even freezing is no absolute guarantee. If you care which is which (fabricated versions are often more expensive, aside from any other consideration) check out the package to make sure.

Considering the taste and "mouth feel" of fabricated potatoes, no wonder the family in the TV commercials prefers Stove Top Stuffing.

Innovative Ingredients

From the consumer's point of view, one of the most worrisome aspects of modern "foods" is what they're made of. Even when they are derived from real food, the end product has been so processed that without artificially coloring, artificially flavoring, and preforming, it wouldn't be recognizable. Manufacturers say these "new foods" are developed solely to satisfy the consumer's insatiable appetite for something called variety.

It never seems to occur, even to the consumer, that the sales appeal of "new" may be due to lack of satisfaction with the old overprocessed product. Today's supermarket contains thousands of "foods" that Mother Nature would throw up her hands at and that, more and more, are displacing real food. Maybe the void the consumer is trying to fill with novelty products is simply a natural and healthful desire to return to real food.

Preprepared Onions

In the world of the food manufacturer and fast-food restaurateur, the more an item can be preprepared, the better. No longer do the manufacturers and restaurateurs buy bags of onions to slice, dice, chop, or mince by hand. Instead containers labeled powdered, granulated, ground, minced, small chopped, chopped, special large chopped, large chopped, sliced, and ¼-inch diced, as well as toasted onions and extruded onion rings, come all ready to use in canned foods, gravies, sauces, crackers, cheeses, meat loaves, hot dogs, onion rolls, dips, pizzas. Consumers who use dry soup and dip mixes, which are full of chemicals and additives of various kinds (as the labels plainly state), might not object to this type of product, but the average person, trying to eat more sensibly by putting together lunch from a salad bar, might want to know that the bowl of apparently fresh onions came in a 55-gallon drum. (See also Chapter 9, Forever Fresh— The Sulfite Story.) Want sliced onion on your hamburger or onion rings as a side order? No problem; we'll just open another container. Remember, ingredients like this shouldn't be included when you figure your day's supply of nutrients; nutrients are fragile and many of them may be long gone.

Preprepared Fruit

Fruits also lend themselves to evaporation and dehydration. Dried fruits have been a staple food for ages, but modern food manufacturing has taken this simple product much further. Fruits can now be produced not only in dried slices but in various other forms, including powder and flakes. The uses of this type of product, from the consumer's standpoint, can be misleading.

When a cold cereal advertises that it contains fruit, but a USDA analysis reports that the fruit was "too fine to be distinguishable and separable," the consumer isn't getting what he thinks he is. Some cereals labeled granola contain 1 percent fruits and nuts, which hardly justifies calling them granola.

Pear flake powder would allow a product to claim it contained pears, but the consumer might not think that an accurate statement. Unlike real pears, pear flake powder also contains the additives sulphur dioxide and calcium stearate. How little it resembles the real thing is also illustrated by its flavor, which even the manufacturer describes as "typically bland with no musty, decayed, or other off flavors." I doubt if this was what the consumer had in mind when buying fruited cereal with "pears."

Apples are a popular fruit, but "apple" or "apple-flavored" may not be what you think. What you may get is "Low Moisture Apple Fiber Solids," which consist of "Cell Wall materials (cellulose, hemicellulose, lignin, pectin) as well as Apple Sugars separated from the Juice in the processing of Apple Juice products." After the apple solids are separated, they are "dehydrated and screened to specification. The product is relatively free of peel, stems and seed material." I would imagine it would be relatively free of nutrition, too, and the best the manufacturer can say about the flavor is "bland with no musty or other off flavors," the same taste apparently as pear powder—in other words, no taste at all.

If a powder doesn't fill the processors' requirements, no problem. Manufacturers also offer apples in "dices, wedges, rings, flakes, chips, pie pieces, granules, powder, whatever you want. And if we don't already have the one you want, just give us your specifications, and we'll make it for you."

The consumer cannot help but feel that the nutritional value of this type of product is promotional rather than nutritional. But the consumer doesn't know when he is getting powder instead of real fruit. Products made this way are legally allowed to claim they contain real fruit, with the clear implication that they are healthier and naturally flavorful. The nutritional information on the package is no clue, because it includes whatever synthetic vitamins and minerals may have been added.

Algin—Fabricated Foods from the Sea

Food Processing magazine (Summer 1971) in a special section titled "Foods of Tomorrow," featured "Fabricated Foods from the Sea." Algin, one discovery that makes "foods of tomorrow" possible, is "extracted from giant brown kelp." Its useful property is its ability to cause formation of a gel, which the article describes as "a valuable product development tool."

As the article explains:

Technologists have used this mechanism to create such diverse product concepts as imitation low-calorie spaghetti and spaghetti sauce, fabricated meatballs, artificial caviar, shrimp, soft drink gels, fabricated cherries and blueberries, extruded onion rings, fabricated potato chips, and other previously nonexistent products.

In all of these examples, the fabricated food, whether it is cherries, shrimp, or caviar, consists of calcium alginate, flavoring, and coloring. Although the fabricated foods need not contain portions of the foods being imitated, texture and mouthfeel are very much like the natural food.

In other words, unlike margarine and some other man-made items, algin imitations need not contain even a tiny amount of the real thing; they are totally fabricated.

Another product made possible by algin is instant milk pudding; adding hot milk to calcium alginate "produces a custard-type body when the system cools." No wonder homemade pudding "from scratch" tastes so different.

And if you think the fruit flakes mentioned earlier are pretty far out, algin makes them seem almost wholesome. Algin makes possible "fruit or vegetable flavored particles that resemble the natural food in appearance." (As usual, no claim is made that it tastes like the real thing.) "To fabricate the product, an algin syrup containing sugar, coloring, flavoring, etc., is deposited in a calcium chloride bath to form spheres which resemble fruit or vegetable pieces. The same technique can be used to form artificial caviar."

This disposes of the consumer's hope that large pieces of fruit or vegetable in a food item are some guarantee that it is the real thing. It will have "very much" the "texture and mouthfeel" of real food, and artificial color and artificial flavor disguise it even more. It may end up as the "blueberries" in your blueberry muffin or the "shrimp" in your seafood salad—you have no way of knowing for sure if your palate has been blunted by years of eating processed foods.

These imitation foods are presented to the processors as conferring various consumer benefits. For instance, meat and gravy loaves are neat to eat. "A barbecue or a sloppy joe could be quickly jelled into a loaf suitable for slicing and serving between bread as a sandwich. Such a sandwich would not be messy when prepared or eaten and there would be no seepage of sauce, gravy, or soup into the bread." No delicious, homemade brown gravy to mop up, either—but no matter, there is very little good homemade white bread to mop it up with.

To make imitation shrimp with this method (there are others), "protein source, alginate, flavoring, coloring and other ingredients would be formed into a shrimp shape and dipped into a calcium bath. The calcium-algin reaction provides body and texture, and the result is a shrimp ready to be breaded and prefried." And if you want to keep it from drying out until the consumer buys it, just coat it with an edible algin film formed "by dipping the particular food, such as meat, fish or fowl, in an algin solution followed by a dip in a solution of calcium salt."

Other fabricated foods to look forward to from this one product are gelatinized beer you can serve without a glass, and fabricated cherries you can pop into your mouth with no fear of swallowing the pits. Note the consumer benefits.

Contrary to a popular television commercial of a few years ago, fabricated foods *can* fool Mother Nature. A recent salad dressing commercial shows a distressed man complaining that no one makes a salad dressing that doesn't separate (actually, lots of companies do). His wife immediately comes to the rescue with a *new* salad dressing that won't. Xanthan gum is the secret stabilizer that makes this possible. It's not something you put in a homemade oil-and-vinegar dressing, but commercial dressings use it because "ingredients stay better mixed and more pourable without flavor masking." The big consumer benefit here is that you don't have to shake the bottle before pouring on the dressing.

There are other stabilizers that "protect the palatability of frozen convenience foods during the freeze-thaw cycle," make ice cream "taste" better by providing "smoother texture and full flavor release," and keep the cocoa in chocolate milk suspended. The alert consumer may have already noticed the "improved mouthfeel in powdered juice drinks," or a "long-lasting foamy head" on beer. Both come to you compliments of propylene glycol alginate.

Thickening agents of this sort are used in ice cream, yogurt, soups, baby food and formula, soft drinks, and many, many other foods. You don't use them when you make these foods at home; obviously, they are not inherently necessary in the manufacture of these products. In fact, most high-quality commercial products don't use them. Among the yogurt makers, Dannon and Colombo manage to make creamy, smooth-textured yogurt with great "mouthfeel" without a drop of these additives.

As far as we know, the additives are not harmful, but how can they be as good to eat and as nutritious as real food? If this trend continues, home cooking will disappear. How can it possibly compete when homemade dressings with real oil and vinegar separate, ice cream melts quickly, and homemade chocolate milk ends up with a layer of delicious chocolate sediment at the bottom of the glass? Real fruit and real vegetables will soon taste peculiar to palates accustomed to the totally artificial, and may even become harder to find and more expensive to buy. Even more serious is the fact that no one really knows what health problems will show up years—and generations—from now from ingesting these unnatural foods. The study of nutrition is still in its infancy, and many medical schools still fail to include even an elementary nutrition course in their curriculum.

CHAPTER 4

Surimi—
The Great Pretender

Among Japanese products familiar to the American consumer, cars, TV sets, and computers probably head the list. Most Americans are totally unaware of an even more ubiquitous but harder to recognize import that is growing faster than any of these. Surimi, a fabricated Japanese paste, is proving a bonanza to our food industry; Americans are consuming it at the rate of over fifty million pounds a year.

If you think you have never eaten surimi, you are probably mistaken—understandably so, since it masquerades as more familiar foods or is euphemistically labeled as seafood, or something that sounds equally acceptable but is as uninformative. If you have eaten "seafood" salad, Sea Bites, Sea Stix, Krab Newburg, King Krab, Sea Tails, and similarly designated "foods," you have eaten surimi.

The FDA, describing many surimi products now in the market as "fake crab meat, lobster, shrimp, or scallops," has no real objection to them as long as they are not misleadingly labeled or advertised. If properly identified on the label as "fish," "Pacific white fish"—which the FDA calls a "fanciful name"—or pollock, the careful consumer, equipped with a magnifying glass, can determine that the can in the crabmeat section of the canned seafood shelf is not really crabmeat as the picture of the crab on the can would seem to indicate. If the product has been repackaged, the ingredients may be deliberately or sloppily mislabeled as a prepared product, as real shrimp, and so on. If it is a prepared product at the deli counter or in the fish case, a simple description such as "seafood," "crab-flavored fish cakes," or "crab sticks" may mislead the unsuspecting consumer, who may not be aware of all the nuances of fabricated food descriptions.

It is even more difficult to recognize surimi when dining out. Menus do not list the ingredients of the foods they serve (perhaps a good thing if you want to continue to enjoy restaurant food), and the glowing descriptions that accompany many dishes are hype rather than fact. No menu is required to identify the seafood salad as surimi (processed and painted to look like a mixture of shrimp and crabmeat) or the lobster newburg as fabricated pollock in fancy dress. Or that the "chicken nugget" is minced real chicken—held together with surimi paste. It hasn't happened yet, but your favorite franks could one day be pure surimi; the Japanese have been making hot dogs like that for over twenty years and, given plenty of mustard and sauerkraut, it's not that easy to tell them from the real thing.

Surimi is so versatile that it can be made to imitate almost any food. In the planning stage is fabricated caviar, little orange-color balls that look like salmon roe but are actually made from seafood gelatin filled with salad oil. As we have seen with chicken nuggets, surimi is not confined to fishy-tasting products. Frank Kanawa, a vice president of JAC Creative Foods, one of the manufacturers processing raw surimi into finished products, says, "There are thousands of things that can be made from this base." To make this point he served surimi-based "pork" sausage and "pasta" with spaghetti sauce at a West Coast food convention. No one apparently recognized either dish as anything out of the ordinary.

The potential uses of surimi are mind-boggling. William Gilman, director of marketing at Intersea Fisheries, a surimi importer, says, "From a marketing point of view, the sky's the limit. [Surimi] goes into retail stores, to salad makers, food processors, to bars for happy hours, restaurants for seafood stuffing and salad—you name it, you can find someone using it." Vito Russo, a member of the National Fisheries Institute's surimi committee and vice president of Norda, Inc., a food flavorings manufacturer, sees still another use, "as a protein source, the way we use soy."

What Is Surimi?

Although surimi was first introduced into the United States about ten years ago, it has been a staple of the Japanese diet for nine hundred years. Made from cheap fishes, such as pollock, shark, croaker, sea eel, and lizard fish, surimi is minced and formed into over two thousand items—fish cakes, fish balls, fish sausages, and other food analogs—that may be broiled, baked, steamed, or fried. As a staple of the Japanese diet, surimi is an example of Japanese ingenuity, creating a legitimate source of protein and nutrients and adding interest to an otherwise somewhat limited choice of foods.

The surimi imported into the United States is still made from cheap fish—although the price of the finished product is far from cheap at the retail level—but it has been processed beyond recognition. First the fish is mechanically deboned, then repeatedly washed with cold water so that it becomes odorless and colorless. The drained mass is strained and pureed to a paste to which sugar, salt, potassium sorbate, sodium glutamate, and starch may be added. The result is formed into flat rectangular blocks that stack efficiently for freezing, packing, and shipping.

Surimi paste of this sort is not considered edible, but it forms a marvelous base for further processing. It can, for instance, be given the elastic, chewy texture of shellfish. All the food processor has to do is thaw the frozen blocks; perhaps blend the surimi with a little real shellfish; add a number of nonfish ingredients—possibly egg whites, starch, wheat flour, or other binders; natural or (more likely) artificial flavors; sugar and sorbitol; preservatives such as sodium tripolyphosphate—color it appropriately with artificial color; and shape it like lobster meat, crabmeat, shrimp, scallops, or some other real thing. (Since natural crab and other shellfish flavors are often obtained by boiling down shellfish shells, this is an efficient use of what would otherwise be a waste product.)

Imitation surimi products demonstrate the originality and ingenuity of today's food manufacturers. Making imitation Alaskan king crab legs, for example, uses a technique derived from the manufacturing of spaghetti. Kamaboko dough (the surimi fish-cake product) is extruded into continuous filaments, which can then be woven or glued together to resemble crab leg muscles. Streaky artificial red coloring is added to the surface and, without an honest label, the average consumer might easily take the resulting product for real crab legs. The FDA describes the result as "generally wholesome and nutritious, although the severe washing process and dilution with starches and water result in a product nutritionally inferior not only to the original fish from which it was made but also to the seafood it imitates."

One of the immediate problems that occurs to many consumers upon first learning about surimi-based products is the difficulty they pose for anyone who is allergic or who has a health condition that requires avoiding even such innocent ingredients as wheat flour or eggs. It is most unlikely that the ingredients list would be so complete as to include everything that has been added, both in Japan and in the United States, to the finished product. And in spite of the FDA description as "a wholesome and nutritious product," the consumer is tempted to respond, "Compared to what?" At the prices charged for these products, it might seem that the consumer dollar could be better spent on less worked over food.

Manufacturers say surimi products benefit the consumer because ounce for ounce, the consumer gets more nutrients out of a dollar's worth of surimi products than from the real thing. The argument is that surimi foods are generally considerably cheaper and more consistent in quality than real shrimp or lobster, for instance. Marion Burros, the *New York Times* food editor, feels differently. "I resent having surimi crab being passed off as real crab in sushi bars and being charged as if it were real crab." Check it out for yourself next time you pass the canned crab section in your supermarket. I found that imitation (made from pollock) crab was considerably more expensive than some brands of real crab, and though it was clear from a reading of the label which was which, a hurried shopper might easily have bought the imitation. Even when it is cheaper, you may prefer to pass up what is still a luxury fake—$6 or $7 a pound—until you can afford the real thing.

The FDA tries to monitor labels, clamping down on misleading product labeling that suggests a product is the real thing when it is not. When a food that resembles another food is not as nutritious, it must be labeled as an imitation. Since surimi is not as nutritious as the shellfish it often imitates, it should always be labeled imitation, a word manufacturers avoid because it tends to put the prospective purchaser off the product.

A permitted alternative to using the word "imitation" is to add supplements to make the product as nutritious as the real thing. Another is to manufacture and label the product with a vague name, such as "seafood" (as in "seafood salads," "seafood cocktails," "stuffed with seafood"— all names particularly popular on restaurant menus and salad bars). The FDA would still like to see informative labeling that tips off the consumer to the surimi-based nature of the product, but the agency doesn't pretend to be able to police this area very thoroughly. James Green, an FDA spokesman, explains the agency's position: "With only a thousand investigators around the country, it's physically impossible to go after minor economic violations of this nature unless there's a health problem involved."

From the consumer's standpoint, an even more serious problem is the growing importance of fish in the diet. The recent discovery that fish may play an important role in reducing the incidence of heart disease is bound to increase the amount of fish consumed. Yet so far as I have been able to determine, no studies have been made as to whether any of the beneficial fatty acids in fish survive this severe processing. Consumers eating "seafood" to improve their health may be doing just the opposite if it is not the real thing. (See also Chapter 3, More Fabricated, Processed, and Altered Food.)

CHAPTER 5

True Stories from the FDA Files

The Food and Drug Administration, the national watchdog over most of our food, is concerned primarily with instances of deliberate deception, usually revealed through misleading labeling or failure to conform to Standards of Identity. Thanks to the FDA investigators, many of these foods are discovered before they get very far into the marketplace, and when discovered, they are usually promptly removed.

Food fraud is not new. The idea of a "baker's dozen," consisting of thirteen items rather than twelve, originated in the days when bakers frequently shortchanged their customers (who couldn't count as fast as the rolls went into the string bag). To prevent being accused of this unseemly practice, bakers took to giving the extra roll or muffin, thus demonstrating the degree to which they were bending over to be honest. Nor is short weight or short count the only ways the customer was cheated. Thoreau, writing in his *Journal,* referred to the then-common custom of watering milk when he said, "Some circumstantial evidence is very strong, as when you find a trout in the milk." The FDA is still confronted with this quaint custom, and it is not, as we will see, confined to milk.

The FDA and the Tuna Fish Caper

A classic case from the FDA files concerns the Lakefish Canning Company, which operated in Minnesota in the 1940s. Like most canners, their factory was near their source of supply; freshwater lakes nearby were rich with carp, which they canned and marketed labeled as freshwater carp, packed in soya oil.

Unfortunately for the company, carp is not a fish highly regarded by Americans, although it is prized in the Orient, Europe, and the Middle East for its white, nonoily meat. The company tried to increase sales by putting recipes on the labels and even tried labeling some of the cans lakefish, an invented species that they hoped would avoid the onus attached to carp. Nothing worked, and by 1950 the company was bankrupt.

It was then that the Price Wholesale Grocery Co. of St. Paul entered the picture, buying up the remaining stock of canned carp and "lakefish." The owner of Price was ill and his company was temporarily being run by his son Norman. Norman apparently knew that carp was a no-no because he promptly relabeled the cans: one batch as "LC light meat tuna," packed for the LC Mercantile Co. of Quincy, Illinois, the other as "Veteran light meat tuna fish," packed for the Gordon-Brewster Co. of Rochester, New York. Approximately 22,320 cans were relabeled in this fashion and shipped out to retail stores.

Unfortunately for Price, an alert housewife who bought the "tuna" was suspicious of it and got in touch with the FDA district office in her city of Minneapolis. FDA investigator Hugh J. Hennessey was assigned to the case. He confirmed that the can's contents were not tuna and soon discovered that the firm of Gordon-Brewster did not exist. In the best tradition of the private eye, Hennessey followed the tracks of the suspicious cans and soon found himself at Price wholesalers. Confronted with the false labels (the "tuna" had by then been properly identified as carp), Norman denied any complicity in the matter and said his company was in the business of buying up "distressed merchandise," which in this case had already been labeled. Hennessey was able to prove otherwise, and Norman finally admitted what he had done.

The FDA, through the Price company's distribution records, succeeded in tracing 423 of the 465 cartons Price had bought from Lakefish Canning and sold to retail outlets. Some of the cans had been sold, presumably to consumers who had not complained, but two hundred cartons were recovered and, as is customary in such cases, seized by court order. The Price company was fined, and the cans, with wholesome though mislabeled contents, were donated by the court to charitable institutions.

Once again the FDA had, without fuss, fanfare, or public knowledge, protected the American consumer against marketplace fraud. But that did not stop the practice; as we will see, only continued vigilance on the part of investigators, helped by the consumers who report suspicious foods, keeps our foods reasonably honest.

Some foods seem to lend themselves more easily than others to this type of fraud; among the most frequent appear to be fish, juices, and syrups. Here are some recent examples.

"Flounder" Fillets

Eaten any frozen breaded flounder fillets recently? Are you sure they were flounder? In June 1980 the FDA charged with false labeling Masschusetts Coastal Seafoods, Inc. (which was packing and labeling the article). The FDA said the article's labeling was "false and misleading in claiming that the only fish in the article was flounder . . ." The fish labeled flounder was actually turbot. A default decree "authorized actual or constructive destruction by delivery to a locally recognized charitable institution."

"Pure" Orange Juice Concentrate

The FDA ran into a different kind of problem, though it still came down to improper labeling, with a shipment of more than a million pounds of frozen orange juice concentrate that had been produced in Mexico, reprocessed in the United States by the Texas Citrus Exchange, and shipped to two Florida firms. Routine tests by an FDA laboratory revealed that some of the juice had been artificially colored with turmeric and annatto (allowed color additives but not if not identified on the label) to make it more attractive, and some had been diluted with water, or had been doctored with sweeteners or flavorings to make it taste better. None of these things was actually harmful, but they were not proper additives for pure orange juice concentrate (to be sold at pure orange juice concentrate prices).

The FDA, in a series of meetings with federal and state officials and Citrus Exchange officials, agreed to compromise; it would not confiscate the juice but the juice would be relabeled to properly identify the contents. The result was that the shipment was divided into three lots: the one that contained 100 percent orange juice would be labeled Frozen Concentrated Orange Juice; the one that was 100 percent orange juice colored with turmeric and/or annato would declare the artificial colors; the product that was diluted and so contained less than 100 percent orange juice would be labeled concentrate for orange juice beverage.

Although this compromise made sense, neither too strictly penalizing the packers nor cheating the consumer, it still required the consumer to pay careful attention to the labeling and to the subtleties in terminology. Next time you see "concentrate for orange juice beverage," or anything other than "100 percent frozen concentrated orange juice," be sure that you know you are not buying pure, undiluted juice, and be sure the store has not priced it just as high as the real thing.

"Maple," "Honey," or Whatever

Another category of food that appears over and over again in the FDA reports of seizures and various court actions is table syrups. The process of adulteration is as easy as pouring a different liquid into the bottle, and apparently the profits to be made from substituting other sweeteners for pure maple syrup or honey are frequently too great to resist.

An example was reported in May 1985 as a product the FDA identified as "Table syrups" ("maple-flavored," "cane," and "sorghum"). "When shipped by Anthony Syrup Co., Philadelphia, Miss., corn syrup had been substituted for maple syrup in the eight-case lot, for cane syrup in the twelve-case lot, and for sorghum syrup in the twenty-five-case lot; the labels of the articles were false and misleading as to food contents." In addition, the eight-case lot ("Maple Flavored Table Syrup") failed to conform to the definition and standard of identity for table syrup, since table syrup should contain not less than 10 percent maple syrup and the article contained no maple syrup. The "Ribbon Cane Table Syrup" failed to conform to the definition and Standard of Identity for table syrup, since cane syrup should be made from the juice of the sugar cane, and the article was made with corn syrup, as was the lot labeled Sorghum, Molasses and Cane Syrup Blend, which contained none of those ingredients. This case clearly illustrates the value to the consumer of the Standards of Identity, even though sometimes these standards make for unclear ingredient labeling.

The disposition was reported as "Default—ordered destroyed."

The enormous amount of time and work involved in this case is typical of what goes on behind the apparently simple identification and prosecution of false and misleading labeling.

The charges grew from five years of investigation, during which Oliver Anthony, owner of Anthony Syrup, had purchased over 6 million pounds of corn syrup and 1600 gallons of artificial maple flavoring. So great was the difference in cost between the real and fake ingredients that the U.S. attorney who prosecuted the case said he "could not estimate the profits" that Anthony and his co-defendant, Dewey Garland Clark, had made by the substitutions. The products, which went under such names as Anthone's Pure Sourwood Honey, Anthone's Wild Flower Brand Honey, Anthone's Pure Maple Syrup, Anthone's Maple Flavored Table Syrup, Anthone's Old Fashion Sorghum, and Clark's Farm Pure Sorghum, were shipped to eight states—Texas, Tennessee, Kentucky, Arizona, Oklahoma, Oregon, Virginia, and Utah—from 1978 to 1982. Though the substituted ingredients were not in themselves harmful or unwholesome, the government's case was based on the fact that the label is "a binding statement by the packer or processor that the product is what it claims to be. When it is not, whether because of wrong weight, or unlisted ingredients or outright deception,'' the FDA can seize the product, subject to further resolution of the matter.

Both defendants pleaded not guilty on all thirteen felony counts of violating and conspiring to violate the federal Food, Drug and Cosmetic Act by placing adulterated and misbranded foods in interstate commerce. Subsequently the conspiracy charges were set aside. Anthony then pleaded guilty to six charges and Clark to three. They were both placed on four years' probation and ordered to report every three months to a probation officer. In addition, Anthony was fined $20,000, Clark $10,000; which they were allowed to pay over two years. Several states, after repeated seizures, had embargoed the trading of Clark and Anthony products within their borders.

This resolution of the case was welcomed by the maple syrup industry, particularly in Vermont, and by the honey industry across the country.

In view of this and similar cases, the consumer might be better off, both in taste and pocketbook, buying pure maple syrup and a bottle of corn syrup and mixing it, to taste, at home. Unfortunately, unless you can recognize pure maple syrup or have reason to trust the brand, this may not work either, as we see in the next example.

"Maple Syrup"

Earlier, in March 1981, the FDA reported about the Anthony Syrup Co.'s maple syrup that ". . . the article had had a substance other than maple sirup [sic] substituted for the article . . . the article's labeling was false and misleading, since the article's invoice falsely and misleadingly represented the article to be maple sirup . . . the article failed to conform to the definition and standard of identity for maple sirup, since the article was made with sirup derived from a source other than the maple tree."

Eventual disposition of the "maple" syrup was taken care of by converting it into bee food.

More from the FDA Files

The FDA Food/Economic and Labeling Violations files gives evidence that the consumer is right to question any deviation from the familiar in food items. Here are some brief examples.

Lobster Tails

Frozen rock lobster tails and conch meat from Haiti were being examined because they were suspected of being decomposed; decomposition is usually detected by organoleptic analysis—in other words, by smelling the suspected item. To get his nose closer to the meat, the examiner split the lobster tails open; he found to his surprise not only lobster meat but clams, pieces of metal, and a small stone.

"Vitamin-C-enriched" Cranberry-Apple Drink

The name was right but the label optimistically described the article as containing 45 percent of the U.S. RDA of vitamin C. As the FDA report put it, it "contains less."

When a Fillet Is Not a Fillet

In one case the label read, "IQ Sole Fillet Product of Holland," but the shipment contained Greenland turbot instead. In another, the problem was not the type of fish—it *was* whiting—but the definition of "fillet." Technically, a fillet is a "boneless piece or slice of meat or fish." As the FDA put it, "It is not simply a fish with its head cut off." Consumers who like fish but hate bones will be happy to know they can usually trust "fillet" on the label to deliver the kind of fish they enjoy.

"Sesame" Oils

Sesame oil is expensive; cottonseed oil is not. The FDA found "the valuable constituent sesame oil had been partially abstracted; cottonseed oil had been substituted . . ." And to add insult to injury, "Longevity Brand lot falsely and misleadingly represented that the article would prolong life."

Fake Apple Juice and Apple Concentrate

The label said "PURE Apple Juice," but the product really contained water and other ingredients—and no apple juice at all. The FDA was willing to allow the manufacturer to keep the product and recondition and/or relabel it, but "the manufacturer was unable to get its supplier to fully identify some of the articles' ingredients."

Olive Oil

Once again the oil was less than 100 percent olive; it had been diluted with a cheaper oil but sold as the real thing.

Making Tomatoes Toe the Line

Rules are rules, and standards are standards, but some violations aren't quite as serious as others. This product "failed to conform to the standard of quality for canned tomatoes, since the article contained tomato peel in excess of 1.06 square inches per pound."

Since the tomatoes were still perfectly wholesome food, disposition was donation to a nonprofit charitable organization.

Aloe Vera Juice Blends—Plus

Both the blends—with fresh orange juice concentrate and with fresh cranberry concentrate—contained the type and amount of juice the label claimed. Unfortunately the juice also contained the nonconforming food additive Germall II, a preservative for cosmetics intended for external application.

Saccharin—Not Always Noted

Although saccharin may be used in foods, the law requires that it be shown on the label along with the warning "Use of this product may be hazardous to your health. This product contains saccharin, which has been determined to cause cancer in laboratory animals." Manufacturers are understandably unhappy about having to put this on the label; frequently they don't when they should.

The FDA cites numerous examples where it has been found as the sole or partial sweetener but not so indentified. One such product was a protein supplement drink whose vanilla malt, chocolate, strawberry, and banana flavors were sweetened with saccharin, with no label declaration. The FDA seizure of 190 cases, valued at $2,000, was apparently the last straw for the firm, which sold the company—including the seized goods, which the new owner destroyed under FDA supervision.

What You Can Do

Things are frequently not what they seem; neither can you blindly trust the information on a label. When you open a can, frozen food package, or bottle, pay attention to the appearance of the ingredients then and as you remove them; note any unusual taste or exceptionally watery consistency. Report anything suspicious to the FDA office in your vicinity.

CHAPTER 6

The Search
for the Safe
Artificial Sweetener

Most modern food would not exist if extensive use were not made of salt or sweeteners. Taste tests have proved to food manufacturers that most consumers find totally flavorless food agreeable only if it is made salty or sweet enough. Artificial flavors are usually not enough; but salt or sugar can stand alone.

Ever since sugar was given a bad name as a cause of tooth decay and "empty" calories, chemists have worked overtime to discover a substance that would sweeten food with low or no calories and without causing dental caries. The three most successful of these substances are saccharin, cyclamate, and aspartame. All are far sweeter than sugar, all are man-made chemicals, and all have aroused considerable controversy as to whether they are safe to ingest. Sugar is the least sweet of sweeteners, but it has the most agreeable taste. Saccharin is bitter, but aspartame is not unpleasant. They have all been developed or exclusively produced in the United States by commercial companies: saccharin by the paint company Sherwin-Williams; cyclamate by Abbot Laboratories; aspartame by G. D. Searle & Company. Since the products are highly profitable, attempts to limit or ban their use naturally led to considerable controversy and met with strong objections from the patent holders and manufacturers.

The public was eager for a miracle sweetener that satisfied its sweet tooth without destroying it and allowed dieters to indulge freely, and tended to discount warnings of possible health hazards, thereby unwittingly making the task of protecting public health an even more difficult job. Scientists, consumer advocates, nutritionists, and physicians who spoke up against one or another of the artificial sweeteners tended to be regarded as spoilsports;

43

Artificial Sweeteners Compared to Sugar

	# of Calories Equivalent to 1 Teaspoon of Sugar	Sweetness Compared with Sugar	Present Legal Status
Sugar	16		allowed
Saccharin	1.5 powder 0.0 tablet	300 times	ban moratorium extended
Cyclamate	2.0 powder 0.0 tablet	30 times	ban being reconsidered
Aspartame	2.0 powder 0.5 tablet	180 times	approved

NOTE: Aspartame contains 4 calories per gram, the same as sugar, but because it is so much sweeter, much less of it need be used to achieve the same "sweet" taste.

SOURCE: FDA.

what they had to say was not what the public wanted to hear, and the public proved it. Today 69 million Americans (not including children) are consuming products containing saccharin and/or aspartame; the only reason they are not also consuming cyclamate is that, for the present, it has been banned.

Behind the Present Status

Saccharin

Saccharin was discovered in 1879 by a scientist at Johns Hopkins University. At first it was primarily an antiseptic and food preservative. As early as 1911, however, a scientific board classified saccharin as an adulterant, not suitable for use in foods; in 1912 the board limited its use to products "intended for invalids" but did not strictly enforce this restriction during World War I. During two world wars shortages of sugar led to sugar rationing, and gradually saccharin began to be used as a sweetener in more and more foods.

The 1958 Delaney Clause, which banned any new food additive that was shown by tests to cause cancer, did not affect the status of saccharin (or of cyclamate, which was also in use by then) because the clause did not apply to GRAS (generally recognized as safe) substances. (See Chapter 31, GRAS—Are Food Additives Really Safe?)

In 1968 the Committee on Food Protection of the National Academy of Sciences issued an interim report on the safety of nonnutritive sweeteners. The report concluded that adults probably did not consume more than 1 gram of saccharin a day and that such a small amount was "probably not a health hazard." It advised, however, that additional studies be made.

As the new studies began to produce results, the FDA, which had begun to review the safety of GRAS-listed additives, decided to remove it from the GRAS list with a provisional rating that allowed it to be used until the studies to determine whether it was safe were completed. Meanwhile, world-wide interest in the sweetener had generated studies in a number of countries. As the results came in, one by one, the conclusion was inescapable. There was clear evidence from Canada, Great Britain, and other European countries, as well as from United States scientists, that led to a statement from the FDA in 1977 that "The findings indicate unequivocally that saccharin causes bladder cancer in test animals."

Canada immediately prohibited all uses of saccharin except as a tabletop sweetener and permitted it to be sold only in pharmacies. The FDA planned to follow suit but was forestalled by public protests. Interests that wished to retain the unrestricted sale of saccharin ridiculed the methodology of the Canadian tests, pointing out that the test rats had been fed the equivalent of eight hundred cans of diet soda a day. The public, ignorant of the nature of this type of scientific study and easily confused as to its validity—which is agreed to by most of the scientific community—felt safe because, of course, no human would ingest that amount in that period of time.

This misunderstanding, encouraged by those who were against the ban, led to the Saccharin Study and Labeling Act of 1977, which mandated a two-year moratorium against a ban. It directed further studies, however, and these not only confirmed saccharin's carcinogenicity but also found that the substance seemed to enhance the incidence of cancer caused by other carcinogenic agents consumed at the same time.

In spite of this Congress has repeatedly extended the moratorium.

The present law does its best to protect the consumer with a warning label on all saccharin that advises consumers of its carcinogenity. The FDA's stand in 1986 was still that it should not be used in food and beverages but only as a tabletop sweetener by those who are considered at special risk from sugar, such as diabetics.

Almost no one, even among those who are in favor of saccharin, denies that saccharin causes cancer. The FDA argument for allowing it to be used is that "the risk of contracting cancer from using saccharin is very small."

Cyclamate

Cyclamate was synthesized by accident in 1937 by a scientist at the University of Illinois. By 1986 it was marketed in approximately forty countries, including Canada. Questions as to its safety arose in 1968, when the National Academy of Sciences (NAS) recommended additional studies of it as a food additive. In 1969 NAS's caution paid off with the discovery that cyclamate caused bladder cancer in rats and mice. The FDA removed it from the GRAS list, and soon thereafter, in September 1970, imposed a total ban.

In the fall of 1971 hearings were held before the House Judiciary subcommittee attended by growers, manufacturers, packers, and distributors of cyclamate who were seeking to be reimbursed for losses they claimed resulted from the cyclamate ban. In the course of the hearings, some interesting facts were brought out. First of all, the congressmen gave the FDA somewhat of a hard time on the GRAS list. (See also Chapter 31, GRAS—Are Food Additives Really Safe?) This arose from the fact that the request for reimbursement of losses was based largely on the additive being GRAS-listed and, therefore, presumably safe. It had, the argument went, been used in good faith and with confidence that it was safe; the sudden ban had caught them with "extensive inventories of foods," which could no longer be sold.

Among those making statements to the committee was James Turner, who identified himself as an attorney and as the author of *The Chemical Feast*, "the Nader report on the Food and Drug Administration." He said he felt that Abbot Laboratories (the makers of cyclamate) should compensate those who suffered losses because Abbot had "continuously assured these businessmen that there was no problem with cyclamates" in spite of the fact that their laboratory had informed them on October 8, 1969, that feeding studies done under contract for Abbot showed evidence that did seem to indicate a link between cyclamates and bladder cancer. Although Abbot did not make this information available to the general public, they had actually quickly passed it on to the FDA.

In 1973 Abbot sought permission to remarket cyclamate on a limited basis, for use only in special dietary foods and for specific technological purposes. Three years later the National Cancer Institute, reviewing more than four hundred toxological reports submitted by Abbot, concluded that the evidence neither established nor refuted the carcinogenicity of cyclamate. On the basis that it had not been demonstrated that the additive was "safe for human consumption," the FDA refused Abbot's request.

Efforts to get permission to remarket cyclamate continued unabated until September 1980, when Jere E. Goyan, then FDA commissioner, issued a "final negative decision" on the grounds that the safety of cyclamate had not been demonstrated, that it had not been shown that cyclamate would not cause cancer and would not cause inheritable genetic damage. The decision also said, however, that the evidence submitted "does not conclusively establish that cyclamate is a carcinogen."

Abbot filed again in 1982, submitted fifty-nine new studies and other data. Although there was new evidence that seemed to implicate cyclamate "as a cause of tumors in the urinary bladders of rats and in the lungs, liver, and lymphoreticular tissues of mice," and indications that cyclamate can conceivably cause chromosome breakage, thus conceivably posing a mutagenic hazard, and that it can atrophy testicles, new evaluations were limited only to whether it was a carcinogen. At the present time, at the FDA's request, the National Academy of Sciences/National Research Council is now "conducting an independent review of the carcinogenicity data on cyclamate." Meanwhile the FDA has positioned it on their "up for consideration" list.

The consumer may be interested to know that the FDA's view is that

> critical to the evaluation of food additives are issues such as how the body uses a substance and breaks it down into other forms, and how the substance affects body functions. For example, almost none of the saccharin a person consumes is broken down by the body; it is excreted by the kidneys virtually unchanged. Cyclamate, on the other hand, is metabolized, or processed, in the digestive tract, and its by-products are excreted by the kidneys. Aspartame breaks down in the body into three basic components: the amino acids phenylalanine and aspartic acid, and methanol (wood alcohol).

Aspartame

Inasmuch as aspartame is the newest and most widely used of the artificial sweeteners, it merits its own chapter, which follows.

CHAPTER 7

Aspartame— Help or Hazard?

The newest, and by far the most popular, of artificial sweeteners is aspartame, which is marketed by G. D. Searle & Company under two names. It is called NutraSweet when used as a food additive; Equal when used as a sugar substitute at the table.

It was approved by the FDA, for the second time, in 1981 for use in dry foods and as a table-sugar substitute, but sales did not really take off until 1983, when it was approved for soft drinks. By 1984 worldwide annual sales of aspartame amounted to $600 million, and the Department of Agriculture estimated worldwide use at 414,575 tons. The tonnage figure might not seem large compared to that of sugar (8,000,000 tons) or of saccharine (1,184,500 tons), but aspartame is a newcomer, and its use is growing rapidly. Sugar use, on the other hand, has declined steadily, from 10,100,000 tons in 1979. Tonnage figures are misleading, also, because aspartame is about two hundred times sweeter than sugar, so less needs to be used to achieve the same result.

One of the reasons for aspartame's popularity is that it tastes like sugar—with none of the bitter taste that saccharin has—but contains approximately one-tenth the calories in the amount needed to achieve the same level of sweetness. The American Diabetes Association recommends it as safe for diabetics, and dieters everywhere have greeted it as a boon. At present it carries no warnings (except, as we will see, for those with PKU)—unlike saccharin, which is labeled as a possible carcinogen—and while it is listed as an ingredient on package labels, the law does not require that the amount contained be specified.

How Safe Is Aspartame?

In the spring of 1985 two scientists—Dr. William Pardridge, an associate professor of medicine at the University of California, and Dr. Richard J. Wurtman, director of the clinical research center at MIT—testifying before the Senate Committee on Labor and Human Resources, urged that labeling requirements for aspartame be amended to include the quantity. Dr. Pardridge's concern, based on research, was that children might suffer brain damage from excessive intake of aspartame. Dr. Wurtman informed the committee that aspartame consumed at the same time as carbohydrates would have double the effect on the brain as aspartame alone. Since children often have a soft drink along with french fries and a hamburger or hot dog, the likelihood of this combination is considerable.

In June of the same year Dr. Louis Elsas, director of the division of medical genetics at Emory University, said that both pregnant women and infants should not consume foods containing aspartame because of the danger of it causing brain damage to the fetus or the infant. At present foods containing aspartame are supposed to carry a warning for people with phenylketonuria (PKU), an inability to metabolize phenylalanine, one of the amino acids that make up aspartame. It is important for victims of PKU to be diagnosed at birth—screening of newborns is required by all states—so that the victims' consumption of phenylalanine be strictly controlled. About 1 out of every 15,000 newborns are found to have the disease; it does not develop after birth. Overconsumption of phenylalanine can lead to permanent retardation, so only limited amounts of even high-protein foods that contain it naturally, such as meat, eggs, cheese, and milk, can be eaten. The dietary regimen of PKU victims has now been made even more difficult to adhere to due to the fact that more and more products contain aspartame. A victim of this disease must constantly check and keep track of the quantity being consumed. Obviously this is presently impossible in the absence of quantitative labeling of aspartame on every food and beverage that contains it.

In addition to PKU victims, certain other consumers are considered at risk; these include people with advanced renal disease and about 1,750 pregnant women with hyperphenylalaninemia (high blood levels of the amino acid, which could prove toxic to the unborn child). And Dr. Elsas is concerned because unborn children of this group are at risk if aspartame is consumed during the fetal stage. "A small change in the phenylalanine level in a pregnant woman's blood," says Dr. Elsas, "is magnified by the placenta into the fetal blood, and the fetal brain will concentrate that level further. High levels in unformed or forming brains could cause irreversible damage. No one knows what degree of elevation in the mother's blood may cause brain damage in the fetus.''

In January 1985, the *Journal of Clinical Investigation* published one of Dr. Elsas's studies, which found that the effects of phenylalanine on two groups ranging in age from eight to twenty-four years was to affect their reaction time and to reduce the production of adrenalinelike chemicals in the brain. A later study confirmed these results. Dr. Elsas offered some encouragement in that all the brain changes reverted to normal within a three-week period, but he said it "took longer for full mental function to return.'' He concluded that anyone over the age of six months should limit aspartame consumption to moderate amounts and should get their blood checked if they had any adverse symptoms.

Dr. Wurtman had previously questioned the safety of aspartame, saying the FDA had misled the public by playing down the concerns voiced by such scientists as those at the national Centers for Disease Control. The CDC had received more than six hundred complaints from consumers claiming adverse effects, such as dizziness, headaches, blurred vision, or epileptic seizures, after consuming aspartame. Detailed investigation of two hundred of these complaints led the CDC to suggest that the adverse effects from aspartame consumption, especially neurological and behavioral—which comprised 67 percent of the complaints—indicated the need for a systematic study of its safety. The CDC report said, "The number of instances of persons challenging themselves several times with aspartame-containing products and reporting symptoms with each rechallenge suggests that some individuals may be sensitive. The only way to clearly determine this is through focused clinical studies that should concentrate on such symptoms as headaches, mood alterations and behavior changes.''

This was by no means the first time the safety of aspartame had been questioned. The original FDA approval, in 1974, had been withdrawn when Dr. John Olney of Washington University said his studies indicated that consumption of aspartame might have caused cancerous brain tumors in animals. Another factor in the withdrawal of approval, as reported in the *FDA Consumer*, were "challenges over the validity of the company's data [which] kept aspartame from being marketed.''

The two amino acids found in aspartame, asparic acid and phenylalanine, are found naturally in many foods high in protein. If the quantity of an individual's aspartame intake should be limited, consumption of aspartame plus a high-protein diet poses an additional risk and makes the total amount consumed that much more difficult for consumers to monitor.

Another possible health hazard occurs when aspartame decomposes and exposes consumers to excessive levels of methanol. The FDA states, "At high enough levels, methanol is a poison and can cause blindness. It also is metabolized into formaldehyde, a 'known carcinogen,' critics charge. (Some inhalation tests in animals show that formaldehyde produces nasal tumors)." The danger of decomposition of aspartame seems to stem primarily from the fact that it is sensitive to high temperatures—one of the reasons it was not immediately used in baked products. For example, beverages stored for long periods at high temperatures might contain NutraSweet that has decomposed. The FDA does not perceive this as a danger to consumers, since it says that in studies "the levels of methanol resulting from the use of aspartame in carbonated beverages did not pose any safety issues because they were well below levels of exposure expected to produce toxicity."

If, however, you find your soft drink doesn't taste quite right, it may be that the aspartame has broken down somewhat. It is less stable in liquids than in solids and, since soft drinks might have been stored for a while in high temperature warehouses—Searle quoted "typical storage periods" of up to 52 weeks and up to 130 degrees Fahrenheit—the drinks, while still supposedly safe, may lose much of their sweetness.

The FDA has set 50 milligrams per kilogram of body weight as an allowable daily intake, estimating that actual average use would be about 8 to 10 milligrams. By the spring of 1984 a national survey revealed the average intake at that time was 19 milligrams, and the maximum level was 28 milligrams, both well over the estimated average use. By January 1985 the FDA reported average consumption to be 30 milligrams, with many consumers ingesting above the 50-milligram intake the FDA had established as the safe allowable maximum. In commenting on these consumption figures at that time, Dr. Wurtman said consumer levels of consumption could easily reach amounts that have been linked in animal studies to adverse effects on brain chemicals. Also, since his studies showed that high levels of aspartame may trigger a craving for carbohydrates by depleting the brain of a chemical that measures carbohydrate satiety, dieters may be exacerbating rather than solving their problems. And since, as we have seen, there is possibly danger that a carbohydrate/aspartame combination will increase the adverse effects of aspartame on the brain, this craving may lead to other complications.

Children may be especially at risk, partly because of their smaller size. Dr. C. Keith-Conners of Children's Hospital in Washington, D.C., reported in February 1985 the case of two children who suffer extreme agitation when they consume the amount of aspartame equivalent to that in a six-ounce serving of Kool-Aid sweetened with NutraSweet. He said one of the children becomes so agitated that he has to be restrained. The other, who reacts with aggression to sugar intake, becomes even more so when given aspartame.

Searle and Company has said that six hundred complaints are very few, considering that more than 100 million people now consume aspartame, although they concede that "a few people may be allergic or sensitive to it." The FDA has joined Searle in taking the position that aspartame is the most extensively studied food additive in history and that its safety has been clearly established. In February 1985 Dr. Sanford Miller, then head of the FDA's Bureau of Foods, said, "I don't know of any substance in recent years that's been looked at with the intensity of aspartame. No one has yet come up with the slightest evidence to show we were wrong in approving it."

As more studies are done, Dr. Miller might perhaps reconsider whether possible dangers from aspartame have not been indicated by more than "the slightest evidence." For one thing, Dr. Walle Nauta, an MIT psychologist and head of a public board of inquiry that reviewed safety concerns in 1980 at the request of the FDA, has said that had the panel known how widely aspartame would be used, it would have issued stronger recommendations. He told the publication *Common Cause* more specifically that use of aspartame in soft drinks "never figured in our decision-making." Dr. Nauta's panel did not investigate the validity of the tests but only their results, so the question of whether the results were valid was never considered. In July 1985 *The New York Times* reported that several scientists were conducting studies of aspartame or its components and that their preliminary data have indicated that aspartame may be responsible for a range of problems. Searle says their own studies contradict this and that it is conducting further studies to confirm their conclusions. The FDA's Center for Food and Applied Nutrition considers the claims against aspartame unfounded.

In 1981, when Dr. Arthur Hill Hayes, Jr., then FDA commissioner, granted approval of aspartame, several of the agency's scientists and an independent board of inquiry (that had been set up to evaluate Searle's studies of aspartame's effect on animals) had reported that Searle's research did not adequately answer questions about the carcinogenicity of aspartame. Testifying before Congress, Dr. Alexander M. Schmidt, a former FDA commissioner, said some of the Searle experiments were "poorly conceived, carelessly executed, or inaccurately analyzed or reported." In spite of these opinions, Dr. Hayes, Jr., granted approval.

More recently Dr. M. Adrian Gross, senior science adviser at the EPA (Environmental Protection Agency) and a former pathologist at the FDA, wrote to Senator Howard M. Metzenbaum, as a member of the Committee on Labor and Human Resources, to point out that despite the experiments' shortcomings, "at least one of those studies has established beyond any reasonable doubt that aspartame is capable of inducing brain tumors in experimental animals." Searle's Dr. Frank M. Sturtevant, a pharmacologist who is director of the office of scientific affairs at the company, has explained that some of the data that had been given to Dr. Gross for review was incorrect. The correct tabulations, he said, show "no statistically significant increase in brain tumors in experimental animals."

Although even some proponents of aspartame seem to think that consuming too much may cause serious illnesses, the possibility of limiting intake of aspartame to "safe" levels grows increasingly dim as it is approved for use in more and more foods. Almost all "sugar-free' soft drinks now contain aspartame; many even feature the fact that they contain only aspartame, with no saccharin added. Dr. Wurtman points out, in this connection, that a 2-liter bottle of Diet Coke contains about 1,200 milligrams of aspartame, which means a seven-year-old child, weighing about forty-five or fifty pounds, will exceed the allowable daily limit suggested by the FDA by drinking just one bottle. Pudding mixes, gelatine desserts, breakfast cereals, hot chocolate, and bubble gum—all of which are consumed in considerable quantity by children—contain aspartame. The latest approved use for aspartame is in vitamins, both adults' and children's.

How to Avoid Aspartame

Since new products are constantly being added to the list of aspartame-sweetened items, the only way the consumer can limit overall intake is to examine the package and read the label. If "sugar-free" is prominently displayed, read the label to find out what sweetener has been used. If it is a "diet" food, find out what accounts for lower calories. It could be less fat but it might be aspartame. Searle has made it easier to detect aspartame by recommending that the consumer look for a little blue swirl device that identifies products containing 100 percent NutraSweet. Locating this device on a package makes it easier for the consumer who wishes to avoid this additive. Remember, you need to try to estimate the amount of aspartame you may be ingesting daily in order to determine whether you are within the FDA's suggested "safe" levels. If you or someone in your family is especially sensitive to this—as to any other substance—the safe level might be considerably lower than that suggested by the FDA. Dr. Wurtman, who is, in addition to his position at MIT, a consultant to Searle (on products other than aspartame) is of the opinion that ½ gram to 1 gram a day should be safe for those adults who have no special sensitivity. Even this amount, however, may need to be lowered if consumed in conjunction with a high-carbohydrate diet. Generally speaking, however, Dr. Wurtman does not believe that moderate amounts are harmful to most normal people.

PART TWO

High Tech
in the
Kitchen

CHAPTER 8

Forever Foods— The Food Processor's Dream

From prehistoric time man has tried to preserve food so that it would not spoil into inedibility. The hunter soon learned to dry his meat and fish so that his efforts could feed himself and his family for longer than a few days. The women of the family did the same with plants, roots, and fruits and vegetables. As time went on, preserving by means of salting, smoking, and corning were developed. In cold climates, winter made freezing sometimes a viable alternative and the Eskimos developed a unique method of preserving fish by hanging it out in the sun to rot and then freezing it. They considered the end result a great delicacy and Stefansson, the noted Arctic explorer, reported that it tasted much like Roquefort cheese.

Today, with much of our food produced far from where it will be eaten, the food processor's search is increasingly for foods that will last as near to forever as possible. When food was grown locally—remember the vine-ripened tomatoes and tree-ripened peaches of the old farmers' markets?— we ate it in season, and except for winter root vegetables like turnips and the hardier fruits, like apples, we did without when it was not in season. Today a much wider variety of foods is available year round—shipped sometimes from halfway around the world. This has led to the development of produce grown not for flavor or increased nutrients but for the ability to withstand the rigors of shipping and transporting and of being picked green. And more and more fresh produce is processed to keep it "fresh" long after it would otherwise look its age.

One result of "fresh food processing" is that the consumer is exposed more and more to methods of preservation that are or may be hazardous to health. The use of sulfites is one such example (see Chapter 9, Forever Fresh—the Sulfite Story), the problem with nitrites and nitrates is another, as are all the chemical preservatives that are pressed into service in the pursuit of eternal freshness. When did you last see a stale loaf of brand bread? Even the consumer can now process foods to make them last longer; milk exposed to radiation in your microwave oven will stay ''fresh'' weeks longer than untreated (only pasteurized and homogenized) milk.

Two of the most recent developments—irradiation and aseptic packaging—seem straight out of Buck Rogers. (See also Chapter 13, The Nuclear Pantry—Irradiated Foods.)

The Aseptic Package

In 1982 the following appeared in an advertisement in a Houston, Texas, newspaper:

> Week after week it stays fresh and delicious—with or without refrigeration!
>
> Here's the milk you can buy now and drink later—weeks and months later if you wish it! It comes in an extraordinary new carton made possible by advanced technology, so you can keep it in a cupboard or keep it in a refrigerator . . . you just refrigerate after opening.

The product being advertised was low-fat milk that, in its new carton, will keep, unrefrigerated, for as long as six months. Aseptic cartons of this type are now routinely used for fruit juices and similar beverages and come in handy single-serving sizes with their own straw attached. Since they do not require refrigeration until opened, they can be stocked on any supermarket shelf, in an office desk, or a child's lunchbox. It is only a question of time before the technology will be adapted to solid foods.

Europeans have had this technology in their food markets for over twenty years, but it could not be used in the United States until the FDA approved the use of hydrogen peroxide to sterilize the polyethylene surfaces that come in contact with the packaged food. Hydrogen peroxide? Right. The same antiseptic that Grandma poured over your knee when you scraped it. The solution foamed interestingly, and the scrape was cleansed. The same antiseptic qualities are now put to work in many other ways as a food preservative. Among other uses, for example, it is one of the chemicals you may get on your ''fresh'' fish.

The use of aseptic packaging is growing so rapidly that by 1981 the Dallas firm had produced more than 15 billion units of aseptic packages, which they were distributing in more than seventy countries worldwide.

Whenever a preservative is used, the question of safety arises. The FDA regulation approving hydrogen peroxide in flexible aseptic packages has established a residue level in food that must not exceed 10.1 parts per million, or the equivalent of 100 parts per billion. This level was established on the theory that the hydrogen peroxide residue would dissipate to 1 part per billion or less within twenty-four hours after the food has been packaged. Up to now approval has not been granted for other plastic coatings due to lack of determination as to the amount of hydrogen peroxide that these materials would allow to migrate into the packaged food.

The object of all this, of course, is to create "commercially sterile" food, which the FDA defines as food that has been processed to the point that it is free of microorganisms that could harm public health or that might cause a nonrefrigerated food to spoil during storage or distribution. Food that is to be aseptically packaged is sterilized separately; then, after cooling slightly, it is put into the package that has been sterilized with hydrogen peroxide. All this must be done under sterile conditions, that is, in a "commercially sterile" environment.

It would be helpful to be sure this new packaging is really safe, but given the history of other food additives and residues, and the FDA's own cautious acceptance of hydrogen peroxide, it might be better to take the poet Alexander Pope's advice, "Be not the first by whom the new is tried," at least as far as feeding it to children. Meanwhile, bottles, cans, and cartons aren't all that inconvenient.

CHAPTER 9

Forever Fresh—
The Sulfite Story

Sulfurous compounds, or sulfites, have been added to foods and beverages for almost a century. Food processors have found sulfites invaluable in many ways: as preservatives, to prevent browning, to inhibit bacterial formation, to control fermentation, for their antioxidant action, and for similar purposes. Sulfites have been traditionally added to such foods as dried fruits; maraschino cherries; corn syrup; raw, frozen, and dehydrated potatoes; shellfish and other seafood; fresh fruits and vegetables; salad dressings; pickles; wine and beer. Since they are now used in dough conditioners, they may be found also in finished packaged goods, such as cookies.

The safety of this additive was first questioned in 1907 by Dr. Harvey W. Wiley, chief of the Bureau of Chemistry, the government agency that preceded the formation of the FDA. He objected to the use of sulfur dioxide in the processing of dried fruits, contending that it not only spoiled the flavor of the fruit but also was actually harmful to humans who ate it. The fruit packers objected that it had not been proved harmful and that dried fruit would look much less attractive to the consumer if it were not used. Unfortunately, Dr. Wiley was overruled and sulfur dioxide and other sulfites continued to be used.

Four years later a USDA study confirmed Dr. Wiley's contention that sulfur dioxide in food could cause destruction of blood corpuscles, anemia, backaches, and lethargy in certain individuals who had a sensitivity to the chemical and who ate it over a period of time. The study received little publicity, however, and was generally unnoticed or ignored.

Today—seventy-six years later—the label on a package of a popular brand of raisins includes the words, "prepared with sulfur dioxide for color retention," and sulfur dioxide is still routinely used in processing all dried fruits, except those that are "organically" prepared. Knowing that sulfur dioxide and sulfites are still on the GRAS list is proof that the FDA considers them "generally recognized as safe," and processors may still use them freely.

Once again, however, the sulfite controversy is in the news as the dangers of its use are illustrated by an increasing number of adverse consumer reactions and as nutritionists discover other harmful effects. For some time, for example, lowered sulfite levels have been recommended for use in foods high in thiamin, such as beef, because they have a destructive effect on this essential B vitamin. And now it has been discovered that asthmatics and others with sulfite sensitivity may have life-threatening reactions upon ingesting foods treated with sulfites.

Dr. Alice S. Huang of the Harvard Medical School, writing in *The New England Journal of Medicine* (August 23, 1984), reported her personal observations of a group exposed to sulfites:

One of us has experienced transient itchy palms within 15 minutes after the ingestion of many different commercially prepared foods probably containing sulfiting agents, such as chili soups, sandwiches, salads, jalapeños and pizza. An especially severe attack occurred after ingestion of Chinese pickled green turnips and dried shrimps used to flavor bean curd soup. Besides the initial palmar and plantar pruritis, this attack was characterized by generalized uticaria beginning at the extremities and genitalia, leading to facial and laryngeal edema, severe abdominal pain, and fulminant diarrhea. The pain and macular rash gradually subsided over one to two hours.

A threshold level of sensitivity was determined after a dental appointment. The initial symptoms of palmar pruritus were evident after an inoculation with 1.8 ml of lidocaine hydrochloride containing 0.5 mg of sodium bisulfite per millileter. In the past, only 1.0 of this local anesthetic had been given to [me], without eliciting any reactions. Thus, as little as 0.9 mg induces symptoms.

Dr. Huang concluded that we should all be aware when sulfites are present in foods and medications. Following this excellent advice is practically impossible at present, since the consumer has very little way of knowing what foods or beverages have been treated with sulfite; neither medications nor many foods list this information on lables, nor—until 1985—was there a proposal to ban it from salad bars, where it is freely used to keep the salads "looking fresh." Dr. Huang said further, "Not only are labeling requirements essential, it is inappropriate to use life-threatening preservatives when other, safer agents are available.''

Further study has discovered that sensitive persons can have what is known as a Type I hypersensitivity reaction shortly after eating sulfited foods. Ironically, the treatment for this reaction is epinephrine, in which sodium bisulfite is used as a preservative. Epinephrine, the drug of choice for asthma, is routinely used by and for asthmatics, who are particularly prone to bad reactions from sulfites. In other words, a person having a sulfite-induced asthma attack could be treated with an injection of medication containing the very substance that is already threatening his life. This would seem to be a clear indication that sulfites should be banned from prescription and nonprescription drugs.

One sulfite sufferer, B. Carolyn Knight, has written a book, *Canary in a Coal Mine*, about her eleven-year battle with sulfur sensitivity. In spite of intensive research, neither she nor her doctors had been able to track down the cause of her severe illness. As it turned out, she was particularly sensitive to the potassium metabisulfite her father used to control fermentation in his homemade wine.

The National Restaurant Association, to its credit, has taken the sulfite problem seriously. First, they issued informative literature (see Facts about Sulfites) to help sulfite-sensitive individuals who are eating out. Then they supported the suggestion that a ban be placed on the use of sulfites in restaurant and produce markets. In the meantime many restaurants have voluntarily discontinued sulfiting foods in their kitchens. This action is similar to the way Chinese restaurants voluntarily cut back on the use of monosodium glutamate when consumers discovered "Chinese restaurant syndrome."

How to Avoid Sulfites

1. The National Restaurant Association recommends that you avoid the following major food categories if you are or suspect you are sensitive to sulfites or if you have asthma:

   avocado dip and guacamole

   baked goods

   dried cod

   fruit (cut-up, fresh, dried, or maraschino-type)

   fruit juices

   potatoes (cut-up, fresh, frozen, dried, canned)

salad dressings (dry mix)

salad bars

sauces and gravies (both canned and dried)

sauerkraut

cole slaw

shellfish (fresh, frozen, canned, dried), including clams, crab, lobster, scallops, and shrimp

fresh mushrooms

wine vinegar

wine, wine coolers

beer

cider

2. Many of these food groups may be safe if they are prepared at home. Cole slaw, for example, is probably safe if freshly made from cabbage and homemade mayonnaise in your own kitchen. On the other hand, gelatin desserts, even if made at home from unflavored gelatin, may contain sulfite. Fruit juices, if freshly prepared at home, are free of sulfites, and in any case not all commercial fruit juices contain them.

3. Take-out food eaten at home is subject to the same problems as restaurant food. When ordering, ask whether the restaurant uses sulfites.

4. Processed foods frequently do mention sulfites on their labels, but you may not recognize them as such. They may be listed as: potassium bisulfite, potassium metabisulfite, sodium bisulfite, sodium sulfite, or sulfur dioxide. Since sulfites are also used in processing items that may be listed in the ingredients, such as beet sugar, even this list is not a completely reliable guide.

5. It is thought that the majority of sulfite reactions occur from eating restaurant food, but the solution to this problem is not simple. Even if you ask at a restaurant whether sulfites are used in the food, the restaurateur may honestly say no. What he may not realize is that some of the processed foods that he uses as ingredients in his freshly prepared dishes, such as corn sweeteners and prepared fruit pie mixes, may contain the additive.

A tragic incident that vividly illustrates the restaurant's and the diner's problem was recently related by Jeffrey Prince, a director of the National Association of Restaurants. According to Mr. Prince, a diner, knowing she was sensitive to sulfites, asked the restaurant manager if sulfites were used in any of its food, especially in its french fries. The manager checked the plastic bag in which the potatoes had been delivered, but no sulfite preservative was listed on the label. What neither the manager nor the diner had any way of knowing was that the french fries had been repackaged in smaller quantities by the distributor; the original package had listed sulfites but the smaller package did not. The diner, reassured, ate the french fries and died.

6. Since fish is often processed right on board the fishing boat, and since fillets are sometimes dipped in sulfited water at that time to keep them fresh and to preserve their whiteness, you might want to shop at a fish market that does its own filleting. There is no way you can protect yourself against the probable sulfiting of scallops and shrimp unless labeling of fish containers is required to state that sulfite has been used (and you have access to the original container, which is not usually on display). Perhaps there should be a law requiring fish markets to post which fish has been sulfited—though the market's proprietors might not always know.

Facts About Sulfites

Certain individuals are hypersensitive to sulfiting agents used in processing specific foods, beverages, and drugs. These people experience adverse reactions of varying degrees of severity.

Asthmatics or other individuals with this hypersensitivity should avoid consuming items which contain sulfiting agents. They can identify these items by reading labels on packaged foods and by inquiring about their presence in foods eaten away from home.

Sulfur dioxide and several forms of inorganic sulfites that release sulfur dioxide when used as food ingredients are known collectively as sulfiting agents. They are marketed as "vegetable fresheners" or "potato whitening" agents and are used to eliminate bacteria, preserve freshness and brightness, prevent browning, increase storage life, and prevent spoilage of certain food products. They are also used to improve the quality or texture of finished baked products.

According to some studies, 5% to 10% of all asthmatics are hypersensitive to sulfiting agents. They may experience reactions ranging from relatively mild to severe. Symptoms may include difficulty in breathing, flushing, hives, gastrointestinal disturbance, and, possibly, anaphylactic shock.

SOURCE: National Restaurant Association and Food Allergy Committee of the American College of Allergists. Co-Chairmen Sami L. Barna, M.D., and Robert J. Dockhom, M.D.

Limited Sulfite Ban

On July 8, 1986, the FDA finally banned the use of sulfites on raw fruits and vegetables. The FDA release stated, "The ban eliminates their GRAS status when used on raw, packaged, or unpackaged fruits and vegetables." This means, however, that sulfites may still be used in many other foods, such as dried fruit, nuts, lemon juice, maraschino cherries, vegetables, canned soups, baked goods, and other processed foods. In the case of most of these foods, sulfites are required to be listed on the label. I checked my cupboard against this list and found sulfite only in the raisins; there was so sulfite listed on the frozen lemon juice, grape juice, or canned soups. Apparently it is possible, by careful selection, to purchase some of these items sulfite-free. If you wish to avoid sulfites, examine each type of item separately; do not assume, for example, that all of a certain brand of soup are sulfite-free; check each variety you plan to purchase. Sulfite is not, however, invariably identified on the label, as, for example, when it is used on shrimp and other seafood and in wine and beer.

A notable exception to the ban is raw prepared potatoes, which, of course, includes frozen potatoes. French fried and hash brown potatoes account for the bulk of potato consumption in the United States, including their use at home and in restaurants. The FDA's position is that potatoes accounted for only 6 percent of the complaints received, compared to 28 percent for salad bars, but one cannot help but wonder how many people who feel ill after a meal think of possible sulfite-sensitivity or relate their illness to such a common food as a french fried potato. Frank A. Young, FDA Commissioner, further explained that potatoes are more complicated to deal with than are other fresh vegetables and fruits.

Representative Ron Wyden and Senator Albert Gore, Jr., who sponsored the original legislation in Congress requiring the FDA to evaluate and possibly regulate sulfites in food, are among those not satisfied with this limited ban. As Senator Gore put it, "The FDA has chosen to ignore the Congress and the clear wishes of the American people by failing to protect those Americans highly vulnerable to sulfites other than those in fresh fruits and vegetables." And the FDA admitted in its own release, ". . . there is no known level at which sulfites do not pose a health risk to susceptible people."

Possibly the most serious effect of the limited ban is that it may lull consumers into a false sense of safety. To minimize risk of ingesting sulfites, it is still necessary to approach salad bars, in particular, and prepared foods, in general, with caution; especially such foods as pickles, seafood, dried fruits, and frozen potatoes, which may not be prepared by the restaurant, delicatessen, or market.

What finally led to the ban, seventy-eight years after Dr. Wiley sought

---

Sulfites Before Congress

In a hearing before the House Energy and Commerce Subcommittee on Oversight and Investigation, under the chairmanship of Representative John D. Dingell (D. Michigan) on March 28, 1985, a ban on the use of sulfites in food was urged by members of Congress, scientists, and people who said they or their loved ones had suffered from inadvertent exposure to chemicals.

Among the reported allergic reactions to sulfites was that suffered by Medaya McPike, a 10-year-old girl from Salem, Oregon, whose parents were among the witnesses calling for a ban. Medaya's father, James McPike, said the girl had had an asthmatic reaction the previous month after eating a meal of guacamole and tostada in a restaurant. The meal contained sulfites and as a result of ingesting it, she had fallen into unconsciousness and died five days later.

"If sulfites are safe, as the Food and Drug Administration indicates by giving them a status of 'generally recognized as safe,' then why is our 10-year-old daughter dead?" Mr. McPike asked. "How many more, just like our 10-year-old Medaya, will have to die before the FDA will do something to regulate or eliminate this additive from our food?"

---

it, were findings from the Federation of American Societies for Experimental Biology. They described five hundred alleged adverse reactions, including thirteen deaths, which were possibly due to sulfite-treated foods, mostly food served in restaurants. William Grigg of the FDA ascribed the increase in reported adverse reactions to proliferation of salad bars, which led the agency to conclude that sulfite sensitivity now puts at risk a greater proportion of the population. "Sulfites can cause reactions in up to a million sulfite-sensitive people, mostly asthmatics," Mr. Grigg explained. Unfortunately, this is still true. The next step, to close the loopholes that still expose people unwittingly to the consumption of sulfited foods, would be to extend the ban to all foods. As Representative Ron Wyden of Oregon has explained his position, "There is just no reason to taint foods with sulfite just to keep them pretty."

What Are the Symptoms of Sulfite-Sensitivity?

If you experience nausea, diarrhea, hives, flushing, weakness, swollen tongue, difficulty in swallowing or breathing, or fainting shortly after eating, you might suspect you are sensitive to sulfite and should perhaps see your

---

Sulfite Labeling

A release from the FDA (September 6, 1985) indicates how the requirement that "labels of products containing sulfites as preservatives (must) state that sulfites were used," is enforced.

"The Food and Drug Administration today warned that 'San Francisco Herb Co.' brand dehydrated vegetable mixes and fruit mixes distributed to wholesalers and retail stores in eighteen states—and sold by catalog as well— may contain undeclared sulfites that can cause reactions in sulfite-sensitive people. The mixes are being voluntarily recalled by the manufacturer, Hansmar Inc. of San Francisco.

"The various product mixes are packaged in one-pound plastic bags as: Mixed Vegetable Flakes, Vegetable Soup Blend, Vegetable Stew Blend, Fruit Mix, and Fruit Galaxy Mix. Besides California, they were distributed in Alabama, Arizona, Iowa, Kansas, Maryland, Michigan, Missouri, Montana, Nebraska, New Mexico, New York, Ohio, Utah, Virginia, Washington State, Wisconsin, and Wyoming. Some of the mixes may have also been mailed to people ordering from the company's catalog."

---

doctor. If your reactions are severe, you might want to seek emergency treatment. It is thought that most people are not sulfite-sensitive, and several of the above reactions are reactions that could occur from other things to which you are allergic, or they could be due to entirely different causes. About 5 percent to 10 percent of those who have asthma will have a reaction, but one-third of the people reporting symptoms did not have any known allergies.

The cause of this special sensitivity is not known; it has not even been definitely established that it is an allergy, although one of the more severe reactions—anaphylactic shock—is an allergic reaction. One theory is that the sensitivity is due to a deficiency of an enzyme called sulfite oxidase that aids in the metabolizing of sulfites.

Is Sulfite Sensitivity Serious?

Sulfite sensitivity reactions vary from merely uncomfortable to severe to life-threatening to death. There have been hundreds of documented reported reactions (and obviously not all those reacting have reported it) during the two years from 1982 to 1984. This comparatively small number might not have caused particular concern except that during that period four (and maybe more not reported) of the people involved died as a result. By July

---

Allowable Sulfite Levels and Food Safety

When a food additive is "generally recognized as safe" (GRAS), it may be known to be toxic but the FDA has determined that the toxicity will not occur under a certain level of ingestion. Food processors using these substances must adhere to these levels, and FDA food inspection includes spot testing to ensure compliance.

In the case of sulfites, the allowable levels have proved inadequate protection to sulfite-sensitive individuals. Two sulfite-related deaths that occurred in July 1985 were traced to the ingestion of white wine and to hash brown potatoes. In both cases, laboratory analysis showed the sulfite content of the wine and the potatoes was within the allowable levels, 242 parts per million for the potatoes and 92 parts per million for the wine.

It is difficult to understand how the FDA can set "allowable levels" for an additive for which they admit "there is no known level at which sulfites do not pose a health risk to susceptible people." (FDA Release, 7/8/86) Perhaps now that sulfites have been taken off the GRAS list it will be more closely regulated. Perhaps not.

1985, the number of deaths attributed to sulfite ingestion had risen to thirteen. By September 1985, the number of adverse reactions reported had risen to six hundred and the total number of deaths to fifteen.

Among the causes from reported reactions were: eating from a salad bar; eating a meal consisting of eggs, home fried potatoes, and fruit cup; eating hash brown potatoes; drinking wine; eating a meal of guacamole and tostada. These all involve known uses of sulfites, such as adding them to foods to keep them crisp, to retard oxidation (raw foods turning brown or spoiling, for instance), and to keep berries red, spinach green, and potatoes white.

Whom to Notify If You Think You've Had a Reaction

In order to evaluate the percentage of the population at risk through the use of sulfites, it is important for everyone to report any reactions either he or persons he is with experience. Write to: Dockets Management Branch, Dockets No. 81N034, U.S. FDA, Fishers Lane, Rockville, MD 20857.

Describe the incident, tell where and when it occured, and list the foods you ate at the time. Do not list just the foods and beverages you think were involved; put down everything you ate and drank.

The Sulfite Lesson

The history of sulfite use in food—from its original inclusion on the GRAS list to its present extremely limited ban—sends a clear signal to concerned consumers that they cannot take for granted the safety of their food. As late as September 6, 1985, the FDA stated in a release, "Sulfites are harmless to most people but may cause hives, nausea, shortness of breath, and sometimes life-threatening shock in up to a million people who are sensitive to the substances." In spite of this indisputable hidden threat to "up to a million" of innocent Americans, sulfites were, and still continue to be, permitted to be used in our food.

Measured by the cost-benefit ratio, the FDA apparently feels that the cost of loss of the profits to be reaped by keeping tired, nutritionally deficient food looking "fresh" and "pretty" outweighs the benefits of health and life to the one million people at risk through ingesting sulfites. If the public disagrees and makes its wishes known, the use of sulfites may finally come to an end.

CHAPTER 10

Bland Is It— Artificial Flavors Take Over

Do you find you don't enjoy your food as much as you used to? Does everything seem to taste the same? Do you long for certain favorite dishes, only to be disappointed when you eat them at that expensive new restaurant? Are you one of the restless millions of Americans eating hotter and spicier foods in an effort to find the elusive flavors food used to have?

If so, don't blame yourself. The food you are eating today isn't the same food you remember. Partly because of the way it is raised, partly because of the way it is processed, partly because of the way it is distributed, and partly because of the push for greater and greater profits, most of the taste has been lost somewhere between the harvest and the dinner table.

Once it is lost, flavor cannot be regained. And if food is harvested before it has developed, flavor can never be fully realized. When fruits are picked unripe for the market, their full flavor hasn't had time to develop; some melons, such as cantaloupe, will ripen eventually, others, like honeydew, will never mature. In neither case will they taste like a tree-ripened melon if picked green.

Vegetables also have a peak period of flavor, but some varieties have been bred more for marketing than for eating. The average store tomato will turn red but it will never truly ripen; to fit it for its hard life it has been bred into a barely edible, totally tasteless, tennis ball-like product, so even if it were picked ripe, it wouldn't have much taste or "tomato" quality. When home gardeners choose their seeds, they avoid the varieties the catalog describes as "withstands shipping well" or "good commercial varieties." Those are the ones you find in the market; they add color to your salads but little else. (Use red peppers or dried apricots instead and get more nutrition.)

The consumer can improve the present poor quality of some fresh produce. If everyone stops buying some of the worst of it, such as out-of-season tomatoes—canned tomatoes have much more flavor—we will see a return to the real thing. Just as with processed foods, when there is a choice between products with real natural flavors and those with unreal "natural" flavors or artificial ones, choosing not to buy inferior produce would have a real impact on the market. The recent proliferation of low-salt, low-sugar, and "all natural" items shows that manufacturers are taking consumers' wishes seriously.

Why has our food reached its present sorry state? The name of the game is profits. And it isn't only fresh fruits and vegetables that are affected; processed food is in an even sadder state.

Trade advertising emphasizes the cost effectiveness of all additives, whether a given flavor, a food enhancer, or a food coloring. Modern "efficient" food manufacturing relies on chemicals to achieve the results that used to come from long, slow ripening (of cheese), rising (of yeast bread), smoking (of meat), curing (of hams), and range feeding (of beef), and all the other ways that man has learned over thousands of years to make his food mouth-wateringly delicious. Modern methods shortcut the old ways, which are too time consuming and, therefore, too expensive. The result is "food" with almost no natural taste; no wonder when it has been extruded, spray dried, irradiated, stabilized, emulsified, watered, injected, dissolved, pasteurized, homogenized, bleached, and loaded with chemicals and additives to make it last as close as possible to forever.

When it comes to the base product, blandness is actually the aim of the industry. The less taste a finished "food" has, the easier it is to add artificial flavor to it. For instance, as one of the trade magazine notes, certain yeast extracts are recommended because

> they can serve as a flavor foundation, providing a base upon which delicate and mellow flavors can be formulated. Tomato, vegetable, mushroom soups, and seafood chowders are examples. . . . Also, they can act as outstanding flavor contributors as well, imparting all of their rich, brothy taste to chicken and beef flavored soups. In these heartier soups they serve well as flavor blenders, too, making for a full-bodied, zesty yet mellow tasting product.

An example of an application of this product is described, with mushroom soup used as the example. "A relatively high use level is suggested, since it supplies almost the entire brothy character of this soup. Because of the mouthfeel properties contributed by the mushrooms, it is not necessary to use the premium grade product." (In other words, it makes "good" soup with lower quality ingredients, an obvious saving in manufacturing costs.)

And later on: "Its lightness in color does not offend these soups (cream of mushroom, cream of celery, and cream of other vegetables). A slightly cream colored character often imparts the impression of butterlike richness." The suggested ingredients for the mushroom soup are: "Basic Broth: Mushrooms (canned, including stock), Non-fat Milk Solids, Autolyzed Yeast Extract, Tomato Paste, MSG. Other Ingredients: Wheat Flour, Corn Starch, Butter." Among the "Suggested Variations" is "partial or total replacement of butter with hydrogenated vegetable oil."

A discussion of chicken soups suggests, "If no chicken broth or chicken solids are added, and the formula depends entirely on chicken fat for natural chicken flavor, use the premium grade product to impart added body." The Onion Broth recipe, using the yeast extracts, says it produces "a beef-like onion stock made without the use of any Extracts." In this case, presumably, the ingredients list would give some indication, if read carefully, that meaty, beef-like flavor did not come from beef or any other meat.

In itself yeast is not undesirable (except to those who are allergic to it), and it probably adds B-complex vitamins (if they are not destroyed in the processing), but when it is used to help replace the chicken or beef needed to make a true broth, the result is a fabricated version of real chicken or beef broth. Recently it has been discovered that chicken soup has certain especially beneficial qualities. The consumer who feels under the weather and eats this kind of chicken soup to get this beneficial effect may never know why it didn't work. Read ingredients lists on soup labels; there are some good real soups. Or try making your own once in a while.

If, by chance, natural flavor survives in a food, it merely complicates the formula from the processor's point of view, because natural flavors vary and aren't "uniform." Uniformity appears to be one of the most desirable qualities a "food" can achieve—if only from the manufacturer's viewpoint. Processed cheese is valued because, among other things, it is so uniform. Blending ensures uniform "taste," and all the rest of the processing, up to the point that it is poured into uniform cartons, keeps it uniform in texture, color, and shelf life. No surprises could be the motto of the food industry as well as the motel that originated the TV commercial.

Surimi (see Chapter 4, Surimi—The Great Pretender) is about as close to their ideal as food processors have been able to get so far. The raw product is cheap; it has no pronounced taste or flavor to compete with the artificial flavors; it will take on almost any desired form, and can be successfully colored and flavored to pass as the "real" thing. Best of all, it can be called *natural,* a term most consumers still find reassuring.

The manufacturer's desire for a uniform product is flattered in advertising, with such copy as this from an ad for lemon flavoring:

If Mother Nature was perfect, she would create sweet lemons . . . and bland lemons . . . as well as sour lemons. But because professional cooks, bakers and beverage makers demand different flavors, they call us for our flavor expertise. We respond with natural, natural-artificial and artificial flavors that improve on Mother Nature . . . Your customers always remember the way it tastes, and [Brand X] flavors always taste the way they remember.

The food processors know their "formulations" are tasteless but still want them to have consumer appeal, so they try to imitate nature. (As we saw when we talked about meat, they even have to add flavor to animal feed because it tastes so awful to the animals that they won't touch it otherwise.)

In the old days, explorers and caravans were sent in search of new spices to make the limited menus and often spoiled foods palatable. The spice trade became so profitable that companies grew up that sold nothing else. Many of them are still in business today, with one important difference: the spices and flavorings from exotic places have been joined by the products of food chemists—artificial, laboratory-created flavorings that are shadowy imitations of the real thing. More than one generation has grown up never having tasted real vanilla and thinking watered ham is what real ham tastes like.

"Natural Flavors"

Just because a product label says it's natural doesn't mean it is. The government does not define *natural,* nor are there any regulations as to when the term can or cannot be applied to food. A look at the flavor industry shows how hard it can be to decide where the line has been drawn between natural and artificial. To make it even more difficult, the two are often combined, as when a natural flavor is beefed up with an artificial one. Most natural flavorings are made by companies that also make artificial ones, and it is sometimes difficult to tell which is which even from the sales literature of these companies.

The government allows flavors to be called natural even though the foods to which they are added do not naturally contain them, and even though their function is to "enhance" other flavors rather than to add flavor themselves. Because of these labeling laws, the consumer who wishes to avoid artificial flavors cannot depend on labels.

A natural flavor, at least to my way of thinking, is something directly derived from its source; vanilla from the vanilla bean, cocoa from the cocoa bean, coffee from the coffee bean. If it has been processed one bit more than is absolutely necessary, is made in a laboratory, does not occur in nature, or is combined with an artificial flavor, I no longer consider it natural.

The "Excessive Sweetness" Natural Flavoring

There is a curious flavoring on the market described as "a unique blend of natural ingredients specially formulated to reduce excessive sweetness in candy and other confections. It is stable under the acidic or alkaline conditions associated with most foods. It will not cause inversion of sugar nor will it promote rancidity. It is stable at temperatures encountered in candy manufacturing.

As the sales literature suggests: "It may be used effectively to reduce excessive sweetness in confections such as: creams, cake icings, fondants, fudges, marshmallows, liquid centers, chewing gums, nougats, caramels, cake fillings, hard candies, toppings."

The consumer may wonder whether it wouldn't be simpler just to use less corn syrup, or less of whatever sweetener is making the product excessively sweet, but the sweetener is used to "excess" in food processing because it performs other functions. The Technical Bulletin for the product, which the consumer never gets to see—they aren't classified, but the manufacturers don't send them to consumers—explains:

> Some candy and other confectionary applications require use of specific types and concentrations of sweeteners in order to achieve desired appearance, consistency, storage stability, or other physical characteristics. Because formulation latitude is restricted in such applications, excessive, objectionable sweetness can occur.

One side effect is, of course, that the consumer doesn't realize what a lot of sweetener the product contains and so consumes much more corn syrup or whatever than he would if he knew what he was eating. Since most consumers are trying to cut down on their intake of sweets, hiding excessive sweetener does a real disservice; the fact that it is done to add consumer appeal benefits only the manufacturer.

It would be helpful if, in addition to listing each type of sweetener separately, the total amount of sweeteners were listed. Until labeling laws are changed to require this, you should note the first three ingredients; if all are some form of sweetener, the total percentage is bound to be high. Unfortunately, thanks to this particular additive, you can no longer rely on your sense of taste to tell you when a product is too sweet. By the way, knowing the name of the additive that masks excessive sweetness will not help you to spot it; the flavoring just described would appear on the ingredient line simply as "natural flavor."

The Natural "Flavor Enhancer and Improver"

Among the most used additives are the "flavor enhancers"—a name that ignores the fact that there often isn't any flavor to enhance. Manufacturers discovered long ago that, given the right degree of saltiness or sweetness, many consumers will accept a flavorless food as "tasty." However, not all foods lend themselves to this simple solution.

A product described as "Flavor Enhancer and Improver" is described by its manufacturer as "a unique, multifunctional blend of flavor ingredients designed to add sweetness, enhance flavor, and reduce objectionable bitterness. This is available as 'natural and artificial,' and 'all-natural' compositions as well as in liquid and powder forms."

The layman may not understand the description, which is written for the trade, so a translation seems in order. "Add sweetness" refers to its being about twelve to twenty times as sweet as sucrose; it boosts the sweetness of sorbitol, mannitol, and dextrose, and "effectively supplements the sweetness of sucrose and aspartame."

"Reduce bitterness" refers to "the unpleasant bitterness of saccharin." It also "prolongs flavor," which is further explained as meaning that it "can extend flavor impression and produce long-lasting effects." And it enhances flavor in that it "brings out full flavor and smooths out harsh notes." The all-natural version may, of course, be listed, under present government regulations, as "natural flavors"; the other as "natural and artificial flavors."

Natural Chocolate—Artificial Color

A Natural Chocolate Extract, from the same company, is almost natural—made from cocoa bean extractives, natural vanilla extract, and alcohol. But just when you think you are home free, the last ingredient turns out to be "artificial color." And one of the suggested uses is "as a cocoa extender.

Natural chocolate extract may be used to replace 25 to 50 percent of the cocoa in foods.'' In making chocolate ice cream, the manufacturer suggests: ''to compensate for the cocoa powder replaced, corn syrup solids may be employed.''

Why not use only real cocoa beans? The bulletin explains, ''. . . when used as a cocoa extender, Natural Chocolate Extract affords significant savings in periods of high cocoa prices without sacrificing flavor quality.'' Don't complain, though. Natural Chocolate Extract also offers flavor characteristics ''superior to artificial chocolate flavors.''

"Natural" "Vanilla" Flavoring

One of my pet peeves has always been the substitution of the artificial flavor vanillin for natural vanilla. Now the consumer has another problem, a product described as ''a blend of natural flavors specifically designed to replace pure vanilla extract. It contains no vanilla extract and offers substantial savings when used as a partial or total replacement for pure vanilla.''

Among its uses are in ''most products in which vanilla is used as either the main or a background flavor. Such products include vanilla flavored bakery products, beverages, candy, yogurt, syrups, and toppings . . . also performs well in foods flavored primarily with chocolate, butterscotch, cream, maple, butter pecan, caramel, nut, and other flavors.''

And what can you learn from the labels of foods containing this product? At present, very little. ''For a nonstandardized food which contains the word 'vanilla' in its name (e.g., Vanilla Yogurt), up to 50 percent substitution of pure vanilla is suggested. . . . The name of this product would then be modified, for example, to Vanilla Yogurt with Other Natural Flavors. The ingredient line would declare 'natural flavors,' or 'vanilla and other natural flavors.' ''

The same company makes ''compound vanillas,'' which are natural and artificial vanillas; these come in five versions, one of which may be had ''regular,'' with ''a brown vanilla-like tint,'' and the other ''white,'' which has no added color. (The totally artificial vanilla concentrates also come colored or ''white.'')

Incidentally, if you believe, as some experts will insist, that vanillin is just as good as real vanilla, consider the product ''artificial vanilla bean aroma.'' The sales brochure says, ''The product imparts a rich, true vanilla bean note to your imitation flavored products.''

It is easy to buy pure vanilla extracts to use at home, but be sure to avoid the imitation vanilla extracts that are now sold on the same shelf. If no one buys them, they will soon disappear. Meanwhile everyone will praise your puddings, cookies, and other real-vanilla-flavored homemade items and never know that your secret is the real vanilla.

Other Artificial Flavors

There is a wide range in the quality of artificial flavors. How good one is depends on how close it is to the real thing. In order to arrive at an artificial flavor, the food chemist attempts to break down the flavor's elements and then to reproduce them in the laboratory. The artificial flavor is then constructed from the most important elements that have been isolated and artificially created. To use imaginary numbers, suppose the real flavor is made up of 250 different elements. The artificial flavor may be a blend of chemical equivalents of 25 or 40 or even 100 of these elements. The result may be recognizable—a chocolatey or cherrylike flavor, for instance—but it will lack the subtleties and nuances of the true flavor, causing a diminution of the pleasure of eating real, full-flavored food. Even the best artificial flavor cannot compete with Nature—no matter what the ads claim.

Scotch Whiskey Flavor

The advertising of artificial flavors is an art in itself. One bulletin is headed: "[Brand X] Scotch Liqueur Natural Flavor with 0.1% Artificial Topnote." The first paragraph extols the real thing: "the exquisite soul-satisfying taste of the original secret formula has been pleasing sophisticated palates for generations." Then it smoothly leads into the hard sell. "Great tastes are worthy of emulation. . . . The smoky notes of peat-fired malt barley which give Scotch Whiskey its characteristic flavor have been wed to aromatic spices and flavor oils to simulate the sublime taste. When added to a base of fine Scotch, this outstanding flavor clearly resembles the unique original flavor." When this product was first introduced, a sample was offered to prospective purchasers in the form of a piece of candy described as a "flavored non-alcoholic soft cream candy center, enrobed in a smooth chocolate coating. One taste will transport you to the Isle of Skye, the home of world-famous liqueurs."

Crabmeat or Crabmeat Flavored?

When you reach for a can of crabmeat, what you may get is a fish with: "natural & Artificial Crabmeat Flavor. . . . This special flavor, created by our flavor experts, utilizes reaction techniques developed during many years of research . . . captures the delicate balance of fresh, juicy and meaty flavor notes found in real crabmeat.'' It may even have the ''mouthfeel'' of the real thing, but instead of crabmeat, it could be our old friend surimi. Flavor chemists feel about surimi the way a sculptor feels about a block of fine Italian marble; the possibilities for creative expression are infinite. Artificial crabmeat flavor is only an example of what can be done with this marvelously versatile and amenable paste.

"Aspartame Plus"

Aspartame is, of course, an artificial sweetener (see Chapter 7, Aspartame—Help or Hazard?); and it is very popular with manufacturers because of its pleasant taste. Unfortunately, from the manufacturers' standpoint, it is more expensive than some other sweeteners. As an article in the February 1984 issue of *Food Engineering* put it, ''Its high cost and degradability worry some consumers and food people.'' Ottens Flavors has come up with a solution which the Ottens's Vice President—Research and Development Richard J. Mangiere says, ''Prompted us to test Ottens Plus along with aspartame as a sparing agent.''

Ottens Plus is described by Mr. Mangiere as an artificial flavor that tastes sweet when used with sweet-tasting food systems. He says, ''Ottens Plus flavor potentiators are blends of natural and synthetic flavor materials, nondescript when used alone . . . but pleasantly sweet and synergistic when used with sugar.'' What it does is increase sweetness but reduce the amount of sugar—a more expensive natural ingredient—that is needed by up to 30 percent. It works especially well with artificial flavors also, with aspartame as well as with cane sugar. As Mr. Mangiere sums up its benefits, ''What is most important . . . is that the sweetness level is maintained and there can be up to a 20 to 30 percent cost savings.''

The consumer, already worried about whether aspartame is safe, and confronted now with still another additive, may wonder whether it wouldn't be simpler—and safer—if we all went back to real sugar. It could be eliminated from unnecessary foods (such as salad dressings, soups, and other processed foods), and we could reduce our intake of sweets and eat more fresh and dried fruits instead.

Tofu Flavors

As the consumer becomes more health-food conscious, certain natural foods that were previously found only in health food stores have now become generally available in supermarkets. This is a definite help, but growing sales have attracted manufacturers who have no commitment to the product as a health food but see it only as a potential profit-maker. To accommodate this new market, the flavor food scientists have developed "flavoring systems" especially for tofu. Tofu has traditionally been eaten by vegetarians in the form of analogs, most commonly meat, with natural flavorings and seasonings. Now, thanks to modern technology, the consumer who wishes to avoid artificial flavor has to be as wary of tofu as of any other processed food.

As tofu is incorporated into food processing, it has been developed into a base, which the manufacturer describes as having the following favorable characteristics:

- excellent shelf life due to extremely low bacteria count
- product stability during repeated processing cycles, e.g., freezing/thawing
- simple process of manufacture
- wide variety of possible applications

In addition, okara, the hull of the soybean (from which tofu is made) is a by-product that is usually discarded or "bulked off" for animal feed. Okara is high in fiber and contains protein; manufacturers use it "in various bakery products."

Among the artificial flavors a tofu eater may now encounter are artificial pork, for the meatball analog; artificial English Cheddar cheese, for the cheese spread analog; artificial coconut flavor, artificial evaporated milk flavor, and artificial vanilla flavor for the okara snack bar. The moral is that tofu buyers should check the ingredients list on the label, just as with any other processed food.

"Buttery" Baked Products

Butter seems to be a popular flavor to imitate, but apparently the imitation is not entirely satisfactory since margarine manufacturers are now making a point of adding "real butter" in an effort to achieve a better-tasting product. Since the real thing is an expensive ingredient, however, artificial butter flavor is popular with manufacturers of bakery products. It is a little surprising that they do not brag about using artificial butter flavor, since it would probably appeal to the many consumers who are trying to limit their consumption of butter because of its cholesterol content. Sometimes, as with other flavors, natural and artificial butter flavor are combined to create a flavoring that, as one food processor puts it, "adds the true rich taste of farm-fresh butter . . . [and is] delicious and convenient to use while cost effective."

The wide range of artificial/natural and wholly artificial bakery flavors is impressive. The list put out by just one company includes, to name just a few: Butta (Butter), Butta Almond, Butta Pecan, Butta Orange, Cream (Sweet), Donut, Peach, Pineapple, Raspberry, Danish, Piña Colada, Sour Cream, Coffee Cake, and Carrot Cake. Many of these flavors—even the more unusual-sounding ones, like coffee cake—are available as "natural flavors," so do not assume your favorite product is necessarily using the wholly artificial version. (The label may give you a clue.)

The same company, of course, makes many types of nonbakery flavors. For instance, not specified and listed under "Food Flavors, natural; artificial; and, natural and artificial," as well as Flavor Enhancers, are: "beef (roast, rare); beef (roast, well done); chicken (roast, white meat), and seafood enhancer."

Essential Oils

The name "essential oils" sounds as if it couldn't be anything but natural. Actually today they, like other flavorings, come natural, natural-and-artificial, and modified. Among the artificial the most popular flavors are peppermint, spearmint, and citrus, all of which can be customized, say the manufacturers, "to achieve the desired overtones, mouth-feel and aroma."

Fruit Flavors

Food scientists are proud of their artificial fruit flavors, as the following two glowing catalog descriptions show:

Natural & Artificial Cherry Flavor Concentrate . . . a well rounded flavor with a sweet wild cherry profile . . . a tart berry flavor, bottom notes.

Artificial raspberry flavor . . . true raspberry notes . . . highly concentrated but not perfumey and will give a pleasant, real fruit flavor profile.

Protein Hydrolyzates

The yeast extracts referred to, especially in connection with soup, in the early part of this chapter are technically called protein hydrolyzates. They are variously referred to as flavors and flavor enhancers, and are added to many foods, including instant dried soup mixes, canned foods such as vegetables and beef stew, hot dogs, canned chili and similar prepared foods, cocktail sauces, cheese products and spreads, spice mixes, and dried gravy and sauces. They are made in various forms and may be identified on the label as autolyzed yeast extract, hydrolyzed vegetable protein (HVP), hydrolyzed casein (milk protein), and hydrolyzed plant protein (HPP). The consumer will recognize one of the most familiar forms—hydrolyzed soy sauce.

Technically protein hydrolyzates are naturally occurring amino acids, which, as you probably know, are the chief constituents of proteins. As in soy sauce, they tend to make foods quite salty. If HVP and monosodium glutamate are both listed among the ingredients, consumers on low-salt diets should reconsider whether that particular food is a desirable addition to the menu. Dieters may find this product used as a vitamin supplement in high protein formulas, because of the B-complex vitamins it contains.

Although the composition may vary, depending on the source—which is sometimes soybeans or peanuts, sometimes grain, such as wheat or corn (identified as hydrolyzed cereal solids)—soybeans are most commonly used. This might lead the consumer to think the proteins are fairly complete, though, in fact, a possible protein imbalance is one of the questions some nutritionists have regarding the safety of this product.

In addition, their high content of glutamic acid has led to some concern that ingesting them, especially in the form of hydrolyzed casein (which is comparatively high in glutamic acid) might adversely affect the central nervous system and especially infant brains and the brains of adults with brain-type illnesses.

Beef-flavor compounds that are neither protein nor yeast hydrolyzates nor yeast autolyzates have been developed and may be used instead of the other flavor enhancers. If you wish to limit your intake of foods that contain the hydrolyzates or autolyzates, look for them in the list of ingredients as, for instance, "hydrolyzed vegetable protein and other natural flavors." There are many processed foods, including canned soups, that do not use them.

Future Flavorings

Unless the consumer takes action against artificial flavors, here is the picture painted by a respected, high-quality firm in the business:

We're dedicated to product development that extends the frontiers of flavors and seasonings far beyond where they stand today. Recent areas

Natural Flavors—A Wide Choice

Manufacturers who use artificial flavors can seldom claim that they do so because those flavors are not available in natural formulations. Here is a list from just one manufacturer of the natural flavors they offer. (Note: many of these flavors are offered in a number of different ways; generally I have listed them only once.)

apple cinnamon
almond extract
roasted almond flavor
apple flavor
apple butter spice oil
apple cider flavor
apple essence
bacon flavor
background for bread
bar-b-que flavor
wild berry flavor
boysenberry flavor
butter emulsion
butter cinnamon flavor
butterscotch flavor
cappuccino flavor
celery flavor
bleu cheese flavor
nacho cheese flavor
romano cheese flavor
cheesecake flavor
cherry extract
black cherry flavor
cherry cola flavor
chicken flavor
chili lemon flavor
chocolate flavor
cinnamon extract
cinnamon maple flavor
coconut flavor
coffee flavor
cognac flavor
cream flavor
creme de cocoa flavor
custard flavor
Danish pastry flavor
eggnog flavor

fig concentrate
fruit cocktail flavor
ginger extract
grape flavor
hazelnut flavor
clover honey flavor
Karmo flavor
lemon emulsion
lemonade emulsion
oleo lemon butter emulsion
oleo lemon, lime, orange emulsion
flavor for key lime
malt flavor
milk flavor
cooked apple
smoked almond flavor
anise extract
apricot flavor
apple cherry flavor
apple cinnamon flavor
apple raisin spice flavor
banana flavor
brown sugar
beef flavor
blueberry flavor
butter flavor
butter almond flavor
buttermilk flavor
butter vanilla flavor
caramel flavor
cheese flavor
Cheddar cheese flavor
Parmesan cheese flavor
Roquefort cheese flavor
cherry flavor
red cherry flavor
sour cherry flavor

cherry vanilla flavor
background flavor for green chili
cinnamon emulsion
cinnamon flavor
cocoa flavor
coffee concentrate
coffee cake flavor
cola emulsion
crème de cassis flavor
hot curry flavor
dairy flavor
dill flavor
fat flavor
frangelico flavor
mixed fruit flavor
ginger ale flavor
grapefruit emulsion
honey flavor
Kahlúa flavor
kirsch flavor
lemon oil
pink lemonade flavor
lemon sugar flavor
lime extract
Madeira emulsion
maple flavor
mint flavor
molasses flavor
mocha extract
mushroom concentrate
oil nutmeg
fried onion emulsion
oleo orange flavor
peach flavor
peanut butter flavor
background flavor for pecan pie
background flavor for pepperoni
background flavor for pistachio
pork flavor
punch flavor
red fruit punch flavor
raisin concentrate
raspberry flavor
rhum du beurre flavor concentrate
rum flavor

rum butter flavor
background flavor for sausage
shrimp flavor
sour cream flavor
spearmint extract
brown sugar flavor
background flavor for sweet potato
tarragon flavor
tea and lemon base flavor
background flavor for teaberry
turkey flavor
walnut flavor
wine flavor
sherry wine flavor
yeast flavor
background flavor for nuts
onion flavor
onion and garlic powder
passion fruit flavor
roasted peanut flavor
peppermint extract
space flavor—sweet pickle
pineapple flavor
plum flavor
prosciutto spice flavor
citrus punch flavor
tropical punch flavor
raisin spice flavor
black raspberry flavor
root beer flavor
oil rum Jamaica
rum cream flavor
seasoning flavor
smoke flavor
sour cream and onion flavor
strawberry flavor
sweet and sour flavor
taco flavor
tea base flavor
tomato catsup spice flavor
tutti-frutti flavor
black walnut flavor
sauterne wine flavor
Worcestershire sauce flavor
vanilla flavors

Artificial Spray-Dried Flavors

The reader might be curious to know what sort of flavors appear on the artificial—but not the natural—flavor list of the same manufacturer. Here are just a few of the artificial flavors available. All the natural flavors are also available as artificial; I have tried to list only those not available as "natural flavors."

bourbon	cereal
cinnamon, sweet	graham
grape cream	Hawaiian sweet bread
honey graham	lemon mint
oatmeal raisin	pumpkin pie
sugar cone	vanilla cream
cranberry	red currant
seedless white grape	watermelon
sauterne	milk
condensed milk	malted milk
beef stick	pork
pork fat	pork sausage
potato	fresh potato
fried potato	fresh tomato

of our research include aroma synthesis, discovering flavor components from traditional foodstuffs and the development of unique combinations of natural and synthetic ingredients. . . . We're creating flavors that work in texturized proteins, low sodium foods and dietary products. We're researching new ways to stabilize flavor systems to survive in aseptic packages and microwave ovens.

It is hard to resist the enthusiasm in this sales literature or to think of dampening the excitement of the food scientist who has succeeded in developing, for the candy and bakery manufacturer, not just chocolate, but "bitter chocolate, cocoa extender, milk chocolate, semi-sweet chocolate"; and for TV dinners, not just beef, but "rare roast beef and well-done roast beef." Or, as another flavor manufacturer puts it: "Absinthe to zucchini. We offer flavors limited only by the imagination. They are available in standard and customized forms. Whatever the category—citrus or savory, natural or artificial. . . . Vast is our list of standard flavors."

The descriptive literature of flavor manufacturers inspires the reader with new respect for nature's skill. In order even to approximate natural flavors,

Artificial or Natural—These Flavors Run the Gamut

This list comes from just one manufacturer who offers flavors in "water-soluble, oil-soluble or oil-dispersible forms, and as powders for use in soy-based and soy extended products, gravies, sauces, casseroles, soups, snack foods and in restructured meats."

Bacon Flavors
Cured Bacon
Lean Bacon (Canadian)
Extra Crisp

Beef Flavors
Rare Roast Beef
Well-Done Roast Beef
Beef for Stew
Beef for Soup
Fried Beef
Corned Beef
Beef Barbecue

Chicken Flavors
Cooked Chicken
Roast Chicken
Fried Chicken
Chicken Fat

Ham Flavors
Baked Ham
Cured Ham
Smoked Ham
Spiced Ham

Hamburger Flavors
Medium Cooked Hamburger
Char-Broiled Hamburger
Meat Loaf

Hot Dog Flavors
Seasonings
Meat Flavor Blend

Pork Flavors
Roast Pork
Pork Chop

Steak Flavors
Medium Cooked Steak
Char-Broiled Steak

Turkey Flavors
Cooked Turkey
Roast Turkey

Fish Flavors
Anchovy
Catfish
Crab
Lobster
Mixed Seafood
Salmon
Shrimp
Tuna
Whitefish

Seasonings
Beef
Bologna
Chili
Curry
Enchilada
Hot Dog
Nacho Cheese
Oil-Soluble Smoke
Pepperoni
Pizza
Pork
Poultry
Seafoods
Smoke Powder
Sweet Sausage
Taco
Water-Soluble Smoke

And, if by any chance, you want something not on the list, the company will be happy to develop it for you.

the flavor chemist must try to isolate and analyze the components; even apparently simple flavors are found to be extremely complex. One manufacturer describes the tools and methods used in developing flavor systems: ". . . Our computerized library contains detailed information on flavor components, their characteristics and chemical analysis from 10,000 formulas covering our entire array of product." Another tool is "The Sensory Profile . . . a road map of sensory evaluation . . . identifies and denotes the intensities of the flavor and aromatic components in your flavor target . . ."

It seems that the priorities of processed food manufacturers are lowered costs, the development of more profitable "new foods," and ways of making these new foods acceptable to the consumer. Natural flavors are expendable; their loss is accepted as an inevitable part of the manufacturing process. Whether foods that have lost their savor have also lost vital elements that are necessary to health will not be known for generations. The danger, meanwhile, is that we will learn to prefer the fake over the real; in many instances we already do.

CHAPTER 11

Forever Beautiful—
The Dubious Magic
of Food Colors

The food processors know it's no use making food last forever if it doesn't look pretty; making food look pretty is what artificial color additives are all about. Let us see what this means to the consumer.

From housewife to professional chef, anyone who prepares food knows that its appearance can contribute greatly to the eater's enjoyment of it. The Japanese, who have developed food presentation to a fine art, spend years learning to cut, slice, and shred meat, fish, and vegetables, and the recently popular nouvelle cuisine leaned heavily on looks, convincing diners, for a time, that an artful arrangement of three fanned-out snow peas, a dab of beet puree, and a pink peach half accompanying two paper-thin slices of rosy baked ham was worth three or four times the price of the usual sirloin-steak-and-baked-potato-with-tossed-salad dinner. Sometimes appearance takes precedence over flavor, and a beautiful-looking plate of food may be totally tasteless.

Nature herself apparently realizes the appeal of color, for foods are naturally colorful. Witness the deep purple of eggplant, the bright reds and yellows of tomatoes, and the emerald green, red, yellow, and purple of peppers. A bowl of fruit, with apples, plums of every description, grapes ranging from green to red to purple so deep it is almost black, is a picture that has often caught the artist's eye—even without the tropical banana, mango, pineapple, and papaya. No cook worth his or her whisk would serve yellow turnips with sweet potatoes, or cabbage with mashed potatoes. Even the comparatively bland-looking New England boiled dinner has rosy corned beef providing visual excitement, with the orange of boiled carrots as a grace note.

The Instability of Natural Colors

Botanists and food scientists have analyzed how nature arrives at her colors: the reds of fruits and vegetables are often due to lycopene; chlorophyll is responsible for the green of lettuce and peas; anthocyanins contribute purple; and so on through the spectrum. But these natural colors are transient under many circumstances. A green leaf turns to the brilliant colors of a New England autumn, revealing golds that were always present in the leaf but were masked by the green chlorophyll that is no longer there. As vegetables and fruits ripen, their color becomes brighter—green peppers turn red, flowering kale turns purple. On exposure to air, some colors change or are lost entirely—peeled apples turn brown; so does iceberg lettuce when the core is cut; exposed hamburger turns gray. The function of artificial colors and chemical additives is to disguise or prevent these natural color changes, thereby fooling the consumer into thinking an item is fresher than it actually is.

Neither does natural color serve only to please the eye or to indicate ripeness or freshness. The more we learn about nutrients, the more we find that color is nature's clue. Dark green leafy vegetables signal the presence of certain nutrients; for example, the darker the orange or yellow of carrots and winter squash, the more vitamin A they contain. And many consumers recognize that the brown of whole grain bread indicates its nutrient superiority to white (though that can be misleading since the color of brown "wheat" bread and "black" bread is often due to food coloring). Artificial colors simulate the presence of nonexistent nutrients—in fact, as we will see, they are often used for exactly that purpose. Thanks to artificial flavors, we can no longer trust our sense of taste, and now we can be misled in judging nutrient value.

The Problem with Processing

Processing tends to destroy natural colors, bleaching and dulling them so that foods lose much of their appeal. As primitive man learned to process his own food by cooking, drying, and smoking, he became familiar with the natural changes that resulted. But as food preparation became more sophisticated and increasingly moved out of the home, some of these changes were resisted. For hundreds of years, up to the present time, color additives have been used to deceive the consumer, as when bone meal was added to bread when white bread became more desirable than black. Sometimes poisonous colors were used, even though they were added for no more important reason than to make a product more attractive, as when red lead was added to hard candies.

The consumer's attitude toward color in food seems to justify the food processors' concern. Before they learned that the practice destroyed nutrients, home cooks routinely added sodium bicarbonate to fresh peas to retain their bright green color—a few restaurants still do. The secret of bright green cooked broccoli is still cherished in home kitchens. (Steam it no more than 12 minutes; do not, under any circumstances, take off the cover until time is up. Once the cover is off, it must stay off; re-covered, the broccoli will turn a dull olive green.)

Color is sometimes used to create food novelties. Recipes in magazines suggest adding all sorts of vegetable colorings to create exotic dishes out of ordinary ones, such as adding beet juice to make pink boiled rice out of white. In the East shisu, or purple perilla, is still routinely used to give foods a handsome reddish tint.

Certain natural seasonings are used because they add color as well as taste, as is the case with curry. Saffron rice gains its golden hue from the saffron stamens, although a similar color—but different taste—can also be achieved with turmeric.

For some reason certain colors have been inseparably linked in our minds with certain foods, even though they never are that color in their natural state. Consumers expect mint jelly and pistachio ice cream to be green (a color originally achieved through a mixture of Blue No. 1 and Yellow No. 5), though left alone, they would be clear and cream-color, respectively. Maraschino cherries, the delight of every child, would lose all their appeal if they were their undyed, bleached, and colorless selves (instead of dyed, originally, with Red No. 1), and we still happily reach for iced birthday cakes topped with blue, green, yellow, and pink flowers, and hunt through the rainbow of jelly beans for our favorite artificial colors.

Manufacturers strongly resist the idea of banning artificial colors, and the FDA record of protecting the consumer is clouded by endless extensions and delays, by which bans on colors of proven toxicity have been delayed for years before finally being imposed. It is only recently that the consumer has become aware that insistence on colorful food may exact a price in health; "no artificial colors" is now beginning to take its place on the label along with "no artificial flavors."

The Colorful Chemicals Take Over

As the commercial food processing business grew, the problem of retaining the look of "natural" food colors became more difficult and more pressing. One can almost sympathize with the food processor who first viewed with dismay the results of the processing. Dull, drab vegetables spilled out of the can; white potatoes turned gray; winter butter was pale instead of golden yellow (this was eventually rectified by the addition of Yellow No. 3 or Yellow No. 4). Unless colored, peach and most other ice cream flavors—except chocolate, of course—showed no hint of how they would taste. Sausages were gray (although the flavor was not affected), and white foods were often not truly white. Egg noodles failed to look rich with eggs (they often weren't, but that wasn't the point), and lemon ice was colorless (remember the lemon ice sold by the little penny candy store in a pleated paper cup? It was refreshingly tart/sweet with the fresh flavor of real lemons, but it wasn't any color at all).

In the beginning, adding concentrated natural colors helped retain some of the otherwise lost color, but food processors soon found that natural colors often could not withstand the rigors of modern food technology. Exposure to air, heat, water, cutting, peeling, mashing—everything seemed to affect them unfavorably. Over and over again the manufacturer found that natural colors were unreliable; sometimes they faded, sometimes they turned strange shades during processing. And on top of all that, the natural sources of colors—seeds, fruits, spices, and herbs—became increasingly costly.

The discovery of coal tar dyes saved the day for the food industry. Coal tar dyes were cheap, stable, reliable, and colorful as all get out; unfortunately, as it turned out, they also tend to be extremely toxic. First invented by European chemists, they soon made their way to America, where they flourished. In 1940 the FDA certified 251,000 pounds of coal tar dyes as safe for use in foods, drugs, or cosmetics. Thirty years later, in 1970, the annual amount used had grown to 3,735,000 pounds. Even though many had already been found to be unhealthful and others were suspect, over 95 percent of these certified food colors were being used in food. Today the consumer who wants to avoid artificial colors has a problem: in 1984, 8.8 million pounds of artificial colors were used in food, drugs, and cosmetics; of that total the bulk—approximately 8 million pounds—went into your food.

Advantages and Disadvantages

The development of artificial colors revolutionized the food industry, gave a boost to the development of fabricated foods, and allowed even more intensive processing. It no longer matters what the base product looks like (see Chapter 4, Surimi—The Great Pretender); when it reaches the consumer it will look like a real, and familiar, food. In addition, from the manufacturer's point of view, artificial colors have, as we have already noted, a number of marketing advantages. They increase sales of both "natural" and man-made "foods," and they help raise the profit margins considerably. They are abundant and reliable. As one manufacturer of artificial colors puts it in a sales brochure:

> Unfortunately, nature is both fickle and inconsistent. Natural spices and plants used for their food coloring values vary with seasonal factors, harvest times, and geographic location.
>
> About 300 different carotenoid compounds have been identified in nature. A hundred or so have been synthesized in the laboratory. . . . Three . . . are identical with nature's own.
>
> . . . You can count on color uniformity from batch to batch, the year 'round. . . . And you can depend on a continuous and abundant source of supply.

From the consumer's viewpoint, however, there are no advantages. The function of artificial color is purely cosmetic. It is not used for the purpose of adding nutrients, or even energy. The manufacturer uses food colors because the consumer insists on them, otherwise, he claims, certain food products wouldn't sell. He may have a point, but maybe those products *shouldn't* sell if they have to be gussied up to be acceptable. In any event, the consumer has a right to know that there is no reason to be sure that even the colors still permitted in today's food are safe, and that many manufacturers would probably have to improve the quality of their ingredients if they were denied the crutch of artificial colors.

While it is true that some color additives may accidentally contain vitamins, such as the E and A in laboratory-synthesized beta-carotenes, this is not why they are used, and these vitamins are easily available and possibly more beneficial when obtained from natural sources. Furthermore, these additives confuse the consumer, because the food processor is allowed to list them on the label as nutrients rather than as artificial food colors. Neither does the label reveal even more important information, such as when the brand of canthaxanthin (a beta-carotene red coloring) used may be in the form of a crystalline chemical compound that comes in a matrix of "gelatin, sucrose, modified food starch and coconut oil; BHT and BHA and ascorbyle palmitate as antioxidants; sodium bisulfite and parabens (methyl and propyl) as preservatives."

Aside from the consumers who wish to avoid additives, or at least would like to know which ones they are ingesting, these hidden additives might also be objectionable to certain groups—such as vegetarians who wish to avoid gelatin, and those who are staying away from highly saturated fats such as coconut oil because of cholesterol content. It may be argued that the amount of these additives contained in medicines and in the portion of pizzas, barbecue sauces, russian dressings, fruit punches, bloody mary–type beverages, cakes, simulated meats, dehydrated soup mixes, spice mixes, and spaghetti sauce mixes—to list only a few of the suggested "food applications"—that a given consumer eats in the course of a year might be too small to pay attention to. The fact is that no one knows how much an individual consumer is eating. Since there is no way of measuring a person's total intake of additives from all the many food items in the average diet, it may be that all these small amounts add up to a harmful large amount. And one would have to add those ingested as well in drugs, medicines, and vitamin supplements.

Even if these additives are not harmful (and at present they are supposed not to be), the consumer is kept in the dark about their very existence in foods and is unable to exercise free choice as to whether to eat them.

Benefits Versus Risks

When you compare the benefits of artificial colors to the risks the consumer runs in ingesting them, the risks win hands down. The only reason the FDA bans any colors is solely that they have been shown, beyond any doubt, to be dangerous to consumer health. Unfortunately, many previously permitted artificial colors have been found to cause cancers of all sorts, as well as kidney and liver disease, allergies, gene mutations, birth defects, behavioral disturbances in growing children, and other equally serious and unpleasant illnesses—either in animals or humans. As more and more natural colors disappear from our increasingly chemicalized foods, we are ingesting more and more artificial colors and can look forward to possibly accelerated instances of these undesirable side effects. The enormous increase in their use, to approximately 8.8 million pounds, obviously exposes more and more consumers to larger and larger quantities. Artificial colors are ubiquitous; it takes real care and effort on the part of the consumer to cut down on them in daily food; avoiding them entirely is almost impossible.

In a 1984 information release, the FDA reported that it had permanently approved or terminated more than a hundred color additives on its "provisional" list (see Chapter 12, How Safe Are Artifical Food Colors?). That leaves only a handful that may now be used in food, which means that more than 75 percent were terminated, presumably because they were proved harmful to humans. You might think that an additive like color, where the consumer's risk-benefit ratio could be expressed as, for example, cancer versus green-colored mint jelly (the flavor is not affected one way or the other) would not be allowed until proved safe. In fact, colors that had been used before 1960 were generally approved until proved unsafe, and meanwhile we unwittingly ate them. (See also Chapter 31, GRAS—Are Food Additives Really Safe?)

The FDA does not appear to see the danger as a serious problem. It has granted extension after extension for tests to determine whether a color is safe or unsafe—and it is still granting extensions to this day. In 1984 the FDA position was clearly stated when it granted an additional extension for the eleven remaining (at that time) provisionally listed color additives: "The continued use of these color additives for the short time needed for the adequate evaluation of the data and for the preparation of the Federal Register documents will not pose a hazard to the public health." Twenty-five years (so far) is surely not a "short time," and how much longer it will take to establish whether the remaining colors are truly safe is yet to be determined.

The present state of testing may not be adequate for the much larger amounts we are now ingesting; neither, as is always a problem with animal tests, may they extrapolate successfully to human reactions. In addition, we are now consuming these artificial colors along with greater and greater quantities of other chemicals, many of which previously did not even exist and which may interact with them in ways of which we know nothing. Many diseases, such as cancer, have long, slow reaction times, and no manufacturer will be content to wait up to twenty years to be sure a color additive is not a carcinogen. Infants, young children, the ill and the elderly, as well as those with special ethnic backgrounds, genetic traits, and allergies may not be represented in the animals used for testing, yet they are exactly the human beings who may be at greatest risk.

When you think that all this testing and government expenditure and risk to the consumer is simply so that a colorless jelly bean or gelatin dessert can be prettily colored, or, even worse, so that inferior or highly processed food products can be made more physically attractive, you cannot help wondering whether we have our priorities straight.

Some Uses of Added Color

One serious disadvantage of artificial food colors, as we have already mentioned, is that they may be used to mask the use of inferior ingredients

---

Catsup by Any Other Name

An example of how difficult it is for the consumer to know whether he is protected by food laws is catsup. Real catsup need not list ingredients allowed under its standard of identity; only additional optional ingredients need be listed. Added color is not allowed as an ingredient under either circumstance. So far, so good. But under the same law, imitation catsup, which need not comply with the standard of identity, "may contain added colorings as long as it is properly labeled, i.e., "imitation."

---

and to create the appearance, rather than the reality, of good food. Used together with artificial flavors, it is possible to fool the consumer into thinking a product that contains no butter is "buttery," and one that has no eggs, or very few, is rich with them. Artificial strawberry flavor plus strawberry color can disguise the total lack of any real fruit. Small potatoes left over from last season may be dyed red in the spring so that they resemble "new" potatoes, which command a premium price. (The FDA doesn't act against this practice because it claims lack of proof that it is done to deceive the consumer, although it is hard to imagine any other reason an inexpensive old white potato that was salable at a lower price in the fall had to be dyed red for higher-priced spring sales.) Yellow potatoes were dyed to give them the deeper look of "yams" (there aren't any real yams grown in America, but most consumers and even some food writers think the moister, orange-fleshed sweets are yams) until the practice was banned in 1968.

The Food, Drug and Cosmetic (often referred to as FD&C) Act of 1938 specifically prohibits the use of a color additive in foods, drugs, or cosmetics "if it will deceive the consumer, conceal inferiority or damage, or otherwise result in misbranding or adulteration." In 1960 this law was reinforced by the Color Additives Amendments. The amendments required the FDA to write a regulation for every individual color additive allowed, "specifying its physical or botanical or chemical identity, the products or kinds of products in which it may be used, the quantities that may be used, and (any) other conditions of use necessary to protect public health."

In spite of these laws and of numerous amendments, inadequate testing, legislative foot dragging, and generous interpretations of the law have consistently put the public at risk from colors that tests indicate may be unsafe. It is sometimes difficult to actually "prove" that an additive causes cancer or some other serious illness; someone can always dispute the methodology and question the validity of the conclusions. The consumer needs to be more aware of how decisions are reached that allow such additives into food, and to have more of a say as to what degree of risk is "acceptable." Provided with the knowledge that a prettified food may cause cancer, the public may prefer to adjust to the appearance of naturally colored food.

Since there are now so many fewer permitted colors, it is inevitable that much more of one single color is being consumed. The safety of the still permitted colors thus becomes even more critical and the possibility of adverse effects on human health more liable to occur. (See Chapter 12, How Safe Are Artificial Food Colors?, for lists of artificial colors presently used in food.)

CHAPTER 12

How Safe Are Artificial Food Colors?

By definition color additives are "any dyes, pigments or coloring substances that are used in foods, drugs, or cosmetics." Some, such as saffron and turmeric, have a dual additive function, both as a color and as a flavor additive, and must conform to the regulations governing both groups.

The first artificial food color, mauve, was invented in 1856. By 1900 eighty artificial colors were being added to foods. When the United States passed the Pure Food Law in 1906, all but seven of the eighty were determined to be harmful and were banned from use in food. By 1971 some of the original seven dyes had been discarded but others had been added, and ten colors, including two blues, a green, three reds, a violet, and two yellows, were allowed. At that time 90 percent of the colors used in foods were artificial. Today it is estimated that 95 percent of added food colors are artificial.

The Federal Food, Drug and Cosmetic Act of 1938

In 1938, in response to concern expressed about the increased proliferation of artificial colors, flavors, and other additives, the Federal Food, Drug and Cosmetic Act (FD&C Act) was passed. The law specifically "prohibits the movement in interstate commerce of adulterated or misbranded food"; it does not, however, protect the consumer against food manufactured and distributed only within a given state. And although the act was intended to protect the consumer from harmful additives in food, as well as in drugs and cosmetics, it did not require prior proof of food additive safety. Under the law it was up to the FDA to determine which substances were "poisonous or deleterious," and to see that foods already containing such substances were taken off the grocery shelves. Fifteen food colors were included among the substances. Colors were given numbers, such as FD&C Yellow No. 1, for easy identification. (This system has proved to be generally confusing, and at the present time an effort is being made to devise some better method.)

Even in those early days additives were invented faster than the agency could deal with them, and, since the time for testing averaged two and a half years, consumers continued to ingest many colors that had not yet been determined to be safe. The extent of the potential danger to the consumer was pointed up by a congressional survey conducted in the 1940s: of the 704 chemicals known to be used in foods at that time, only 428 were definitely known to be safe. Eventually even 428 turned out to be an overoptimistic number. In 1950, for example, three "listed" colors were "de-listed" when a number of children became ill after eating candy and popcorn colored with them.

Gradually, it became evident that all colors would have to be tested for safety, and in 1960 the Color Additives Amendments were added to the original FD&C Act. The amendments required "that colors used in foods, drugs, and cosmetics be safe for their intended use." Under this law two hundred additives already in use were put on the "Provisional" list, an interim category where they would stay until tests resulted either in their being moved to the "Permanent" (approved) list or in their being "terminated." Some colors stayed on the provisional list for decades, but, happily, only two used in food—Blue No. 2 and Yellow No. 6—still remain there today. The "intended use" phrase adds another factor to consumer confusion; it results, for example, in some colors that may be used in drugs and cosmetics but not in food. Red No. 3, on the other hand, is listed as Permanent for food but Provisional for external drugs and cosmetics.

The FDA, which has been criticized frequently and strongly by consumer organizations for its numerous and lengthy extensions of testing (at present, for instance, Blue No. 2 has been listed as having an "indefinite" extension), says "extensions were granted for various reasons: the extra time needed for certain animal tests requiring up to three years to complete; the development of new criteria for evaluating the safety of chemical substances; and the lengthy litigation concerning cosmetics color requirements."

One attempt to improve the situation was the passage of the Food Additives Amendment in 1958 which required the industry to prove the safety of chemicals added to foods. If the evidence (usually from animal tests conducted by the manufacturer) passed FDA muster, the "acceptable" amount that could be used was set; sometimes other conditions were imposed. (See also Chapter 31, GRAS—Are Food Additives Really Safe?)

Some consumer groups feel there is no such thing as a safe artificial food color. For example, in December 1984 the Public Citizen Health Research Group filed a petition asking for a ban on ten "provisionally listed" color additives used in foods, drugs, and cosmetics. The colors were Red No. 3, Yellow No. 5, and Yellow No. 6, allowed in food, and Orange No. 17, Red No. 8, Red No. 9, Red No. 19, Red No. 33, Red No. 36, and Red No. 37, allowed only in drugs and cosmetics. The petition alleged that enough scientific evidence had already been produced to support a ban on all the additives. In a letter to the group, FDA Commissioner Frank E. Young said that a continued extension of provisional listing of the colors is necessary for a careful evaluation of recently completed testing. "I have concluded that the public health will not be endangered by the continued marketing of these color additives while these scientific, legal, and policy issues are addressed," he wrote. Mr. Young's letter also pointed out what he said were a number of factual errors in the petition and its supporting documentation, and outlined the FDA's reasons for disagreeing with the conclusions drawn by the petitioners.

"Certified" Colors

As with so many government terms, the consumer confronted with FDA's "certified food colors" appellation probably does not understand what that designation means and interprets it as more reassuring than it is.

Certification in itself deals only with compliance to regulations and is required only of certain colors. Artificial colors that may be used in food must conform to certain standards of purity of manufacture if they are to be permitted to be added to food. Certification means that the composition of a particular batch of colors requiring certification conforms to these standards. Lack of certification is not in itself meaningful to the consumer, although "certified colors" are always presented on the label as a plus. It is assumed by the FDA—but has no bearing on the process of certification— that the colors have already been tested for safety.

As we have noted, old testing methods frequently allowed dyes to be certified (which assumes safety as well as purity) that were later found to be dangerous. In addition, many dyes, such as Butter Yellow and Red Dye No. 1, that were found to be toxic early in the century, continued to be allowed to be used for years. Red Nos. 4 and 32 (the Reds seem to be especially toxic), Orange Nos. 1 and 2, and Yellow Nos. 1, 3, and 4 were subsequently taken off the certified list, and, though even colors that do not require certification may still be considered safe, these colors were removed from the certified list because they had been found unsafe. Even certification is no proof that adequate studies as to safety have been done (so far as our technology permits); neither does decertification for reasons of proved toxicity necessarily mean that the dye is banned. Past experience would seem to indicate that as long as artificial colors are used in food, future tests may indicate that eating them has put the consumer at risk. The consumer might well be excused for considering that the only safe artificial color is one that has been banned.

Ironically, violet coloring, which was used to stamp meat that had been inspected by the Department of Agriculture (USDA), was discovered to be a carcinogen in Canadian studies but, in spite of that, was allowed in the United States for an additional decade. It has been replaced by another coloring that is at the moment still allowed. (When you trim the fat off your lamb chops and similar meat, you may notice it; might as well make a point of removing it rather than taking the chance of eating it.)

Not all colors that may be used in food are required to be certified. Many are "exempted from certification because, in the form in which they are used, batch certification is not considered necessary to protect public health." In 1980 there were twenty-five certification-exempt color additives permitted in food; most of them were natural or synthetic vegetable compounds (from beet powder, caramel, beta-carotene, grape skin extract, fruit or vegetable juices, paprika, saffron, and similar familiar sources). Some, such as cochineal extract, which is derived from the tiny dried bodies of a brilliantly red insect, are of animal origin. The idea, possibly, was that a color was probably safe if it came from "natural" sources. At present, however, three natural colors—cochineal, paprika, and turmeric—are viewed "with caution," although they are thought probably to be safe.

The Trouble with Testing

It is often difficult to establish that a color additive is harmful, even with sound scientific methods. In addition, the tests themselves are often not accepted as meaningful by the FDA on the grounds that they have not been properly conducted.

An example of an artificial color that consumers were exposed to and ingested in a wide range of foods for many years, in spite of adverse test results, is Amaranth, which was known as Red No. 2 (not to be confused with Citrus Red No. 2, or monoazo). As has often been the case, we owe our knowledge of Amaranth's toxicity to European scientists, in this case Russian researchers, who found that it apparently caused cancer, prevented pregnancies, and caused stillbirths in some rats. No action was taken at first because the methodology of these studies was questioned. Our own scientists, however, had had reservations about Amaranth's safety for over twenty years, and the FDA's Center for Toxicological Research eventually reported a significant increase in rat cancers in its tests done in 1971 (though even in this case it later contended that studies had not established that Amaranth was carcinogenic). In spite of all these studies, the case against Amaranth was never considered proved (the industry resisted banning it because it was the most widely used food color at that time, accounting for about one-third of all the food colors used). It was put on the provisional list pending further tests and was finally withdrawn because it had not been "proved safe," but not until 1976.

In spite of frequent lack of agreement among scientists concerning the safety of food additives, there is no doubt that the technology needed for testing and analysis has improved since the beginning of the century, and the methodology of testing has been refined (even if it is not always adhered to). We have learned to distinguish more closely between colors suitable for clothing and those appropriate for food. Cosmetics fall somewhere in between, but even there, safety standards are much stricter than they used to be. The more we learn, however, the more difficult testing becomes. Before thalidomide made the world aware of how dangerous ingested materials could be to the fetus, the possibility of causing birth defects was not generally considered. Even today, for instance, only one artificial food color has been tested to determine whether it causes birth defects in animals. The FDA has stated that it intends to do further testing in this area but so far does not seem to have done so.

Food Colors Worldwide

Food colors have become the subject of international concern, and the Food and Agriculture Organization works with the World Health Organization (both part of the United Nations) on a Joint FAO/WHO Expert Committee on Food Additives. The twenty-third report of this committee, which met in Geneva in April 1979, stated: ". . . The growing concern in industrial countries about establishing safety criteria for chemicals in food was shared by the health and food regulatory authorities in developing countries; thus the work of the Committee had a substantial impact on the economies of countries that depended on the export of food."

This international approach to the use of food colors (and other additives) is especially welcome as the United States imports more and more foods to and exports more from an ever-wider world market. The food safety laws worldwide are presently fragmented; there is no agreement even between the United States and European countries. As a result, trade in many food items is compromised, and Americans traveling abroad are exposed to color additives that the FDA has determined are harmful. (The Europeans, in turn, have come to the same conclusion about some of our "safe" food colors.) What is needed, obviously, is a consensus, but the history of artificial food colors in the United States indicates one of the roadblocks in the way. Artificial food colors are thought to be essential to consumer acceptance of many foods—especially those that are fabricated, heavily processed, or otherwise altered. These are the items that have been most heavily promoted and that have the highest profit margins; the truly huge volume of business and millions of dollars they represent will not willingly be abandoned.

Natural colors still considered safe include: beta-carotene, canthaxathine, caramel, ferrous gluconate, riboflavin, titanium oxide, carrot oil, fruit juices, grape skin extract, and toasted defatted cottonseed flour. Natural colors considered "probably safe" are annatto and beet red. Natural but "to be viewed with caution" include cochineal, paprika, and turmeric. All natural colors are capable of being "approximated" by artificial colors. Beta-carotene, for example, may be either natural or artificial; if artificial, the label sometimes says "artificial color (Beta carotene)." This can be confusing to the consumer who has learned to think of beta-carotene as "good stuff" but wishes to avoid artificial colors.

Yellow No. 5 (tartrazine), currently the most widely used color additive, has been required to be identified by name on food labels since July 1, 1982 (drug companies have been required to identify it since June 1980) because it causes allergic reactions from hyperactivity to wheezing to hives in some sensitive individuals. Its use has been permitted in just about every food you can think of, including soft drinks, spaghetti, gelatin and pudding desserts, mixes of every description (drinks, soups, etc.), candy, ice cream and sherbets, imitation jelly, and cereals. Yellow No. 6, attractively known as Sunset Yellow, is presently added to many of the same products. Though now suspect, it is still on the FDA's provisional list.

Federal law does not apply to foods processed and shipped within the same state, so only foods shipped interstate are protected to any extent, unless a particular state happens to have strict laws of its own. Often state or local laws are more stringent than federal. For example, sodium nicotinate, used to keep hamburger bright red (rather than the natural gray color it turns on exposure to air) is allowed in thirty-seven states but illegal in some municipalities, though not in all, and is not banned by the FDA. And even when a dye has been banned because it has been shown to be

---

FDA Permanent Food Color Additives

FD&C Blue No. 1
FD&C Green No. 3
FD&C Red No. 3
FD&C Red No. 40
FD&C Yellow No. 5

All except Yellow No. 5 must be listed on the label, where required by law, not by name but only as "artificial colors." Yellow No. 5 must be specified, where required by law, due to its allergic potential.

An example of how complicated the regulations are is FD&C Red No. 3, which is permanent for use in food but provisional for use in cosmetics and ingested drugs.

---

harmful, the manufacturer is often allowed to continue to put it in foods until the supply on hand has been used up. The consumer trying to keep track must fight for good labeling laws.

"Restricted" Colors

Certain colors are considered harmful, but in spite of this are not banned but "restricted," because they are considered important for "consumer appeal." (It is questionable whether consumers would find foods that contain them so "appealing" if they knew they contained a possibly harmful additive.) Among these is Red No. 4, which was discovered in 1965 to cause harm to animal adrenal glands; it is allowed only to dye maraschino cherries red—the manufacturer pleaded that white maraschino cherries would not be salable. Citrus Red No. 2 is restricted to the skins of oranges, but only when the skin is not used in processing. It replaces Red No. 32, which was finally banned as dangerous, but it is described merely as "less toxic" than 32, hardly a recommendation.

The FAO/WHO Expert Committee of the United Nations, which is very conservative when it comes to negative evaluations of additives, released the following note in 1969: "Citrus Red No. 2 has been shown to have carcinogenic activity and the toxicological data available were inadequate to allow the determination of a safe limit, the Committee therefore recommends that it should not be used as a food color." In spite of this, the United States still permits its "limited" use, and the child who sucks on

---

FDA Provisional Color Additives

*FD&C Blue No. 2
FD&C Yellow No. 6

*In answer to a query as to its safety, the FDA reported it was in the process of "being looked into." The closing date "to allow the agency additional time to consider the results of safety tests," however, is listed as "indefinite." FD&C Blue No. 2 is the only one of the eleven color additives still used provisionally in foods, drugs, or cosmetics that has not been assigned a closing date (the date "when the FDA will decide whether these colors are to be permanently approved or withdrawn from the market." Only the two artificial colors listed here are still on the provisional list for use in food.

---

the peel as he eats a fresh orange wedge or the consumer who candies the peel or uses it as "zest" in cakes and cookies or for homemade marmalade is not protected from this admittedly poisonous food coloring. Incidentally, because this color is still allowed, dyed American oranges are banned in Canada, Great Britain, and other European countries. If the consumer will buy only the greenish uncolored Florida oranges and not the dyed ones, more growers will be encouraged to join the ones who have already discontinued its use.

Orange B, in use since 1966, is restricted to coloring the skins of hot dogs. It replaces Red No. 1, which was used for this purpose until it was established that it produced liver damage in animals. Theoretically, the dye does not get into the frankfurter meat, though that has been disputed.

Color Labeling

Artificial food colors are an ingredient category for which the consumer is not protected by labeling laws. Some standards of identity include food colors, so they do not have to be mentioned on the label. An example of this is dairy products, which are exempted from having to specify the use of artificial color. Butter and cheeses are routinely colored, but the manufacturers are not required to say so on the label. Left to the cow, the color of butter changes with what the cow eats; traditionally, summer butter is naturally golden yellow—if the herd grazes in green meadows; winter butter, a product of cows dining on hay and winter fodder, is pale yellow. The dairy industry decided—and convinced the FDA—that the consumer preferred the golden summer butter and that, therefore, the industry should be allowed to color the winter butter accordingly; the fact that consumers had loved butter in all seasons apparently was not considered relevant. Color was considered so important a factor by the dairy industry that when margarine was first introduced, the butter lobby prevented it from being sold already colored yellow; instead the block of margarine and a little packet of coloring were packaged together and the consumer kneaded the color into the margarine in the privacy of her own kitchen. Getting permission to sell yellow margarine was considered a major victory for margarine manufacturers. (See also Chapter 28 and Chapter 29.)

Food Colors and the Delaney Clause

Although the 1960 Food and Drug Act required that additives could not be used in food until the manufacturer submitted proof that they were safe (an improvement over earlier laws that required instead that the government prove them unsafe), the pace was slow. Manufacturers were given two and a half years to conduct their tests, and even at that, the tests were often incomplete or poorly done. The FDA did not take a particularly tough stance, often accepting as proof data that other organizations and countries thought questionable. Extensions were—and still are—freely granted, exposing the consumer to years more of risk. There was one clause that the FDA did take seriously and that came to be known as the Delaney Clause. It read: "No additive shall be deemed to be safe if it is found to induce cancer when ingested by man or animal, or if it is found, after tests which are appropriate for the evaluation of the safety of food additives, to induce cancer in man or animal. . . ." The effectiveness of this clause lay largely in two words, *cancer* and *animals*. The consumer does not want anything added unnecessarily to his food if it may cause cancer. Animal testing made it barely possible to establish that an additive might cause cancer.

Unfortunately, as most people know, cancer may take a long time to surface. An ingested carcinogen may not reveal its dire consequences until twenty years after it is ingested; how, then, could it be established within a mere two-and-a-half year period that an additive was a potential carcinogen?

The researchers knew the answer: they would feed the animals much higher levels of the product being tested than a human would consume and do so over a concentrated time period. Thus the time factor was offset by the quantity factor and the result could be evaluated in terms of human risk. In spite of the fact that most scientists accept this as a valid research method, manufacturers routinely ridicule the higher quantity, saying humans

---

Restricted Food Color Additives

FD&C Citrus Red No. 2   allowed only for the specific use of dyeing mature but naturally mottled green oranges an orange color

FD&C Orange B   allowed only for the specific use of dyeing frankfurter skins

NOTE: In both instances, as with all additives, the amount that is allowed to be added is specified.

---

would never consume anything like that large an amount. This ignores the point that no one says they would; it is simply a research tool. And if by any chance it sometimes exaggerates the risk, what consumer would not rather have the risk of cancer exaggerated somewhat than the other way around.

Eliminating Artificial Colors

Foods don't need artificial colors. For years gelatin desserts were deliciously made with only natural fruit and other flavors. Today that once wholesome food, so much enjoyed by both adults and children, is loaded with artificial colors and flavors. It would be nice to think that someday we would once again be able to buy beautiful gelatin desserts that contained no artificial colors or flavors but only true fruit flavors, naturally colored. If consumers refuse to buy artificially colored gelatin desserts, manufacturers may be inspired to go back to their original formulas. Until that time the consumer has the resort of the not-too-time-consuming chore of making them at home "from scratch."

CHAPTER 13

The Nuclear Pantry—
Irradiated Foods

Irradiation is a food process that, unknown to the public, has been used for a number of years on certain foods, such as pork, potatoes, wheat, wheat flour, and spices, primarily to kill insects, bacteria, and other organisms and to prevent sprouting (as in potatoes). It has recently been in the news because food processors, having discovered a possible new benefit, are pushing the FDA for wider approval.

In 1984 the primary excuse claimed for its use was the new benefit of extended shelf life. Consumers were told that irradiated fruits and vegetables would last ever so much longer and stay "fresh" far beyond their normal life span. Further research has shown that irradiation does not have this effect on all foods; some fruits spoil much more quickly after irradiation and do so in a sudden and unpleasant fashion. It is apparently true, however, that extended shelf life does occur in some irradiated foods.

In the past few years, as the industry has geared up to "educate" the consumer, several approaches have been tried. The primary benefit of irradiated foods, its extended shelf life, would presumably mean a cost savings to the consumer. When this benefit did not prevent the rise of considerable resistance from nutritionists and scientists, and those consumers who had heard of irradiated food, the process was repositioned as a fumigant and the emphasis subtly shifted to the less controversial idea of food safety. There is considerable appeal to this approach, since the industry, whose dependence on pesticides and insecticides is being increasingly criticized, offers irradiation as an alternative.

How Radiation Is Measured

Radiation exposure is measured by units called rads.

1 megarad = 1 million rads

1 kilorad = 1 thousand rads

A kilorad is a dose roughly 100,000 times greater than a human would receive from a normal chest x-ray.

What Is Irradiation?

Irradiation is a process by which food is exposed to beams of electrons from an X-ray machine or to gamma rays from radioactive material such as cobalt 60 or cesium 137. The amount of exposure is expressed in rads, an acronym for "radiation absorbed dose." Under proposed FDA regulations, up to 100 kilorads (a Krad equals 1,000 rads) per irradiation may be used. For comparison, a mammogram delivers up to a maximum of 1 rad.

Proponents of irradiation claim that it is harmless and that it will control insects and bacteria, reduce costs to the consumer because of extended shelf life, and destroy only a small percentage of nutrients. Those against it claim there is no proof that irradiated food is not harmful, that its extension of extended shelf life is grossly exaggerated and that, in fact, in some foods, it actually shortens it, and that it destroys an appreciable percentage of nutrients.

How Can You Recognize Irradiated Food?

Under the present law, you can't. Neither will you be able to in the future unless you tell the FDA that you want irradiated foods identified on labels.

The besieged consumer, who will be ingesting this unknown product, may find it difficult to determine what the experts think. But whether or not he decides to take a chance on irradiated food, he will feel strongly about his right to know whether a food he is about to purchase has been irradiated. Studies have shown that consumers want more informative labeling and want to know what is in their food. Manufacturers are clearly aware of the consumers' desire for information. They try to profit from it by heavily promoting "nutrition information." Just as margarine packages feature "no cholesterol," cereals proclaim their high RDA quantities of "supplements free," and boasts of "no caffeine" are bannered across cans, boxes, and bags, and featured in ads and commercials. So why, when consumer advocates asked that irradiated foods be so labeled, has the industry strongly resisted?

A nineteen-page form letter signed by Dr. George G. Giddings, Director of Food Irradiation Services for Isomedix Inc., explains the industry's public stand against labeling. He equates the public's negative reaction to words like *radiation* and *radioactive* with *irradiated,* blaming the atom bomb, which led to "radiation and radioactivity [being] suddenly . . . identified with devastation, death and deformity in the collective public mentality. . . ." For this reason, he argues, labeling food as "irradiated" would turn the consumer off, due entirely to an irrational fear associated with the word. Dr. Martin A. Welt, president of Radiation Technology, Inc., which has been seeking FDA approval to treat poultry, fish, and shellfish with irradiation, agrees with this point of view. He does not plan to use the word *radiation* on his labels. "If I put the word *radiation* on the food, even though there's no radiation in the food, people will think that it is radioactive, even if it isn't. I will fight putting the word on." He does, however, intend to send a signal to the truly informed consumer: the packages of foods irradiated by his company will have a radiation symbol—three flower petals in a circle surrounded by a segmented band.

The problem the industry perceives with the idea of irradiated food is not much different from the difficulties recently encountered in selling consumers on microwave ovens. Despite early claims of leaking microwaves and possibly unhealthful effects from exposure to them, the public soon accepted the explanation of how they had been made safe and has generally embraced microwave ovens with considerable enthusiasm. So it would appear that at the very least, the food processing industry is underestimating the American consumer's intelligence. It is doubtful that the public would want information hidden from it on the grounds that such information would be "confusing." An informed consumer is still the American ideal and, to achieve that goal, labeling should be as complete as possible. As Kitty Tucker, president of the Health and Energy Group, put it, "If a consumer walks into a grocery, she knows that canned soup has been canned—but there will be no way to tell if a package or fruit has been irradiated." And no way, therefore, to make a choice.

Are Irradiated Foods Radioactive?

As near as I have been able to discover in conversations with numerous consumers, including those who are only dimly aware of the process, this idea is something of a red herring; not one person was worried about radioactive food resulting from the process. By raising a question that can so easily and positively be answered in the negative, other less harmless questions can be shunted aside. Over and over again industry literature loudly proclaims that irradiated food is safe because it is not made radioactive. Of course it isn't, but the point is no one has ever said it is.

What *does* concern many informed experts and consumers are the dangers of cobalt 60 and cesium 137 being routinely transported through communities, used in irradiation plants near residential areas, and the eventual creation of additional nuclear waste, which cannot be safely disposed of in any manner so far devised by humans. The industry has maintained a discreet silence on these issues. (See the section, Radioactive Waste—A Further Concern, following.)

Is Irradiated Food Safe and Wholesome?

As we have said, irradiated food is not radioactive; the atomic nuclei are not affected. Most of the beams travel through the food, with less than 10 percent remaining inside the food tissues. These emissions or protons set the food electrons in motion, causing chemical changes in the food and destroying some bacteria and insects.

It is at this point that one of the changes that has created controversy takes place in food. As the protons are set in motion, they break many of the chemical bonds with which they come in contact and in doing so create radiolytic particles (RPs). RPs are a form of trace chemicals not found in nature except when living systems and biological materials are exposed to radiation. No one knows what effect ingesting them will have on the human body. As Cheryl Crooks described the reaction in an article in *Health* magazine in December 1984:

> It's not until the negatively charged electrons have finally exhausted themselves and can do no more destruction that they settle down with positive-ion partners and become neutral atoms.
>
> The entire reaction occurs within a fraction of a second. In this time each electron will have traveled a total distance of less than one inch but will have shattered thousands of chemical bonds.
>
> We eat the result.

Dr. Giddings responded specifically to Ms. Crooks's article as follows:

> Permit me to correct the more serious errors [in the article]. The referred to "internal chemical changes" do not "worry" informed qualified scientists because there are so relatively few changes compared with the

amounts of chemical changes occurring during roasting, broiling, canning, etc., and, especially, during digestion of foods, and because the relatively few changes that do occur during ionizing radiation energy food processing are so well understood and benign.

The consumer may have a problem relating to an argument that equates the changes caused by an unnatural process such as irradiation with that of a natural process such as digestion.

As to the question of RPs specifically, a study by the U.S. Army found that irradiated beef contained 65 volative RPs that hadn't been present before irradiation. So the creation and existence of RPs as a by-product of irradiation is not disputed. The question is: how safe is food once it contains radiolytic particles? And what happens to humans who ingest it?

Dr. Walter Urbain, food scientist and professor emeritus at Michigan State University, says that RPs are not only safe but that even if they aren't, they are present in very small quantities. Since, however, we know that even minute quantities of certain substances—down to parts per billion—are considered hazardous, "small" quantity alone is not a reassuring measure. Dr. John Gorfman, professor emeritus of nuclear chemistry at the University of California, strongly disagrees with the notion that the changes are "well understood and benign" or that irradiated food is safe:

They're lying when they say they know it's safe. Only the Lord himself can tell which are carcinogenic and which aren't . . . to really be able to say whether this technique has serious adverse effects on humans would require epidemiological studies of twenty to thirty years on 100,000 or more subjects. That study has not been done. It's not likely to be done. For someone to say that irradiated food is a safe product to eat is disingenuous. We don't know what the long-term safety is.

Dr. Giddings's response to Dr. Gorfman was:

Whereas "the Lord" does not consult to and advise the FDA on the safety of new medicines and medical devices, food additives and processes, etc., imperfect man has devised rather ingenious ways and means of testing for establishing their preclearance safety, and these do not, and cannot possibly include epidemiological studies on millions of humans over decades, which would by their very nature require, among other impossible technical requirements, preclearance approval at the outset (i.e., a "Catch-22" or paradoxical proposition). There are no absolutes; assurance of safety beyond reasonable doubt is the best that one can achieve, and this has most certainly been achieved in the case of this food process.

Beatrice Trum Hunter, author of *Consumer Beware,* has documented the levels of nutrients that remain in irradiated foods with impressive specificity. She finds that vitamins, as a group, are radiosensitive (likely to be affected by irradiation), some more than others, and are destroyed by irradiation. Among the more sensitive vitamins she lists vitamin A and carotene, vitamin C, thiamin and other B vitamins, and vitamin E. Irradiated temple oranges, for example, lost up to 28 percent of their ascorbic acid; corn lost up to 29 percent of its ascorbic acid and 44 percent of its carotene. Whole milk lost up to 61 percent of its vitamin E. She also ascribes nutrient loss and changes in grains and vegetables to irradiation.

As to proponents' claim that even conventional methods of food preservation results in the creation of RPs, Ms. Hunter says: "Among the RPs in irradiated foods are unique radiolytic products (URPs) about which even less is known. These substances are not formed by conventional methods of food preservatives and result exclusively in irradiated foods. The FDA expressed concern that irradiated foods may contain enough URPs 'to warrant toxicologic evaluation.' The long-term biological effects of URPs are unexplored and unknown."

In March 1984 the USDA released a report of twelve studies of irradiated chicken. The report stated, "Two of the studies . . . had some possible adverse findings, which will require careful consideration before the process can be declared safe." Among the findings: mice fed irradiated chicken showed an increase in cancer and kidney disease and a shortened life span; Mediterranean fruit flies (used for generational studies) showed an increase in radiation-dose-related deaths in the second generation when the first generation was fed irradiated chicken.

Meanwhile numerous tests and studies are being conducted to try to settle the question of safety. Since we now know that cancer may occur as long as twenty years after exposure to the carcinogen, and since neither industry, the government, nor the consumer is willing to wait until all the data is in, risk of cancer may be one we will agree to take. Other effects—nutrition, short-term side effects both on adults and on children—may be able to be determined more quickly. As with all tests and studies, however, careful evaluation by a reliable, truly independent, and unbiased third party will be essential—and perhaps hard to obtain. One laboratory under contract to the federal government to compare the effects of irradiation on the protein and vitamin content of enzyme-activated beef was later convicted of falsifying data in many of the tests. And of several hundred studies on the safety of irradiated food, 99 percent were rated inadequate by FDA scientists.

A demonstration study in Florida begun in December 1985 may lead to some more definitive data. Meanwhile the FDA has classified irradiation as a process, not an additive, and therefore not subject to present labeling requirements. Any effort to have it put on labels will involve having it reclassified or otherwise identified as coming under the law.

On July 22, 1984, the FDA responded to a petition filed by Radiation Technology, Inc., that had requested amendment of the food additive regulations to allow pork to be irradiated to control trichinae and other helminths (parasites) in pork. The FDA response legalized irradiation of pork but limited it to the use of gamma radiation for the control of *Trichinella spiralis*. (See Will Irradiation Make Pork Safer?, p. 113.)

The previous February, data from a USDA study conducted by Raltech Scientific Services claimed that mice fed irradiated chicken were found to have a "statistically significant" increase in the incidence of testicular tumors. The Center for Food Safety and Applied Nutrition denied that the study results had established any treatment-related effect that was either biologically or statistically significant. The FDA then asked the National Toxicology Program's Board of Scientific Counselors to review the study data. The result was that the NTP board concluded that available data did not allow the study to be categorized as demonstrating increased risk of cancer and therefore an increased risk had not been determined.

It is interesting to note in passing that there were only 60 cases of trichinosis reported in all of 1984, yet the FDA felt trichinosis was enough of a threat to justify approval of this still very controversial process. (On the other hand, in considering a ban on sulfites [see Chapter 9, Forever Fresh— The Sulfite Story], the fact that 300 people had reported adverse effects was dismissed for years as being too small a number to require any action on the part of the FDA.) Furthermore, an inexpensive new test—far cheaper than irradiation—that can detect trichinosis in pigs before the animal is slaughtered is now available. And if by any chance infected pork reaches the marketplace, it can be rendered harmless easily by thorough cooking, as recommended on all packaged pork and as routinely done by most cooks.

Since irradiation is a process being used or considered by countries throughout the world, the World Health Organization (WHO) formed a special Joint Expert Committee on Wholesomeness of Irradiated Foods to review the studies that had been made through 1981. At that time the committee concluded that foods irradiated with no more than 1 megarad are safe for human use. So far the FDA approval limits irradiation doses to .1 mrad or less, far below the committee's safety level.

There is still further evidence that irradiated food may not be safe and that concern for the public safety calls for more investigation. Irradiated bacon, which had received FDA approval, was found to cause health problems in test animals that ate it; approval was, therefore, withdrawn. Accord-

> ### *Will Irradiation Make Pork Safer?*
>
> Irradiation reportedly eliminates the long-standing hazard of trichinosis in fresh pork. Consumers have always been warned that pork must be thoroughly cooked in order to prevent trichinosis, but they have been assured that pork cooked properly presents no hazard. Irradiation is said to eliminate the danger of trichinosis, but pork will still have to be cooked just as thoroughly as before because of the possible presence of other microorganisms that are not affected by irradiation.
>
> Everything considered, it is hard to see just what the advantage of irradiated pork can be.

ing to the Health and Energy Institute, "A recent test revealed that fruit flies fed gamma irradiated chicken had seven times fewer offspring than those fed thermally processed chicken. . . . A study in India found that children fed wheat freshly irradiated with gamma rays developed blood abnormalities, and similar problems were uncovered in mice, rats, and monkeys. Other animal studies suggest possible harm to the kidneys."

Radioactive Waste—A Further Concern

Gamma radiation, the kind approved for use on pork, is achieved by the use of cesium 137, which is a nuclear weapons waste product, or of cobalt 60, which is produced in nuclear reactors. Since radioactive waste, transported on our highways and through our towns and cities, poses a possible danger due to accidents, leakage, and unplanned exposure, approval of this process would seem to require an environmental impact statement. The FDA, however, has ruled that such a statement is not required since, as quoted in the Federal Register on July 22, 1985, "The agency has carefully considered the potential environmental effects of this action and has concluded that the action will not have a significant impact on the human environment." The Health and Energy Institute (HEI), a private, nonprofit research and education organization, disputed this in a mailing dated July 31, 1985, in which it stated that "food irradiation facilities will use large, dangerous radioactive sources, which pose hazards at both the irradiator and during transport."

Irradiated Food—As of January 1986

At the present time the FDA has approved five uses of irradiation in food.

1. fresh pork—to eliminate trichinosis
2. potatoes— to inhibit sprouting
3. wheat and wheat flour—to kill insects
4. spices and other seasonings—to control microorganisms and insects
5. fruits and vegetables—to inhibit sprouting and increase shelf life

Americans who travel abroad may be interested to know that approximately twenty-eight countries permit the use of irradiation of some foods. These include Belgium, Hungary, Japan, the Netherlands, Israel, Uruguay, Czechoslovakia, and France.

The FDA is currently considering a proposal that would allow the use of irradiation in all foods when insect control is a problem; in fruits and vegetables to prevent sprouting and increase shelf life by slowing ripening; and for wider application for pork (meat regulations must be coordinated with the USDA, which has primary jurisdiction).

Theoretically, the public is notified of FDA proposals and given an opportunity, usually for a period of ninety days, to comment on them. Any proposals regarding irradiated foods are of special interest to the consumer for several reasons:

Food safety—an ongoing concern.

Food labeling—Since industry is opposed to identification of irradiated foods, only a strong public interest and protest will bring about proper labeling.

Cost—If irradiation is approved, the expensive research and development required will be financed by the federal government—which means by you, the taxpayer—but turned over free to industry.

Loss of local government control—It is proposed that state and local governments be prohibited from regulating any aspect of food irradiation independently. This is contrary to most other federal food regulations, which apply only to interstate commerce and not to trade within a state. Since many states have stricter food laws than those of the federal government, the consumer will lose by this proposal.

The Health and Energy Institute claims that the irradiation program is deliberately kept from the public. In a May 6, 1985, series of releases, HEI charged that Department of Energy (DOE) funds to build demonstration food irradiators were requested as part of its nuclear explosives budget in

---

Possible Irradiation Hazards

Aflatoxins, potent cancer-causing chemicals created by funguses occurring naturally in some foods, were produced more abundantly than normal on irradiated foods in several studies. The exact reasons and overall health effects are unknown—but aflatoxins are 1,000 times more potent carcinogens than the banned pesticide EDB, for which irradiation is a possible substitute.

Vitamins A, C, E, and especially B may be destroyed by the process; amino acids and fats in foods may also be altered. The effect of irradiation on food nutrients is probably comparable to that of heat sterilization processes, but if widespread use of irradiation is allowed, many foods may be subject to more than one preservative process before they reach the consumer (fruit may be irradiated to keep it from spoiling before being canned, for example). This could mean a decline in the nutritional quality of our food supply overall.

From an HEI brochure titled *Food Irradiation: What are the Hazards?*

---

secret hearings of the House Procurement and Military Nuclear Systems Subcommittee of the Committee on Armed Services. In addition, HEI claims, "A special food irradiation promotional campaign was launched by the International Atomic Energy Agency and others in December of 1984 with a starting war chest of a quarter of a million dollars. Consequently, many folks are hearing only the glowing promises of the industry, rather than the legitimate concerns of health professionals and consumers."

It is up to the consumer to try to keep informed on this important new process; we have already seen much of our technology rushed into commercial use before we have been able to evaluate it and to assess its affect on our health and well-being. Man's record of improving on nature has not been especially good; perhaps we should go slowly before we take this giant new step toward interfering with something as basic and critical to our health as the very structure of our food.

PART THREE

Real Food

CHAPTER 14

How to Recognize Real Food

Recognizing real food is comparatively easy, and the more real food you eat, the easier it becomes to recognize it. Here are some guidelines:

Choose simplicity. For one thing, real food has a shorter list of ingredients. A whole orange, apple, carrot, turnip, head of lettuce, or potato has no ingredients list. Fake food and processed food, on the other hand, always come with ingredients lists. Since you will inevitably eat some processed foods, choose the ones with the shortest lists; Grapenuts rather than sugared cold cereals; old-fashioned oatmeal instead of gussied-up hot cereals.

Look for fewest "added nutrients." If one product is enriched or fortified, try to find a version that isn't. A few, like milk, must, by law, have certain nutrients added (vitamin D in the case of milk), but most added nutrients are put there to make a better sales pitch. No matter what is added to white bread, it won't match the natural goodness of whole grain whole wheat bread. Natural dietary fiber is better than added cellulose fiber, and butter is more nutritious than margarine.

Buy basic ingredients, not combinations. For instance, when buying frozen vegetables, don't buy the ones in butter sauce or exotic sauces. It's easy and much less expensive to add a bit of butter yourself. If you don't know how to make a cream sauce, take off five minutes and learn. Mastering that one simple recipe will make it possible for you to make curry, cheese, and all sorts of other special sauces, and you can even make a batch of basic cream sauce to keep in the refrigerator and turn into any sauce you want at will.

Prepare food from scratch. You'll be surprised to find that many dishes are quicker to make from scratch than from their "convenience" version. Tests have shown that even a microwave oven is not necessarily a timesaver compared to conventional methods of cooking (and stirring, turning, and resting all take more attention than just heating in a conventional oven). You'll automatically eliminate MSG and numerous chemicals and additives from your diet. Soup is quick to make, and homemade soup is a meal in a way canned soup never can be. A homemade milkshake—even when made from skim milk—with real strawberries or raspberries is a gourmet treat.

Learn to use herbs and spices. If you like food, you'll find this is fun. And you'll save enough money to be able to splurge on something besides preseasoned food that has had all the good taken out of it. You can't go wrong with the basic herbs—parsley, dill, oregano, rosemary, tarragon, thyme, and garlic. Fish with a bit of dill butter or olive oil, a green salad liberally sprinkled with parsley and tarragon, with lemon juice or raspberry vinegar in the dressing, turns a boring diet dinner into a company meal.

Learn some simple food facts. Fast foods are usually high in calories, fat, and sodium. A Big Mac contains 563 calories, mostly from beef fat, but many less publicized processed foods are made with coconut oil, which is much more saturated than beef fat. Homemade hamburgers can be made with leaner beef and cooked to drain off much of the fat. Cokes and similar soft drinks are high in sugar and contain food coloring, flavoring, and other additives; diet soft drinks contain artificial sweeteners. Substitute fruit juices you carbonate yourself with seltzer.

You don't have to become a food chemist to know which foods to avoid; your own palate will tell you once you get away from oversweet, oversalty processed foods.

Avoid food fads. Anytime a "health" benefit is heavily promoted by a food manufacturer, be skeptical. Real food will provide all the fiber you need if you eat a rounded diet of grains, fruits and vegetables, dairy, and meat and/or fish. Cholesterol is not a poison and, unless you have a special medical problem, is a poor reason to avoid the valuable nutrients of real eggs and similar foods (see Chapter 23, What We Really Know About Fats and Cholesterol).

If you want a low-fat diet, achieve it by eating less fat, not by eating chemical substitutes or special "low-fat" versions of real food. It's especially easy to do now that olive oil has been found to be beneficial—even to the extent that some experts recommend eating it in sizable amounts. You needn't substitute margarine for butter; just eat a smaller amount of butter. Substitute yogurt for sour cream; most of the time you'll hardly notice the difference.

If you like chocolate, enjoy it. There are 150 calories in an ounce of milk chocolate and even fewer (121) in cocoa. In spite of what you have heard, chocolate has very little caffeine and does not cause acne.

Ignore food advertising. Now that the government is becoming more and more permissive, advertising claims are getting out of hand. Do not depend on them as a source of health information. Natural cheese is more nutritious than processed cheese, in spite of the advertisements that tell you "each slice is now made from five ounces of milk." This statement is better than the original claim—"five ounces of milk per slice"—but still fails to inform the consumer that processing has reduced the original milk's calcium by one-third and riboflavin by two-thirds.

The Best News of All

With the new emphasis on nutrition, the dangers of chemicalized foods, the difficulty of getting or staying thin, and all the other chores we now tend to associate with food, food has become less and less fun. And, let's face it, there's not much creative satisfaction to be gotten out of putting together a meal by popping a frozen dinner into a microwave oven or opening a couple of cans to arrange on a dinner plate.

If you come home tired and hungry, you don't have to plan anything time consuming or elaborate. Real bread, real cheese and a cup of your own real soup (from your refrigerator or freezer) can be fixed in five minutes. But sometimes the act of fixing a meal can be relaxing and invigorating, a welcome prelude to sitting down and putting your feet up with a tray of good food to restore you.

Real food is fun: it will restore your palate and help you regain the pleasure all creatures find in eating. Real food is creative: your imagination will come to life when opening your cupboard reveals a shelf of herbs and spices instead of processed foods. The aroma of a real loaf of bread; the hearty goodness of a peasant dish of beans or hummus; the sensuous pleasure of a fresh ripe peach or a glistening dish of strawberries kissed with Cointreau—all these are the pleasures that can be had only with real food. The illusory promises of fabricated food will leave you feeling vaguely dissatisfied and cheated—and rightly so, because you will not be truly nourished. But real food will nourish you, body and soul.

CHAPTER 15

Milk Is Real Food

Most of us were brought up to drink milk because it was good for us. The recommended amount was a quart a day, and college football teams in training always found pitchers of milk on their dining room tables. Today, as our diet is coming under increasing scrutiny for its fat and cholesterol content, and as we are discovering that bacterial contamination, pesticides, and cattle feed additives may show up in our food, milk is often viewed with considerably less enthusiasm.

Since whole milk is still a near-perfect food—the first and only sustenance of young animals, including human babies—we ought to be sure all the facts are in before we fault it.

Nutritional Value

Milk contains 3.7 percent fat, 4.9 percent lactose, 3.5 percent protein, 0.7 percent ash (a total of 13 percent milk solids), and 87.2 percent water. It is a particularly good source of calcium and contains phosphorus as well as vitamins A, D, E, and some Bs. Compared to most other foods, milk provides by far the most nutrition at the lowest cost. In addition, it is especially useful for low-meat and vegetarian diets because its amino acids complement many of those found in plants, thus providing the necessary amino acid balance for diets that would otherwise be deficient in this critical area. Milk's vitamin D content is low, so in order to prevent rickets, vitamin D is routinely added. Apparently, it has worked—rickets is seen less often today.

The amounts of the two most important milk nutrients, calcium and protein, are about the same regardless of type of milk; whole, skim, evaporated,

---

Rickets and Vitamin D

We assume from our experience with rickets that there is a direct connection between a vitamin D deficiency and rickets, but, in fact, nutrition is more complicated than the extent of our present knowledge would indicate. An example of this is the fact that breast-fed children do not get rickets, even though mother's milk is comparatively low in vitamin D. This has led Dr. D. R. Lakdawala, of Addenbrooke's Hospital, Cambridge, England, to conclude that "there must be something other than vitamin D in breast milk that protects infants from rickets." Clearly we have not yet sucessfully analyzed the nutrients in real food, and our attempts to simulate them may not be as successful as is sometimes claimed. There may be undiscovered nutrients in real food that are essential to human health and not to be found in the present American diet.

---

or nonfat dry milk all have comparable percentages. There is less vitamin D in skim milk, unless it is fortified, because it is lower in fat, but it contains slightly more calcium.

It is estimated that Americans get two-thirds of their calcium from milk. Two glasses a day provided three-fourths of the old RDA requirement of 800 milligrams for adults and preteenage children. The latest recommendation that women (18 and older), in particular, up their daily calcium intake to 1200 milligrams daily means that at least a quart a day is needed—ideally, more. Actually, no one seems to recommend trying to get your total calcium from milk; there are many other recommended sources, including sardines with bones.

The composition of milk makes it an even better source of calcium than its high-calcium content would indicate, because lactose enhances the intestine's absorption of calcium, as does the added vitamin D. The calcium in milk may, therefore, be more efficiently utilized than the calcium in other foods. It is, of course, not necessary to have such a symbiotic relationship in every food ingested; a truly balanced diet will provide the necessary combination of nutrients automatically.

Milk in the Diet

As we have seen, milk and milk products make a valuable contribution to the diet. There are, however, some possible negatives that have caused many people to switch from whole to skim or low-fat milk and milk products or even to avoid milk altogether.

Cholesterol

Most people have been taught by advertising to be afraid of cholesterol, though a recent study indicates that doctors on the whole have taken a more conservative view. (See Chapter 23 and Chapter 24). As a result, whole milk and whole milk products are increasingly avoided by consumers trying to cut down their cholesterol intake. If whole milk worries you, at least drink skim milk or dry milk, both of which have a low cholesterol content. That will still contribute more real food to your diet than you might otherwise get and may provide some of the unknown but essential natural nutrients that are not to be found in fabricated foods.

While some studies have shown that whole milk apparently raises cholesterol levels and skim milk reduces them, other researchers discount this. The latter claim that the measured reduction should not be taken at face value because it simply masks the fact that cholesterol is continuing to be deposited as plaques on the walls of the blood vessels even though the serum cholesterol count appears lowered. Further research in this area is clearly needed, and it is best not to take any one study as gospel until more facts are in.

Saturated Fat

This is another area (see Chapter 24, A Surprising View of Polyunsaturated Fats) in which advertising and professional biases have clouded the issue, to the confusion of the consumer. For some time government dietary recommendations took a hard line against saturated fats, strongly suggesting that they should be replaced as much as possible by unsaturated fats. As more scientific minds prevailed and more studies were done, the recommendations were toned down until now the latest recommendations are that Americans should reduce all dietary fats and not favor one over the other. You will find many experts who will still not go along with this new position and will insist on the superiority of one type over the other.

An odd side effect of this new position, and one that can increase the confusion among consumers, is that many articles are written by those who feel strongly that saturated fats are harmful no matter what anyone else says. After reporting that the newest thinking recommends lowering all fat intake and dividing it equally between saturated and unsaturated fats, an article may slip back into a statement such as, "So eat less of all fats and try to lower your intake of saturated fat and eat as much polyunsaturated fat as possible." This contradictory summary of all the previous material in the article requires careful reading and analysis on the part of the consumer. Just hold firmly to the fact that an excess of all fats is considered undesirable, but that both saturated and unsaturated fats have value and that they should be consumed in a one-to-one ratio.

The immediate relevance of this discussion is that the fat in milk and milk products is saturated fat. If, however, you eat or drink skim milk, skim-milk products, low- or nonfat cottage cheese, buttermilk, and yogurt, and avoid sour cream, heavy cream, and rich cheeses such as brie, you will be getting comparatively little saturated fat. And even if you prefer whole milk, there are many other foods—such as meat, fast foods, and snack foods—containing saturated fat that are less desirable and more easily eliminated from the diet than milk.

Iron and Vitamin C

Much is often made of the fact that milk cannot be considered a perfect food because it lacks iron and vitamin C. It is quite true that milk lacks these nutrients, but knowing that one can easily get them from other sources makes that no reason to value milk less highly. Whether it is a suitable food for adults is another matter, but on the basis of nutritive content it cannot honestly be faulted.

The Nature of Milk

Because milk is a natural product, it is not always the same. Experts can recognize the type of cow that produced a given sample of unprocessed milk. Some breeds give milk that is much richer, with a higher proportion of cream; others have other recognizable characteristics.

The composition and flavor of milk depends also on the weather, the seasons, the feed, the age and health of the cow, and its lactation and gestation. Its sensitivity to feed is easily seen when a cow gets into a patch of wild garlic. Fortunately—or unfortunately, depending on your point of view—the processing, including pasteurization, homogenization, deodorizing, and blending milk undergoes creates a bland product of great uniformity. As the Department of Agriculture puts it, "These variations are kept at a remarkably low level." Some consumers feel it also denies them the enjoyment and the subtle distinctions our great-grandparents knew.

Raw Milk—Certified Safe

Although annually someone surfaces with a bill to ban its sale on health grounds, raw whole milk that has not been processed is still available in a few localities in the United States. Many health food advocates fiercely resist a ban on raw milk because they feel that, produced under strictly regulated conditions to protect its purity, it is a healthier, more natural product than processed milk. They say, for instance, that pasteurization lowers the vitamin C content by 20 percent and the thiamin content by about 5 percent, that it causes the loss of some biotin and B_{12}, and that it destroys phosphatases, which hydrolyze phosphates. While this seems to be true, it can be argued that milk is not a particularly good source of either vitamin C or thiamin to begin with, and that the nutritional function of phosphates and other milk enzymes is unknown.

Not surprisingly, consumers who drink raw milk find it sweeter and fresher-tasting than processed milk. Whether it presents a health hazard is not clear. If certified—look for the word on the carton—it has been inspected by the American Association of Medical Milk Commissions, but that is a private trade association and its certification is not accepted by the federal government. Actually the regulations for certified milk are even stricter than those for pasteurized milk, and much more frequent testing—daily rather than monthly—is required. Because, however, the government does not accept the certification, raw milk may not be sold across state lines; and some states ban its sale within their borders. There have been some instances of bacterial infection reputedly due to the drinking of raw milk, but they have generally been disputed, and since there have also been many incidents associated with pasteurized milk or milk products, it is difficult to assess whether an extra degree of risk exists with the consumption of certified raw milk.

Many health food advocates feel you are safe as long as you stick to certified raw milk produced by a well-known and regular source and handle it properly, keeping it well refrigerated.

Pasteurization—What It Is

The essence of pasteurization is heating the milk to a sufficient temperature and maintaining it there long enough to kill a number of bacteria. If milk is heated to 145 degrees Fahrenheit, that temperature must be held for 30 seconds. If heated to 161 degrees, it must be held for 15 seconds; 191 degrees for one second, and 212 degrees for .01 second. When used for a dairy product with a fat content of 10 percent or more, or if it is to contain added sweeteners, the temperature level must be 5 degrees higher. This would apply, for instance, to cream and chocolate milk, which require at least 150 degrees for 30 minutes or 166 degrees for 15 seconds. For frozen dessert mixes, at least 155 degrees for 30 minutes, or 175 degrees for 25 seconds is required. The differences are due to the fact that a higher fat and sugar content makes the bacteria more heat resistant.

Ultrapasteurization. A comparatively new process is ultrapasteurization, which increases the shelf life of dairy products markedly. In fact, milk processed this way is often referred to as shelf-stable milk or UHT milk. Instead of the usual pasteurization temperatures, the minimum process requires heating to 280 degrees for two seconds. It is then cooled quickly and aseptically packaged in a hermetically sealed sterilized container. Once opened, UHT milk requires refrigeration like any other milk product. The National Dairy Council says the process is used for milk in some parts of the country but is mostly used for half-and-half, cream, whipping cream, and eggnog.

Some supermarkets carry only ultrapasteurized heavy cream. I do not know if my experience is unique, but I bought some once because I needed it for an organization party and there was no time to shop around. What was needed was whipped cream, normally no problem. But though I whipped and whipped and whipped, the result was simply not satisfactory. I ended up throwing it all out (a couple of quarts of it) and sending out for regular whipping cream (which whipped up beautifully in no time). Food experts complain that ultrapasteurized cream has a cooked taste, which would certainly be understandable.

Incidentally, the labeling laws in this respect are a little complicated. Grade-A milk must be pasteurized, but the label need not say so. However, either homogenization or ultrapasteurization must be revealed on the label.

Homogenized Milk

Homogenization is a process associated with pasteurization (although it is possible to pasteurize milk without homogenizing it), but its function is not to destroy bacteria so much as to create a uniform fluid in which the cream does not separate and float to the top. Homogenized milk is made by preheating the milk and then forcing it, under 500 to 2,500 pounds of pressure per square inch, through a mesh that breaks up the fat into tiny globules and dispersing them throughout the milk, where they stay in suspension. Health food experts claim that this process is unhealthful because it takes the natural fat globules in raw milk, which are too large to do damage in the body (as fat or as cholesterol), and breaks them down into such small-size globules that they pass into the body in ways nature never intended.

Some consumers may remember the problems with unhomogenized milk in the good old days when one or two family members would use all the cream off the top and leave the resulting skim milk for the rest of the family. At that time brands of milk bragged about the amount of cream their "superior" milk contained—visually evidenced by the size of the cream portion at the top. Another contention of opponents of homogenization is that it hides today's much lower cream content (the government lowered the butterfat content requirement in 1975). They say that the reason the dairy industry fights any effort to do away with laws favoring homogenized milk is because a return to the old method would reveal to outraged consumers the small amount of cream that is left in today's milk. Aside from the economic aspects—consumers should pay less for milk that contains less cream—most consumers would probably be content with milk that contained less cream, provided they were satisfied with the taste.

Other Milk

In recent years goat's milk has gained a certain cachet, though most of the milk produced is used for cheese, and goat herds are proliferating, though not on a large scale. Now available nationwide, goat cheese is made in various sections of the country by small establishments. Long known and popular especially in Europe, it has caught on here as a gourmet food and comes in a number of types. The goats are also carefully regulated and inspected, and the milk and milk products conform to all the usual standards.

In addition to whole goat's milk and raw goat's milk, there is low-fat milk, skim milk, half-and-half, light cream (coffee cream), light whipping cream, heavy cream (heavy whipping cream), evaporated milk, condensed milk, sweetened condensed milk, nonfat dry milk, sour cream, and buttermilk made from goat's milk. Federal standards vary slightly for the various items. For instance, except for raw milk, all these forms must be pasteurized if delivered across state lines, but the addition of vitamins A (minimum 2,000 international units, IUs, per quart) and D (minimum 400 IUs per quart) is optional. Only evaporated milk, on the other hand, must be homogenized; it is optional for other types.

Modern Milk

First of all, modern milk is a comparatively safe product. Even our grandparents knew they could buy milk with confidence in its purity. The rise of

---

From the Cow to the Consumer

When the processing plant collects the milk from the farmer, it is usually pumped directly from the farm's stainless steel refrigerated tanks into a tank truck. The driver routinely smells the milk before pumping to make sure it doesn't need to be deodorized—wild garlic or wild onion is quickly detected and could otherwise mean the entire truckload would have to be treated to be palatable. Samples of the raw milk in the farmer's tank are also collected at this time for analysis for antibiotic residues, bacteria count, milk fat content, and for state and local public agency laboratories, who may want to run various tests of their own. This system makes it possible, in the event of an untoward event in the marketing of the milk or the milk product, to trace it back to the source and to locate the problem.

The milk delivered to the processor is blended, much as with sherry, with milk from other sources, so as to create the standardized product the consumer has come to expect from packaged, store-bought milk.

---

veterinary schools in 1884 led to rapid growth and dissemination of information on how to prevent or treat disease in livestock. The USDA established a nationwide Extension Service, which still exists today, to help farmers on the local level. A meat inspection system, set up to assure that only wholesome meat would reach the retail market, had an immediate impact in reducing the incidence of certain communicable diseases and actually practically eradicated many of them. Since diseased meat often infected food handlers and milk and dairy products, all these steps were beneficial to consumers in several food areas.

Another major contribution to the safety of dairy products was the introduction of pasteurization, which destroyed harmful bacteria, such as the ones that caused tuberculosis and undulant fever. Anyone who went to the country for a vacation was able to drink unpasteurized, warm milk from the cow—though not everyone relished it—and they could be reasonably sure that the cow was healthy. And, of course, almost all milk in America came from cows, not from goats, buffalo, deer, reindeer, or horses, all of which have for centuries been main sources of milk for other cultures.

Dairy farming today is very different from that of fifty years ago. Mechanical milking—with the milk literally untouched by human hands and going directly from the cow to the refrigerated storage tank—is the method routinely used. As milk travels from the cow to the carton in the supermarket refrigerator, it isn't once handled directly by humans.

Dairymen are subject to numerous state and local rules and regulations (the federal government establishes guidelines and recommended standards, but the state's own rules are often stricter); the barns, milking equipment, handlers, and overall physical environment, and the animals themselves are regularly inspected and tested.

As dairy farming became big business, dairymen improved their stock through selective breeding (largely by means of artificial insemination), and feed manufacturers supplemented summer grass and winter fodder with increasingly sophisticated animal food products. The result was sharply increased yields. In the 1830s a single cow gave about 1,500 quarts of milk a year; by 1980 the average annual yield per cow was 5,000 quarts.

According to the FDA's standards of identity, a product can be called milk only if it is "the lacteal secretion, practically free from colostrum, obtained by the complete milking of one or more healthy cows, which contains not less than 8¼ percent milk solids-not-fat." (Colostrum is not an unhealthy ingredient in milk but it does not have a desirable flavor and, in any case, is necessary for the health of newborn calves. Restricting it means that milk will not be taken either too early, or too late, in the lactation period.)

If Milk Doesn't Agree with You

Although milk is usually one of the most easily digested foods, there are some people who find it gives them gas, diarrhea, or other similarly unpleasant reactions. The reason for this is probably lack of the enzyme lactase, which is necessary for the digestion of the lactose in the milk. (You may have certain temporary conditions that make it hard to digest milk, but if you have had this problem since childhood, or continuously since adulthood, this deficiency is the likely cause.) Lactose is composed of glucose and galactose, which must be split in order to be properly absorbed by the intestine; only lactase can perform this function.

Most infants are born with the necessary enzyme, which seems to diminish as the child grows older. One theory is that people tend to stop drinking milk as they get older, so the body tends to stop producing the no-longer-needed enzyme. Many nutritionists consider an adult lactase deficiency normal and point out that in nature mature animals—even those that require it as infant animals—do not drink milk. Two African tribes, among them the Masai, drink milk as adults, and among Europeans, Scandinavians tend to be milk drinkers regardless of age. In some ethnic groups the majority—over 70 percent—are known for milk intolerance; among them are those from Central Europe and the Mediterranean areas, Asians, Jews, blacks, and American Indians.

Working Mothers Who Breast-feed

Surprisingly enough, even though more and more new mothers work, more and more of them are choosing to breast-feed their babies. Sometimes, however, it is necessary to pump and store their milk for the next feeding, and a refrigerator is not always handy.

A recent study, reported in the *Journal of Pediatrics,* has determined that breast milk has natural bacteriostatic qualities that inhibit the growth of bacteria. Because of this it appears that it can be safely stored for up to six hours without refrigeration. If your pediatrician agrees, this finding will leave the new working mother freer to attend meetings, travel with the baby, and engage in other similar activities.

If you have a problem with milk, you may find you can tolerate it in small quantities; a spoonful or two in your coffee may not bother you, while a glassful may. If your intolerance is mild, there are several ways you can get around it. Try substituting yogurt for ice cream, buttermilk for whole milk and various hard cheeses and sour cream; cultured milk products contain partially digested lactose, which may be within your tolerance level. Experiment with one lactose-containing food at a time and wait a few hours to see if it bothers you. This may seem like a lot of trouble but it isn't really, and it is worth it; to give up such a good source of calcium without a fight would be to give yourself much more work in the long run. Eating small amounts at a time may allow you to consume a considerable quantity in the course of a day.

If you are very sensitive to lactose, you will have to avoid not only all those food items, but also many more that you would not think of as containing lactose. Here is where labels can be a help. Any creamed dish, creamed soup, dips, or spreads probably contain lactose; so do many so-called convenience foods, such as instant breakfast drinks, protein diet drinks, instant cereals, baking mixes, instant potatoes and many other dried foods, instant cocoa, and ice milk. Avoid all milk products listed on the label, including whey.

Some people find adding the lactase enzyme to what they want to eat works; others simply switch to acidophilus milk (a cultured milk), which may work for you but is not invariably tolerated by those who cannot drink regular milk. Acidophilus milk has a distinctive taste, which may take some getting used to, but it is worth a try. And, of course, you could switch to soy milk and simply eliminate cow's milk from your diet—but this will not provide your calcium requirements.

There is a commercial enzyme product available from your pharmacy, supermarket, or health food store. It is called Lact-Aid and comes either in liquid or powdered form. A packet or several drops added to a quart of milk will predigest the lactose so that your digestive system can handle it. Follow the directions on the package and allow time; it isn't something you can do five minutes before you want to use the milk. Once the milk has been treated, use it any way you would ordinary milk—for puddings, milk shakes, and so on.

If you have diabetes or any other metabolic condition, check with your doctor before trying to deal with lactase intolerance on your own. He may also be able to advise you how to get sufficient calcium without milk or dairy products.

CHAPTER 16

Dairy Products—
A Gray Area

There is a gray area between the real and the fabricated, where most of today's dairy products could be said to fall. A carton of whole milk is still real food, although because of processing it no longer contains all the nutrients it had when it first came from the cow's udder. Unprocessed cheese is still a wholesome food, even though it may be made from this same processed whole milk, and this is true of other dairy products manufactured from the same ingredients. As time goes on, however, more and more processes and additives are entering into the manufacture of milk and milk products, and the consumer needs to be able to judge what the effect is on health and nutrition.

Milk As a Processed Food

As we have seen, milk is now much freer from bacteria and contamination than it often was in the good old days. There is still an occasional incident of illness caused by milk-borne bacteria, but considering how much farther the milk is brought from its source, it is remarkably safe. The cow is an animal that is vulnerable to a number of microorganisms that can be transmitted to humans and cause such serious diseases as tuberculosis and undulant fever. Modern methods of sanitation, inspection, and medication have mostly eliminated danger from exposure to these diseases through milk.

As we have mentioned in the previous chapter, one of the ways milk is processed is through pasteurization. Its primary purpose is to destroy any disease-producing organisms that are in the milk as it comes to the processor.

Milk is an excellent breeding ground for bacteria, and bacteria are everywhere, so even pasteurization is not foolproof; if not properly handled every step of the way—including in the consumer's own kitchen—milk may become contaminated after pasteurization. Unfortunately, however, pasteurized milk's nutritive value has been diminished, and taste and flavor have been compromised.

There is less of a case to be made for homogenization, whose primary purpose is not safety but to reduce the size of the fat globules and distribute them uniformly through the milk. As we have noted elsewhere, some health food advocates think this makes milk a much less healthful product and may be implicated as a cause of heart disease. According to Dr. Kurt A. Oster, a noted cardiologist, homogenization allows xanthine oxidase, a harmful enzyme, to pass through the intestinal walls; without homogenization, it is excreted instead.

Homogenization also makes it impossible for the consumer to compare how much cream (butterfat) the milk contains. Most consumers are not aware that the required cream content of whole milk was lowered in 1975, and without visual evidence of cream content, there is no competitive advantage to producing richer milk. It would be difficult, in any case, to produce milk as rich as it used to be since the Jerseys and Guernseys—famous for their rich, delicious milk—have been replaced by the Holsteins, more efficient factories that produce twice as much milk but nowhere near as much cream. When your grandparents say milk just doesn't taste as good as it used to, they are absolutely right.

Processing modern milk moves it further and further from the original product. Once the milk is taken from the cow, it is handled by mechanized equipment with little or no chance for human hands to touch it. This eliminates one possible source of contamination—dirty hands or clothing—but the equipment itself must be constantly cleaned and sterilized. Cleaning pipes and machinery requires much more than hot water and a bar of soap. Modern technology does it mechanically, without the need to disassemble and reassemble the equipment after every milking or transporting, which is undoubtedly efficient and timesaving, but doesn't allow automatic eyeball inspection of the interior of the equipment. The cleaning materials used are detergents; chelating compounds; compounds for dissolving milk proteins and for emulsifying milk fat; chemical sterilizing compounds, specially formulated to remove milk solids from equipment with a minimum of physical effort; and sanitizing solutions of a chlorine, iodine, or quaternary ammonium chloride. These are all in aid of disease prevention and are presumably safe. Presumably, also, the milk is tested regularly to ensure that no more than an "acceptable" level of cleaning compounds gets into it.

There is a more immediate possibility of chemical contamination in other areas of milk production. To increase the proportion of desirable forage plants to undesirable weeds in the pasture, weed killers are routinely used on pastureland. The flies and other insect pests that used to plague cattle are now destroyed by pesticides and insecticides. These are potent poisons, and the USDA admits they "must be used judiciously. Otherwise, they may be transmitted to milk."

As part of the "judicious use," the use of certain chemicals is forbidden. As the USDA explains, "Cows are not sprayed with insecticides containing chlorinated hydrocarbons since these chemicals can accumulate in fatty tissues and later appear in milk. Similary these insecticides must not be used to control flies around the milking area, where airborne droplets could possibly get into milk." And not only is it the direct-spraying of cows that is risky. The USDA continues: "Contamination of forage crops with chlorinated hydrocarbon pesticides may occur when crops in adjacent fields are treated. To avoid this, spraying is done when air currents will not cause drift." Obviously the USDA takes an optimistic view of the possible. It is not hard to imagine the harassed and busy farmer, having contracted for the spraying of his pastures on a given day, wetting a finger, holding it to the brisk breeze, and deciding to bend the rules a bit. He will be encouraged in his decision by the crop-spraying pilot who has developed a casual attitude toward his dangerous occupation and doesn't really believe that the dust he is spraying is going to do anybody or anything (including himself) any harm. The pilot's work is seasonal, and he cannot be blamed for not wanting his income to depend on the vagaries of the wind. In addition to the farmer and pilot rationalizing the weather, there are those who deliberately flaunt the law. FDA files are full of cease-and-desist orders and recalls, where products banned because of their danger to human health were still being used in food production.

The same technology that the farmer uses for his pastureland is also used by the growers of feed crops, so the cattle get a double whammy, in their own pastureland in the summer and in the feed they eat all winter. A possible side effect of crop spraying is the chance contamination of streams and ground water, as rainwater runoff. Both animals and humans may thus be directly exposed to pesticides and insecticides used on the dairy farm.

How to Recognize Real Milk

Fortunately the government's labeling requirements in this area are a real help to the consumer. Most milk products go back a long way, and the rules governing them were created in a less permissive age. If the consumer will take the trouble to learn what the various appellations mean, there will be comparatively little difficulty distinguishing the real from the fake.

There are many choices—between whole and skim milk, for instance— and you can get exactly what you want *if* you know what to look for. Conversely, you can also identify and avoid the products that appear to be dairy but are not. The following glossary will be a handy guide.

Glossary

fresh fluid milk Always Grade A, pasteurized for home use.

whole milk At least 3.2 percent milkfat and 8.25 percent nonfat milk solids recommended, but some states specify slightly less.

homogenized A process by which milkfat is broken down into smaller globules and remains in suspension, uniformly distributed throughout the milk.

creamline Faintly reminiscent of milk in the days before homogenization, in that it has a layer of cream at the top of the container. I haven't seen any in years, but maybe you have it in your area.

fortified multiple-vitamin and/or mineral "Enriching" additives that are used to "fortify" this product are usually vitamins A and D, riboflavin, thiamin, niacin, and/or iron and iodine. This is not a clear benefit, since these are supplements, so all the arguments against supplements presumably apply and also add to the problems of the consumer who may be monitoring vitamin intake.

With so many foods being fortified without rhyme or reason, it is impossible for the consumer to know how much of the RDAs is being ingested. The USDA yearbook *Food for Us All* says, "unless you rely on fortified milk as a principal source of vitamin D, buy fresh milk without added vitamins and minerals if there is a [cost] difference."

concentrated Milk with a large proportion of its water removed. Since milk is about 87 percent water, concentrated milk presumably provides all the nutrients in a smaller package.

skimmed milk Beloved of dieters and organizations that come down hard on saturated fat, it has been processed to remove most of the fat. Unfortunately, this also removes most of the vitamins A and D.

skim or nonfat milk For a low-fat diet, the less than 0.5 percent milkfat content is helpful; at least 8 percent must be nonfat milk solids, close to or equal to that of whole milk.

fortified skim milk In this version nonfat milk solids must be as high as 10 percent, with less than 0.5 percent milk fat. It qualifies as fortified because vitamins A and D are added.

low fat Contains between 0.5 and 2 percent milk fat solids, so it is not as reliably low in fat as skim milk.

2 percent No more than 2 percent milkfat, usually 10 percent nonfat milk solids.

flavored milk All flavored milk has flavoring and stabilizer added. Read the label if you care whether the flavoring is real or artificial.

chocolate milk Whole milk with chocolate and sweetener.

chocolate-flavored milk Better than it sounds; whole milk with cocoa and sweetener.

chocolate-flavored drink Skim or low-fat milk with cocoa and sweetener; nonfat milk solids may or may not be added.

other flavored milks All the foregoing, sometimes available with flavorings other than chocolate.

cultured buttermilk Cultured buttermilk is usually made by adding bacterial culture to milk. It must contain at least 8.25 percent nonfat milk solids. Uncultured, real buttermilk is the liquid left over from butter making and is still available in a few sections of the country. Most people today have never tasted real buttermilk and probably wouldn't even like it. I do, but I have also learned to like the cultured product.

yogurt Made from whole or skim milk and cultured into a smooth, semisolid product that releases quantities of whey when a spoon is dipped into it. The plain natural product need contain nothing that was not in the milk from which it was made, but reading the labels of various brands will reveal that some manufacturers apparently find the use of a number of additives—not including fruit or natural flavorings—necessary. The popularity of many of these brands would seem to indicate either that the consumer doesn't read labels or doesn't object to additives. Since all the brands are together on the shelf, it is easy to choose the purer product and thus cut down on the daily additive intake.

canned milk All canned milk is concentrated by removing water from milk. It comes in several forms.

evaporated milk Sterilized, with vitamin D usually added.

whole Contains at least 7.9 percent milk fat and 25.9 percent total milk solids.

skim Low fat content is often no more than 0.2 or 0.3 percent milk fat, with at least 18 percent total milk solids. Vitamin A may be added.

sweetened condensed milk An old favorite, often used as a substitute for coffee cream. Contains sugar and at least 8.5 percent milk fat and 28 percent total milk solids.

dry milk A handy supplement to fluid milk, or used alone reconstituted with water. Contains not more than 5 percent moisture.

nonfat dry or dry skim milk Made from fluid skim milk, may contain added vitamins A and D and not more than 1.5 percent milk fat.

whole dry milk Contains at least 26 percent milk fat.

filled milk Not really milk but an invention made from skim milk and vegetable fat, or of nonfat dry milk, reconstituted with water, with vegetable fat added. Ideally, it should be called by a totally different name; calling it milk could easily confuse the consumer who buys it because it appears to be simply less expensive milk.

imitation milk This product needn't contain any milk. It is usually made of several nondairy ingredients processed to a milklike appearance and taste. Among the possible ingredients are vegetable fat, which is not specified and may be coconut oil; protein in the form of sodium caseinate (note the sodium) or soya solids; corn syrup or similar sweeteners; flavorings; stabilizers; emulsifiers; and water. It must be labeled imitation, not because it contains no milk but primarily because it is not as nutritious as milk.

half-and-half A mixture of milk and cream available in both sweet and sour forms. The sour form comes both fluid and semifluid.

cream All cream is higher than milk in fat.

heavy cream Contains at least 36 percent milk fat.

light whipping cream Contains at least 30 percent milk fat.

coffee or light cream Contains at least 18 percent milk fat, generally homogenized.

pressurized whipped cream Sweet cream with sugar, stabilizer, emulsifier, and possibly other additives, in an aerosol can.

coffee whiteners, whipped topping mixes, artificial cream, and most of the aerosol **whipped toppings** Mostly chemical inventions. A quick look at the ingredients on their packages ought to be enough to turn anyone off. The taste of sweet heavy cream freshly whipped is something many of today's consumers have never experienced. Take a small chance (if you think you must lower your cholesterol intake) and whip up just one batch so you can see what you're missing. You might decide to settle for occasional enjoyment of the real thing rather than frequent intake of a poor imitation manufactured by a chemist instead of a cow.

Once you have tasted real whipped cream (and I don't include the "real" whipped cream in the aerosol can, which has neither the flavor, the density, nor the texture of hand-whipped cream), you may find it easy to resist restaurant sundaes and desserts capped with "topping." This is a painless way to cut down on calories and fat and leave room for the occasional enjoyment of the real thing.

Coffee whitener is a term that shows how well the food manufacturers understand their market. No attempt is made here to claim any benefit other than appearance; if you don't like the look of black coffee, you can just whiten it. The fact that you are adding chemicals and a somewhat strange flavor—it certainly is nothing like sweet cream—doesn't seem to bother the consumers who have made this a profitable item. If you are using this type of product to avoid the saturated fat in cream, you have simply traded milk fat for coconut oil, which is even more saturated. (It may be listed in the ingredients as vegetable oil.) Coffee whiteners and lighteners are considered a boon to office workers and retail store clerks because it doesn't have to be refrigerated, but no one seems to have stopped to question what it is they are consuming.

sour cream Can be made most naturally from light cream cultured with lactic acid bacteria, in which case it is called cultured sour cream. It can also be made by acidifying the cream with food grade acids, with or without the use of lactic acid bacteria or enzymes, and is then called acidified sour cream. The cream used must be pasteurized and contain at least 18 percent fat but need not be fortified or homogenized.

Sour cream is also available as sour (cultured) half-and-half, and acidified sour half-and-half, which is allowed to contain 10.5 to 18 percent fat.

Nonbutterfat sour dressing is not sour cream; it need not conform to the regulations for sour cream, but the listing of ingredients must conform to usual labeling regulations.

A study by the Connecticut Agricultural Station analyzed twenty-one different brands of sour cream and seven brands of nonbutterfat sour dressing, collected from food stores over a three-month period. None of the sour creams contained any artificial color or artificial flavor. Surprisingly, in view of the fact that sour dressing is white, three contained artificial color. And it is a commentary on the nature of the product that all but one, Friendship brand, contained artificial flavor.

Only five of the twenty-one real sour creams contained a stabilizer (vegetable gum or carrageenan); but all the sour dressings did. Emulsifiers (mono- and di-glycerides), which help keep the fat dispersed, were in four of the sour creams and all of the sour dressings. Two of the sour dressings contained dextrose or sugar.

The various brands sometimes added a descriptive word to the name, in an effort to make their product more appealing. Among the sour creams were the adjectives "all natural," "grade A," "naturally flavored," and "country packaged." Some variation on *natural* was used by far the most often—eight times. The sour dressing packages kept a low profile except to emphasize "nonbutterfat," apparently their strongest appeal. Since some fat must be used, the consumer can find out from the label that sour dressings contain hydrolyzed vegetable oil.

A comparison of the number of calories in about 2 tablespoons showed 55 for sour cream and 46 for sour dressing, hardly worth giving up the real thing for, and the sodium content was slightly higher for sour dressing— an average of 68 milligrams per 100 grams as against 67. Many of the brands contained considerably more sodium; look for hydrolyzed vegetable protein (which can contain considerable salt) as well as salt on the label.

If you want to eat sour cream, just eat less of it—but enjoy the real thing. If you truly feel you must abstain altogether, why not substitute yogurt?

yogurt An excellent cultured milk product about which almost no one has a bad word to say. It has been a diet staple for centuries in Europe, Africa, and Asia but has become popular in the United States only recently.

You can make it at home easily and inexpensively in a mason jar or an electric yogurt maker, or you can buy live-culture yogurt in almost any market. The milk you use doesn't have to be whole milk. Not all yogurt is alive, so look on the label for something like, "with active yogurt cultures." Inactive yogurt cultures may still taste good (and won't do you any harm) but that kind of yogurt doesn't qualify in my reckoning as the real thing. Ingredients should be something like: "Made from cultured pasteurized Grade A milk, skim milk, and nonfat milk solids." In other words, milk and active yogurt cultures are all the ingredients needed to make real (plain) yogurt; if it contains anything else, ask yourself why it should. Coffee yogurt, for instance, lists sugar even before nonfat milk solids (coffee is the last ingredient), which tells you there's quite a bit of it. You may want some sugar with your coffee, but if you added it yourself, you wouldn't need to add nearly as much in order to be happy with the amount of sweetness. In addition, the more gussied-up yogurts are liable to contain additives.

You can make yogurt at home without adding thickening agents and stabilizers, yet some yogurts apparently require them. And since many yogurts use natural flavorings, like real fruit flavors, why should you settle for artificial flavors, which are laboratory-created imitations of the real thing? Several manufacturers manage to make and sell superb plain yogurt commercially and profitably without additives, so obviously it can be done.

Since yogurt has become so popular, the makers can't let it alone. First they added fruit preserves, then they mixed the fruit in, then they blended fruit until the mixture was practically homogenized. It almost seems as if a new yogurt variation turns up in the dairy case every other day. Try them for the fun of it, if you must, but you can do most of it yourself a lot cheaper and better. For instance, one of the best ways to eat yogurt is to add your own fresh fruit or vegetables. That would eliminate the processing necessary to successfully incorporate new ingredients and would add fresh produce to your diet—with at least some of the nutrients intact.

Another disadvantage to buying yogurt other than plain is that it tends to make you think yogurt is primarily good mixed with sweet things. Actually yogurt is a very versatile product and can add all its good nutrition to a great combination of foods. You can use it to make cheese that is very similar to cream cheese (but richer in calcium and lower in butterfat), and you can do it at home with some cheesecloth, a strainer, and a bowl. Just line the strainer with a double layer of cheesecloth (available in any hardware store), put it over a bowl and dump into the cheesecloth a large carton of plain live yogurt. Pull the ends of the cheesecloth over to cover the yogurt and leave it on the counter for half an hour. The whey of the yogurt will drain into the bowl. Put the whey in a container and refrigerate. Once the whey stops dripping freely, put the bowl of yogurt in the refrigerator. In three or four hours it will be cheese. If it's not convenient for you to be home then, it doesn't matter. It can stay in the strainer all day or overnight. Put the finished cheese in a covered container and store in the refrigerator; it's ready to use. Most people assume yogurt cheese will be a cottage cheese type, but actually it is an excellent cream cheese, very smooth with no curds.

Yogurt cheese can be mixed with cucumbers or onion or any of the other things that make good cream cheese spreads, or dips, if you add a little skim milk. Yogurt is great mixed with a little mayonnaise and seasonings as a salad dressing. It's good in soup (use it instead of sour cream in zucchini soup or borscht—hot or cold), over boiled new potatoes, and as a topping. And that is only the tip of the iceberg. It can completely replace sour cream and is an essential ingredient in the cooking of many other countries. Depending on the manufacturer for ideas will limit your use of yogurt and deprive you of a lot of fun and good food. None of the dishes you can make with yogurt are time consuming, so they are especially good for the busy life of working couples and singles. And because yogurt is cultured, many people who can't drink milk can digest yogurt, making an important and inexpensive source of calcium easily available.

By the way, if you like frozen yogurt, you can make that at home too—with a lot less sweetener than the commercially prepared kind.

When yogurt was first introduced in America, much was made of the fact that Bulgaria, where it is a regular part of the diet, has many extremely aged persons who are remarkably healthy and active. The inference to be made was that eating yogurt regularly would increase your longevity and active years. That has yet to be proved, but no one questions that live-culture yogurt is good for you. Some nutritionists think it aids digestion (unless you have a severe lactase deficiency) and will lower blood cholesterol. It is also sometimes recommended to restore helpful intestinal bacteria that have been destroyed by antibiotics.

Frozen Desserts

ice cream Contains cream, milk, sugar, stabilizers, and up to 1500 possible additives. Contains at least 10 percent milk fat and 20 percent total milk solids.

French ice cream All the foregoing plus egg yolks.

ice milk Popular with dieters because it has 2 to 7 percent milk fat, at least 11 percent total milk solids. Basically made from milk, stabilizers, and sweeteners.

fruit sherbet Water ice with milk added, and various additives, including stabilizers.

CHAPTER 17

All About Real Cheese

Real cheese is made primarily from the milk of cows and goats. The liquid whey is separated out, leaving the curd or milk whey solids, a simple process that can be duplicated at home. Farmer cheese, a popular homemade cheese, is an example of this process. In this instance the home version is superior to commercial farmer cheese because, as a soft, unripened cheese, it should be eaten as soon after making as possible.

Cheese has been known for over four thousand years. As with other very old foods, such as roast pork, it is supposed to have been discovered by accident. The story goes that an Arabian merchant, traveling across the Sahara desert, put milk for his dinner into his saddle pouch and set off on his camel for a day-long trip. The pouch was a calf's stomach, closed at both ends so it wouldn't leak, and the rennet in the stomach lining was mixed with the milk by the rocking stride of the camel. As the sun heated the rennet-milk combination, the milk separated into curds and whey.

When the merchant opened the pouch, he was delighted at the unexpected turn of events. The liquid whey proved an excellent thirst quencher, and the cheesey curds were a welcome addition to his dinner of dates and figs. Many cheeses are still made today in much the same way they were made hundreds of years ago, although naturally occurring bacteria and molds— as in the famous caves where the original Roquefort cheeses were made— have led to more sophisticated cheeses than the original cottage type of the Arabian merchant.

Today there is a wide variety of all kinds of real cheese available, and a more or less successful effort has been made to categorize them. All cheeses are now designated as soft, semisoft, hard, and very hard.

Cheese Classifications

Soft

unripened:

   low fat—cottage, pot, farmers
   high fat—cream, Neufchatel (American)

ripened:

   Bel Paese, Brie, Camembert, hand, Neufchatel (French)

Semisoft

ripened principally by bacteria: brick, Munster
ripened by bacteria and surface organisms: Limburger, Port du Salut, Trappist
ripened principally by blue mold: Roquefort, Gorgonzola, Blue, Stilton, Wensleydale

Hard

ripened with bacteria, without eyes: Cheddar, Caciocavallo
ripened by bacteria, with eyes: Swiss, Emmentaler, Gruyère

Very Hard

ripened by bacteria: Asiago, Parmesan, Romano, sapsago, Spalen

The use of bacteria to produce the various types of cheeses does not mean a cheese is not natural. Most of the cheese-making organisms exist in the air in various localities, such as the spores that make Roquefort cheese in the French caves. Though other blue cheeses are made equally successfully, the French maintain that true Roquefort can be made only with genuine Roquefort spores. The mold cheeses (see list) are so called to distinguish them from other types of cheeses (though not always from one another), but it is not generally known that the holes in Swiss cheese are created by gas produced by bacteria, and that Limburger, a delicious American invention with a pungent odor, is ripened by bacteria.

Other Cheeses

Whey cheeses are usually classified separately from curd cheeses and include Mysost, Primost, and ricotta. Only the last is familiar to most Americans; it is usually used to make Italian dishes, such as manicotti.

Goat cheese has only recently become popular in this country. In addition to the increasing number of imports, cheese from small American goat farms can be found around the country. Many of these cheeses are excellent and are gradually acquiring a reputation for their quality and fine flavor, but most of their products are available only on a local basis or by mail.

Natural Cheeses and Unnatural Cheeses

All of the foregoing are "natural" cheeses, and there are over a hundred varieties. In spite of this wonderful variety, the consumer has to buy carefully to avoid a number of highly processed and imitation cheeses. Usually they are described as cheese substitutes, imitation cheese substitutes, cheese product substitutes, and process cheeses. Of course, such cheeses are sold under interesting names, and they are often intriguingly packaged in tubs or tubes or other handy forms, and are "easy to use," because they are presliced, individually wrapped, or formulated to melt without stringiness. Real cheeses are usually simply packaged and presented and are identified by brand and type without much in the way of hard sell.

Unfortunately, today even natural cheeses are allowed to be much less natural than the consumer would like.

How Natural Is a Natural Cheese?

The FDA does not set standards of identity for cheese substitutes but it does for cheese foods (which is drawing a rather fine line), and it does for seventy-three varieties of natural cheeses. These standards differ according to variety. For instance, according to federal regulations, creamed cottage cheese must not exceed 80 percent moisture and must contain a minimum of 4 percent fat. If it is a dry curd cheese it must contain less than 0.5 percent fat. Cheddar, on the other hand, must contain not more than 39 percent moisture, its solids must be at least 50 percent milk fat, and if it is made from unpasteurized milk, it must be cured for at least sixty days, as must all cheese that is made from unpasteurized milk. This latter requirement has kept the American consumer from enjoying some of the finest European cheeses, because those cheeses are made from unpasteurized milk and do not lend themselves to aging. The European cheese makers have resisted using pasteurized milk because it produces what they consider to be an inferior version of their cheese. However, the American market is a tempting one, and recently some cheese makers have given in.

Cheese regulations are extremely confusing, due to numerous exceptions. For instance, FDA regulations state: "Manufacturers don't have to list required ingredients—such as milk—on the labels of cheese packages" except on some cheeses, including cold-pack cheese (not a natural cheese) and on cottage, Neufchatel, and cream cheese (all natural cheeses). Also, all cheese contains undeclared amounts of salt, "except if the salt is potassium chloride and the cheese is a low-sodium cheese." "All optional ingredients must be listed on the label," except for some, such as artificial colors and some additives. In addition, labeling must indicate if a preservative has been used and whether enzymes were added during the manufacturing process.

If consumers want more complete information on cheese labels, this might be a good time to let the FDA know; it is considering making some changes. Some of the changes already being considered are: listing *all* ingredients, including percentage of milk fat (the milk fat content of cheese can range from 3 to 35 percent. See the chart, Fat Composition of Cheeses, following).

Effective July 1985, amendments for Blue, Cheddar, Edam, Gouda, Gruyère, Limburger, provolone, Samsoe, Swiss, and Emmentaler cheeses require "full ingredient declaration on the lable, permit the use of safe and suitable ingredients that don't change the basic identity of the food, and their composition must be consistent with international standards." If this kind of information is important to you, write the FDA urging this kind of cheese labeling.

Artificial Colors in Natural Cheese

A notable exception to label declaration is food coloring. The Food, Drug and Cosmetic Act specifically allows natural cheeses, butter, and ice cream to contain "undeclared artificial coloring." (It would be comforting if at least only natural colors were allowed.) If you asked why any colors need to be added, you would be told that it is to make the food more attractive to you, the consumer. For instance, milk, which is naturally yellow, might not make a really white cheese, so blue or green coloring is sometimes added as a whitener—just as we used to add blueing to washing machines to make clothes look whiter. Amendments are constantly adding more cheeses to the "whiteners allowed" list; mozzarella and low-fat mozzarella can now add "safe and suitable artificial coloring during the manufacturing process to whiten the cheese." That bright orange Cheddar cheese is another example of gilding the lily.

Fat Composition of Cheeses

Variety	*Approximate % Fat
cream	35.0
Roquefort	33.0
Cheddar	32.8
American	32.2
gorgonzola	32.0
brick	31.0
Swiss	28.0
Limburger	28.0
Parmesan	27.5
Brie	26.1
Camembert	26.0
Neufchâtel	25.0
Edam	23.8
cottage:	
uncreamed	0.3
creamed	4.3

* NOTE: Since these are natural cheeses, there is some variation in the fat content from one batch to another. Percentages given are, however, a fairly close approximation of what you can expect. There may also be a minimal difference between the fat contents of imported and domestic versions of certain varieties.

If you want to avoid artificial food colors in cheese, try Neufchâtel, Gruyère, Roquefort, Limburger, and sapsago. At present, they aren't colored, but some of them may be bleached. Look on the label.

Bleached Cheese

Cheese bleaching agents are "optional" ingredients and, as such, must be declared. If the ingredients include "benzoyl peroxide," or a mixture of "benzoyl peroxide, potassium alum, calcium sulfate, and magnesium carbonate," that cheese is bleached. You'll find bleaches listed especially on labels of Blue, Gorgonzola, provolone, Caciocavallo, Siciliano, Parmesan, Romano, and Asiago. Since there are often several brands of each type of cheese, reading the labels might help you to buy the one—if there is one—that is a little more "natural." Incidentally, vitamin A is destroyed by bleaching, so it is added to all bleached cheeses.

Other Optional Cheese Additives

Other optional ingredients you might find listed on natural cheese labels include:

Water-binding gums, such as gum tragacanth, carob bean gum, guar gum, carrageenan, and gelatin. Neufchatel and cream cheeses apparently always contain it—at least I have been unable to find one that doesn't. Water-binding gum is not an ingredient essential to the making of a true cream cheese; Philadelphia Cream Cheese never used to contain it. When cream cheeses first started listing it, I went out of my way to buy brands that didn't. None of the cream cheeses have tasted nearly as good since they all went the gum route, but today so many consumers have never tasted gum-free cream cheese that they don't know what they are missing.

Preservatives, such as sorbic acid or potassium sorbate, are allowed to be added to wedges and slices of most cheeses, because pieces of cheese are more liable to mold than the whole cheese. This is hard on the consumer, who usually cannot use a whole cheese; it benefits only the manufacturer, not the consumer, because it makes the cheese salable longer and gives it a longer shelf life.

Smoke flavor is added to some familiar cheeses to create a new flavor. Smoked cheese can be delicious when it really is smoked, but usually it is made by the addition of water into which synthetic (sometimes even real wood) smoke has been discharged. If the label says "with added smoke flavoring," that's probably how it was made.

So-called Natural Cheeses

If by *natural* you mean cheese without additives, do not go by the manufacturer's description. The government does not define *natural,* so it is a word without meaning and can be used even though the product contains substances that are not natural—within the consumer's understanding of the word. In addition, the government, as we have seen, specifically allows synthetic colors to be added to what we think of as natural cheeses without identifying them on the label. The vitamin A added to bleached cheeses is synthetic, as is the sodium hypochlorite that may be used in the preparation of cottage cheese. The only truly natural flavors are the ones nature puts in food, but as the label will tell you, many "all-natural" foods have "natural" flavors added.

How to Encourage the Production
of More Real Cheese

While it is not always possible to avoid some of the additives in real cheese, it is much easier not to buy obviously processed or imitation cheese. Manufacturers are quick to spot consumer trends and will respond to an increased demand for the real thing, especially if sales of other cheeses decline.

In addition, since there are additives in natural cheeses only because the government allows them, an informed and concerned citizen can influence regulating agencies to approve fewer additives in the future and to phase out presently allowed ones wherever an alternative exists.

CHAPTER 18

The Vegetable Bonus

The traditional American meat-and-potatoes diet has long ago been replaced by a new lighter, more varied menu. Main-dish salads are now routinely ordered by men as well as women, and the California custom of starting the meal with a salad appetizer is now nationwide. We have even discovered that iceberg is not the only lettuce, and many formerly exotic items, such as avocados and snow peas, are to be found in every supermarket.

Recently the health-oriented consumer has discovered that vegetables not only make for more interesting meals but also improve our health. They provide a wide range of vitamins and minerals in a natural, accessible form. They are rich sources of dietary fiber and, with a few exceptions, are remarkably low in calories. Another plus from the consumer's standpoint is that very little effort has so far gone into developing fake vegetables, although pesticides and preservatives are sometimes a hazard even here. Generally speaking, however, from artichokes to zucchini, what you think you are eating is usually exactly that. Whether you buy your green beans in the produce section, from the freezer cases, or in cans, you will still get honest green beans. Of course, the nutrients in any given portion will vary according to a number of factors—most of which are beyond your control—but at least you do not have to worry about being fooled by look-alike foods. So far not a single vegetable is made of surimi!

Choosing Vegetables Wisely

Fresh Produce

Buying good vegetables is much easier than buying good meat or bread. If you want fresh, raw vegetables, good and bad examples are usually side by side for instant comparison. Asparagus, for example, will contain the firm, dry, tightly closed buds along with loose, gappy, or wet-looking tips. It doesn't take a culinary arts degree to recognize which is better. Iceberg lettuce heads will vary considerably in size, weight, and presence of "rust," with the stem ends of some heads obviously trimmed of outside leaves. A moment's observation and hefting of two heads, one in each hand, will tell you which is the better buy.

Smelling a bag of potatoes will quickly reveal if there is a rotten one among them; salad greens, such as romaine, chickory, or watercress, will look unmistakably wilted if they are old; green beans will be limp instead of crisp, and broccoli will be yellow instead of emerald green. Since you can pick up fresh produce and examine it, there is no reason not to get your money's worth in freshness and nutrients.

Frozen Vegetables

If you want a vegetable that isn't in season or doesn't look good that day, buy the frozen. Experts say that frozen vegetables are often more nutritious than the fresh; modern freezing methods process ripe, freshly picked produce much more quickly than it can reach your market. There is now a very wide variety of frozen vegetables available, and more will be added if there seems to be a demand. For today's busy cooks the convenience factor of frozen food is a distinct plus; the vegetables are already prepared for cooking, and they cook quickly. From a nutrition standpoint, frozen vegetables can be steamed as easily as fresh or, if you want to boil them, require far less water (and that can be used in soups or stews).

To make the most of the food value and your food dollar, always buy plain, unsauced frozen vegetables. Vegetables in butter or "interesting" sauces may contain additives; at the very least you will be paying a high price for something you can easily add yourself. If you want a butter sauce, toos the hot cooked vegetable with a small pat. If you want a simple curry sauce, add a bit of curry powder to melted butter. (Just put the cooked vegetable in a dish, put the butter in the hot saucepan (off the burner), add curry (variations could be dry mustard, garlic powder, minced parsley, etc.), stir with a wooden spoon until the butter melts (a minute). Put the vegetables back, mix with the sauce, and reheat. In a few minutes you'll have a gourmet vegetable.

Raw Vegetables

Crudités were discovered by smart hostesses some years ago, and now almost every cocktail party or respectable buffet has at least one plate of cut-up broccoli florets, carrot sticks, turnip rounds, zucchini strips, and mushroom caps—with or without a nicely seasoned dip. Raw vegetables are easy to prepare (especially with a food processor), low in calories, fun to eat, and not filling. While they are not necessarily more nutritious than cooked vegetables (carrots, for instance, are more nutritious when cooked), they are still excellent sources of nutrients and good for your teeth.

Raw vegetables are especially good for our new eating habit of "grazing." They can be prepared in a free moment (watching the evening news, talking on the phone) and stored in the refrigerator. Snacking on carrot sticks beats reaching for a potato chip. And, of course, raw vegetables are great for anyone on a diet. If you want to feel pampered, mix plain yogurt with minced (the food processor again) onion, garlic, and parsley. It makes a delicious low-calorie dip along with a "cocktail" of tabasco-and-lemon-juice-spiked tomato juice over ice cubes. Most people can diet much more easily if they have a refrigerator full of guilt-free foods to nibble on.

The Fly in the Ointment

Of course there has to be a catch to this halcyon picture of perfect vegetables, and there is. Fortunately the consumer can see that it is eliminated and that only trustworthy vegetables end up in the marketplace. Here are some of the things to look out for.

Sulfites

If you haven't already read the section on sulfites (Chapter 9), do so. And don't miss an opportunity to tell the government, your produce market manager, your congressman, and anyone else who might be concerned that you do not want sulfites used in any of your food. You just might save someone's life by taking action.

Genetic Engineering

All over the country plant biologists have a new challenge: how to "design" crops by altering their genes. Some of the goals they have set themselves are celery with less fiber (just when we are finding out that fiber is good for us), carrots that don't smell musty, vegetables that don't freeze at temperatures below 30 degrees Fahrenheit, and crops that are less "thirsty." An example of how they do this: scientists are trying to create less thirsty crops by introducing cactus genes into them.

How Much Vitamin C in a Potato?

That depends on a number of factors. Here are the results of just two variables: when the potato is harvested and whether it is fresh, cooked, or processed.

Mean Total Vitamin C Content in Potatoes Harvested in Autumn 1960 and Sampled Periodically (Estimated on Fresh Weight Basis in mg.) Per 100 gm. of Potato

	Raw	*Fresh, Peeled, Cooked and Mashed*	*Reconstituted Flakes*
October 1960	29.3 mg	18.8 mg	8.0 mg
February 1961	11.7 mg	8.2 mg	3.1 mg
May 1961	10.6 mg	6.8 mg	2.1 mg

SOURCE: U.S. Plant, Soil and Nutrition Growing Laboratory, Ithaca, New York.

If the plastic tomato, which is all you can buy most of the year, is an example of what plant biologists come up with, I shudder to think of future vegetables. A beefsteak tomato, with all its commercial drawbacks (it's too big, not uniformly shaped, and tends to crack), is still unparalled in flavor. Since flavor is what good eating is all about, it seems to me the tradeoff is not a good one. The food manufacturer and processor may make more money with genetically altered crops, but I am skeptical about their ability to improve the quality of life; that doesn't even seem to be one of their objectives.

There is also the fact that these experiments have a life of their own and tend to be tried out long before anyone can make even an educated guess as to their effect on the total environment. Once again, man is proposing to alter and tamper with basic natural laws without an inkling of possible harmful effects.

Dr. Garth Youngberg, director of the Institute for Alternative Agriculture in Greenbelt, Maryland, is quoted in *The New York Times* (3/16/86): "Is this [genetically altering crops] going to make farming more expensive, more intensified, and less diverse? Will it mean even fewer farmers or less nutritious food? Nobody knows. More needs to be done to answer these kinds of questions." Unfortunately for the consumer, only a few concerned scientists are asking these questions and none of the plant biologists seem to be attempting to answer them; they simply do not concern themselves with anything except the challenge of being able to do what no scientist has been able to do before. Whether it will destroy our food or our health or our family farmers is simply not part of what they think about.

Many of the scientists who developed the atom bomb and made the whole world vulnerable to nuclear destruction lived to rue the day and to confess with horror that they had not thought through the consequences of their research. Perhaps it is time the ordinary nonscientific consumer began to keep closer tabs on where the natural curiosity of the research scientist and the commercial interests of the food processor may be leading us and to demand a slower and more thoughtful march into the future.

Vegetables and Our Health

The more we learn about the importance of vegetables to a healthy body, the more we find things they are good for. As we have already seen, they are a source of natural nutrients, minerals, and fiber. In addition, they seem to have a preventive effect on various diseases, such as cancers of the lung, esophagus, colon, and larynx, to name just a few. Soybeans seem to actually lower serum cholesterol, even in those who have not responded well to a low-cholesterol diet. In a 1985 study at University Hospital in Linköping, Sweden, patients with chronic bronchial asthma showed significant improvement when put on a vegetarian diet. An Australian study done the same year indicated that eliminating meat, chicken, and fish from the diet might lower high blood pressure; the higher the percentage of vegetables eaten, the greater was the drop in systolic pressure. We have long known that carrots are good for night vision (due to their high vitamin A content) and have recently discovered the great benefits of olive oil. Seventh Day Adventists, a religious group, have been the subject of numerous studies, all of which appear to confirm the health benefit of a vegetarian diet. As a group, they have much lower than average incidence of, for example, heart disease and cancer.

It is not necessary to be a vegetarian, if that does not appeal to you. With the allowed three or four ounces of meat or fish recommended for keeping one's weight down, and with the wider variety of whole grain products and interesting vegetables available, a more vegetarian way of life would seem to be a perfectly pleasant way to be healthier. It would be easy enough to try it for a month or two and see how you feel.

Home Gardeners Have a Nutrient Edge

As we have seen, food composition can, at best, provide only a rough guide to the nutritional content of foods. What even home gardeners may not know is that not only do such factors as maturity, season, soil composition, and weather affect nutrient levels, but also one variety of a given crop can have a higher nutrient content than other varieties of the same food. Seed catalogs and garden groups, such as the National Garden Bureau, Willowbrook, Illinois offer this kind of nutrition information.

For example, we have found that vegetables that contain vitamin C will have a higher C content if they are harvested in the sun, then stored in the shade. On the other hand, according to the U.S. Plant, Soil, and Nutrition Growing Laboratory in Ithaca, New York, a growing food crop can lose vitamin C in unusual darkness or reduced light but make up the loss if it is again exposed to sunlight. But the home gardener can minimize even this loss by growing Orlando Gold carrots, for instance, which are 50 percent higher in vitamin C content than even the above-average Imperator.

Here are some examples of how nutrients in the diet can be enhanced by choosing the best variety of vegetable for the home garden.

Item	Variety	Higher than Average Nutrient Content
carrot	Imperator	carotene (vitamin A)
	Orlando Gold	50 percent higher than Imperator
cauliflower	Early Snowball	vitamin C
kale	Dwarf Scotch Kale	vitamins C, A, riboflavin, niacin and calcium
lettuce	Red Sails	6 × vitamin A, 2 × vitamin C, 3 × iron as crisp head lettuce
sweet potato	Centennial	both contain 18 mg/100 gr caro-
	Julian	tene
	Goldrush	{these two varieties next highest
	Allgold	
acorn squash	Jersey Golden	3 × vitamin A
scallop squash	Sunburst	2 × calcium as tomatoes
Oriental squash	Kutu	100 percent more phosphorus and calcium, vitamins A, C
tomato	Caro-Red	10 × vitamin A
	Caro-Rich	10 × vitamin A
	Doublerich	2 × vitamin C

SOURCE: National Garden Bureau, Willowbrook, Illinois.

CHAPTER 19

Tracking Down Real Fruit

Fruit is completely real food. If you grow your own and never use insecticides, pesticides, waxes, or other profit enhancers, it's as good a food as you can eat. Fruit is high in nutrients and fiber; the sweetness of many fruits makes it easier to cut down on other sweeteners, and fruit has fewer undesirable ingredients or diseases, such as oxalic acid in vegetables or alflatoxins on peanuts. Most of the trouble with fruit is man-made, and what man has done can be undone if the consumer wants it that way. Whole fruit is not a laboratory product, but man does rely heavily on laboratory products to produce fruit commercially.

You may feel you are unlikely to be fooled into eating anything but completely real fruit, and to some extent, this is true, particularly with whole fruit. An apple or an orange chosen from the produce department might be considered the real thing, with the reservation that some fruits are more real than others; fruits contaminated by possibly harmful substances, or with nutrient contents that have been reduced from that found in the untampered-with ripe fruit, are not quite the same as the apples with which Solomon wished to be comforted.

Fabricated fruit that the consumer tends to accept readily as the real thing is the sort found in foods such as "fruited" cold cereals, where fruit "flakes" allow the claim of fruit to be made without any of fruit's nutritional benefit and with the fruit "flavor" created in the laboratory, not the orchard, vineyard, or bush.

If you feel I am drawing too fine a line, my defense is that the practices I describe are unnecessary, exist only to cut costs, and can be done away with or used with more discrimination if the consumer demands it. At least you have the right to the information needed to make an informed choice. When your food choices are made in the dark, based on advertising hype rather than facts, the amount of fake food you ingest is beyond your control. With knowledge you can at least eat more real food and limit your intake of fake foods to those "foods" that you have deliberately chosen because you like them in spite of what they are. Knowing what has been done to your food makes it possible for you to take whatever steps you desire—to cut out nonfoods entirely or to eat less. Mothers especially need to know what their children are really eating, since children are so much more vulnerable to poor nutrition and to toxicity.

Behind the Scenes with Some Real Fruits

Apples

Apples are good food. One a day won't automatically keep the doctor away, but it will provide valuable fiber and other nutrients. It isn't true that it is "nature's toothbrush" and can replace the more conventional teeth-cleaning method on a camping trip; there's too much fructose in apples for teeth to go unbrushed after eating one. On the other hand, eating an apple removes some of the plaque (but not between the teeth) and is certainly better than sugared desserts.

However, the apple itself isn't what it used to be. A New York State book of apples, *The Apples of New York* (1905), reveals an incredibly diversified orchard, with six hundred varieties colorfully illustrated and lovingly described in its pages. Apples in those days had names like Maiden Blush, Opalescent, Sheep's Nose, Wealthy, King David, Ben Davis, Arkansas Mammoth Black Twig, Twenty Ounce, and Thompkins King, though the McIntosh, Rome Beauty, and Delicious were already among them. In the late 1800s the USDA listed eight thousand varieties nationwide, but by 1940 a leading cookbook listed only thirty-four. Today there are only a few apple varieties, and most people don't get beyond Delicious, McIntosh, Granny Smith, and Rome Beauty (for baking). The once aptly named Delicious apple is now a mealy, mushy disappointment. The Mac somehow lacks the crispness and tartness of the original. Only the Granny Smith and a few newcomers that may or may not be around awhile longer are really good eating. And the Granny Smith, from South Africa and Australia, is bound to have lost some of its nutrients in its travels.

The reason for the decline of apple varieties is the same as the reason for the decline of quality and the increase of blandness in fresh produce in general: breeding for good marketing qualities rather than taste and concentration of producers. When *The Apples of New York* was published, small apple orchards dotted the state's landscape; every orchard had its special apple, developed and grown by the owner. It was possible to work one's way upstate, picking up a basket here and a basket there, until one had a sampler of over fifty different varieties, all unique to the grower. Today apple-grower cooperatives and large orchards limited to a few states, plus the development of storage technology, such as Controlled Atmosphere (CA) apples, have extended the apple-eating season through most of the year, but we have lost the taste and tang of the Garden of Eden.

Apples are a good example of how nutrient tables can be misleading as a guide to nutrient content. Usually listed as a moderately good source of vitamin C, the ascorbic acid of a given apple is a matter for conjecture; the consumer would have to know a lot more about it than how good it looks in the store. For instance, the amount of ascorbic acid may be large or very small, depending on whether it is a summer, fall, or winter apple (not the season in which you, the consumer, necessarily purchase it) and whether it is eaten just-picked from the tree or after several months of storage. A large summer apple contains about 22 milligrams of vitamin C (if eaten whole, unpared, and in season); a fall or winter apple, under the same conditions, has 14 to 15 milligrams. Store it for more than a couple of weeks and the C content may drop to half that. So when the consumer figures the vitamin C intake for the day, the apple may rate as eleven to twenty-two milligrams worth, with 11 milligrams the more likely figure for most of the year over most of the nation.

The Poisoned Apple

The consumer who has tried to raise apples may have been as appalled as I was to discover that it is considered necessary to spray the trees with insecticides at least eighteen times a summer, to eliminate any insect, disease, or pest that might result in less than picture-perfect fruit. (The spraying must be carefully planned so as not to kill the pollinating honey bees, or the fruit would not be merely imperfect, but nonexistent.) Knowing of this routine spraying, you might equally routinely peel the apple before eating it (though at the sacrifice of some nutrients and fiber)—but peeling won't always be enough protection.

On August 28, 1985, United Press International carried a startling news item. It quoted the Environmental Protection Agency: "Eating an apple a day treated with the chemical daminozide could cause cancer over a lifetime.'' The agency added it was urging its science advisory panel to prohibit the use of the allowed pesticide because of findings that lifetime consumption can cause up to one cancer death per 10,000 individuals. The news item revealed that apple, peach, pear, nectarine, sour cherry, Concord grape, prune, and other fruit, Brussels sprouts, tomato, canteloupe, and peanut growers routinely use the chemical to promote growth, extend storage life, and enhance color. In the case of peanuts, it causes the growth of short, erect vines that are easier to harvest. It does not enhance flavor or produce any consumer benefit. The kicker was: ''the chemical penetrates the fruit and cannot be washed off.'' Neither does rainfall dilute it while the fruit is still on the tree. In fact, exposure to water makes it even more dangerous.

The following day an article in *The New York Times* adopted a milder tone. The headline ''Fruit-Chemical Ban Weighed'' lacked the urgency of the UPI release and waffled even further. Daminozide was described as ''a chemical widely used to regulate the growth of apples and, to a more limited extent, other fruits.'' It did add, ''The regulator daminozide is a suspected carcinogen,'' noting it was known as Alar and manufactured by Uniroyal, Inc.

In the case of apples, Alar is used primarily on Red and Golden Delicious, Stayman, and McIntosh apples, but that applies only to apples grown in the United States, so the consumer has no way of knowing what is happening to, say, Granny Smiths. The ''value'' of this risky chemical is that it ''promotes uniform fruit size, delays ripening so harvesting can take place at one time, intensifies the color of red apples and extends shelf life by two to three months.'' None of these benefits is a consumer benefit, yet the risk is entirely the consumer's. The apple manufacturer is concerned with appearance (redder apples with greater consumer appeal), not taste or wholesomeness, and with an apple that is cheaper to process. Extended shelf life is often promoted as a consumer benefit, but it actually benefits only the manufacturer whose product continues to be salable long after nature would have retired it. It appears that other chemicals produce the same benefits but ''none are as effective.'' The consumer might understandably ask whether consideration has been given to the possibility that these other chemicals are possibly less dangerous.

Many chemicals can be made safer by cooking or washing the treated food, but daminozide becomes more even dangerous, degrading when cooked or mixed with water into UDMH, a chemical that is an even more potent carcinogen (the UPI compared it to its relative, hydrazine rocket fuel). So not only are whole apples suspect, but also applesauce, apple juice, cider, canned apples, baked apples, and all the other hundreds of delicious foods made with apples. All these foods used in cooked dishes or subject to pasteurization have enhanced carcinogenic possibilities. Nor can you avoid it by selective buying; to take one example, it "is used on an estimated 50 percent of the apple harvest." (The *Times* follow-up reduced this to 38 percent.)

As it turns out, the FDA is well aware of this product. It has even established a tolerance level for it—30 parts per million—and its 1985 tests, based on more than two hundred samples of raw apples and apple juice concentrate, found levels acceptable, ranging from a trace to 5 parts per million. The manufacturer disputes the agency's findings, but the EPA hopes to put through a ban; consumer reaction could speed the process, which otherwise could take many more years. The issue is simply what risk is the consumer willing to take when the only benefit is an increase in manufacturers' profits. Consumers finding this particular risk unacceptable can let the FDA know. (Write FDA, 5600 Fishers Lane, Rockville, MD, 20857.)

These are only a few of the interesting things that are done to apples and other fruit, but they indicate why fruit, while it is real, may not be quite what you think it is and should certainly be thoroughly washed and peeled, whenever possible, for whatever good it may do.

Oranges

If there is any fruit even more ubiquitous in the American diet than the apple, it is the orange. Along with other citrus, it is much in demand for its high vitamin C content, and it lends itself to a multitude of uses, both raw and cooked.

Orange production is limited to certain states, primarily Florida and California, so oranges must be transported to their market in other parts of the country. Inevitably most of them are not tree ripened; picked green, they are ripened, when needed, with ethylene gas, almost—but not quite—the same way nature ripens them on the tree. With this technology it might be possible to pick oranges long before they have developed taste and sweetness (unlike some fruits, citrus fruits do not continue ripening once they are picked). The state of Florida controls this tendency to pick fruit before its time with laws that prohibit picking until a satisfactory sugar-acid ratio has been reached in the tree fruit.

There is, as most consumers know, considerable difference between Florida and California oranges—varieties, flavor, and juice quantity, among others—but one difference the consumer may not be aware of is color. California oranges look like oranges; they are an attractive bright orange, a colorful addition to the fruit bowl. Florida oranges aren't nearly so pretty; the warmer Florida nights keeps the color from developing, and even fully ripe oranges are on the green side. Americans have been trained to expect certain cosmetic standards in their produce, and since Florida growers feel the naturally green orange would lose out to California fruit in the market-place, they color their fruit with artificial colors. Incidentally, Texas citrus growers also use artificial color, for the same reason. Red Dye No. 2 has been used since 1959, though it is not described as safe, merely "less toxic" than previous red dyes.

Under the circumstances, citrus zest and peel should not be used. Since this is an important natural flavoring for baking, preserves, and other home and commercial cooking and has certain medicinal uses, it means giving up a naturally delicious and useful product for a trivial reason. One argument for continued use of citrus dyes is that they are used only on the peel, which is not usually eaten—a specious argument given the many uses of the peel in edible products. Flavedo, the outer orange portion of the peel, is used, for instance, in manufacturing frozen orange juice. The consumer's intelligence is so underrated that it never occurs to the citrus manufacturer that money spent on dyeing his produce might be better spent on educating the consumer that ripe Florida fruit is sometimes naturally green. After all, "golden" Delicious apples are often more prized than the red variety, and Ugli fruit has made a virture of its appearance by immortalizing it in its name.

Other countries have been quicker to respond to the dangers of food dyes. Canada and Great Britain, for instance, will not import artificially colored oranges, and as far back as 1964, the British Food Standards Com-mittee recommended that all coloring of citrus fruit be prohibited.

To taste the difference, order a box of tree-ripened fruit from a Florida grove next Christmas. Specify that the fruit must not be artificially colored or waxed. (It's probably too much to ask that it also not be sprayed with a fungicide.) You will then be able to recognize the more natural oranges in your produce market—and enough of these mail orders might even get the message across to the producers.

Incidentally, the vitamin C content of orange juice is an excellent example of how little you can depend on nutrient composition tables.

First, as is true with all plants, the amount of vitamin C in oranges varies along with a number of factors. As with apples, late-season oranges have less C than mid-season fruit; and the variety makes a difference. Valen-cia oranges, the variety most used for frozen orange juice concentrate, have less than certain other varieties.

A Consumers Union study revealed that frozen orange juice has less vitamin C than does fresh-squeezed. This is understandable because it is so much more processed. When the juice is first extracted at the processing plant, it contains considerable air and oxygen, which if left in the juice will destroy much of the vitamin C, color, and flavor. To prevent this the juice is deaerated. It is then pasteurized, destroying more of the heat-sensitive vitamin C; and home reconstituting causes the juice to lose more. In the meantime so much flavor has been lost that it is concentrated further to create a product with about 60 percent solids, to which are added fresh single-strength orange juice. (The water that has been removed in the concentration process—and that now contains some of the volatile flavor essences of fresh orange juice—is passed through an essence recovery unit, and the recovered essence is added back into the juice. This process is also used to enhance the flavor of other juices.) The desired end product will contain about 48 percent solids. At this point peel oil (which has been extracted and run down the outside of the fruit—possibly picking up some daminozide or other pesticide along the way) may be added. A considerable quantity of our frozen juice comes from Mexico and South America and is further processed here (See also Chapter 5, True Stories from the FDA Files). The pesticides that are used in other countries are beyond our government's control.

If this description leads you to consider squeezing your own juice from now on, you will find that the frozen juice industry takes the bulk of the orange crop; the few fresh juice oranges left for the home market are both limited and expensive. In addition, things are rough enough at breakfast without having to squeeze orange juice. It is a good idea, however, to eat fresh whole oranges oftener and to drink some of the juice with carbonated water as a replacement for soft drinks.

Unless its from Florida, where state law prohibits the practice, frozen, canned, and bottled orange juice may also contain added sugar if the flavor doesn't seem up to snuff, though not to Florida orange juice since that state now prohibits it. Canned and bottled juice has long been known to have less vitamin C than frozen, with longer storage time added to the depleting processes. If you drink orange juice "reconstituted from frozen," you have let the manufacturer do part of your job (mixing the water into the frozen juice), and he may choose to use more water than you would; he may also need to store it longer than you would have to. And then it may sit for a couple of days longer in your refrigerator. With every day that passes away from the tree, more nutrients may be lost from this valuable food source.

Real—And Fabricated—Fruit Drinks

Government regulations control the labeling of fruit beverages, but barely; most consumers are not clear about what the various terms mean and so cannot tell when they are being charged pure fruit juice prices for a container of water, heavily sweetened and artificially colored and flavored, at a few pennies cost, to approximate the real thing.

Here, according to the government's standards of identity, are some definitions:

fruit juices—must contain at least 30 percent juice. Since water is the major component of fruit, this does not mean the consumer is being ripped off by the 70-percent-water content

fruit ades—orangeade, limeade, etc., must contain at least 15 percent juice. For some reason lemon-and-lime ades are an exception and need contain at least 12.3 percent juice

fruit drinks and punches—except lemon-and-lime, must contain at least 10 percent juice; lemon-and-lime at least 6 percent

fruit-flavored drinks—may contain less than 10 percent juice

artificially flavored products—need contain no juice

The Manufacturer's View of Additives

Even the most "modern" palate would not settle for the taste of water plus 10 percent or less natural fruit juice. So the less juice, the more additives, artificial flavors and colors, preservatives, and, above all, sweeteners must be added to make a drink salable. Imitation orange drinks, which taste tests have shown many consumers prefer to real orange juice, and which is a totally man-made product, has been carefully engineered to have consumer appeal.

Coke, which makes no pretense at being natural anything, is another example of the problem of engineering a product to suit the public taste. In the summer of 1985 Coca-Cola made a major marketing gaffe when it based its new product strategy on taste tests that showed people prefered the "new" Coke to the "old." The outcry from consumers was so great that Coke reversed itself at great expense and brought back the "old" Coke. Although, as many consumers were then quick to point out, they didn't, really bring it back; Coca-Cola substituted corn syrup for what was possibly the one natural ingredient in the "old" Coke—the sugar. Using corn syrup may have saved a few pennies, but it made a difference noticeable enough for consumers to comment on.

Imitation orange drinks seem here to stay and so do many other instant soft drinks, which seems to mean that many consumers are still not reading the labels. These foods do not pretend to be real juice—although they do claim to be good for you—but they are promoted as if they were satisfactory substitutes for the real thing because of their high vitamin C content, and many mothers serve them to their children because they believe this to be so. Dr. David Reuben in his book *Everything You Always Wanted to Know About Nutrition* says some of these drinks contain more artificial color than vitamins, yet they advertise that you should feed them to your family instead of a fresh orange.

The advertisers of these products have a lot to be ashamed of, if only in sins of omission. Tang, for instance, was heavily promoted in its introductory days as a beverage that was fed to the astronauts. While this was perfectly true, no one bothered to point out the enormous technological problems involved in designing foods for space travel and the fact that some normally important considerations had to be set aside. The astronauts got their drinking water by processing their own urine, but no one has bottled and sold that particular space food as superior to pure natural well water.

Dried Fruit

Dried fruit has been a staple food for centuries and is a rich source of nutrients. Years ago, the season for fresh fruits was short and drying was a simple method of preserving these desirable foods for out-of-season enjoyment. Plums (prunes), grapes (raisins), figs, dates, peaches, apples, and apricots were thus made available to be eaten year-round. The commonest method was sun-drying; it is still used today to some extent. However, since there is objection to the occasional insect attracted to and dried along with the fruit, sun-dried fruit is often sprayed with insecticide to prevent this "contamination."

Since Dr. Wiley's time (see Chapter 9, Forever Fresh—The Sulfite Story), sulfur dioxide has tended to drop out of the limelight. Except for Beatrice Trum Hunter, writing in *Consumer Beware* (where she describes Dr. Wiley's position in considerable detail), even most health food advocates have until recently protested only mildly, if at all, the industrywide use of sulfur dioxide in drying foods.

Rodale Publications, usually on the side of organic, untreated foods, even gives what Ms. Hunter describes as "the poisonous fumes of sulphur" a pat on the back because "it helps vitamin C from being baked out of the fruit along with the water,'' though adding, ''There's a drawback, however. Studies have shown that 1 in 20 asthmatics may be sensitive to the substance, so if you have the condition, avoid sulfured dried fruit.'' As we found out in the discussion on sulfites, this is an understatement.

In 1962 the Joint FAO/WHO Expert Committee on Food Additives, a somewhat conservative organization that frequently refuses to comment on substances because they have not been proved sufficiently dangerous, reported, ''As the standard of diet improves, so the intake of sulfur dioxide rises. The affluent society consumes more wine, cider, and beer, more soft drinks, fruit juices, fruit pulp, dried fruit, and the many other good things that require the presence of this permitted preservative. Since wine alone may contain from 100 to 450 ppm of sulfur dioxide, it is clear that this one commodity can readily provide the full maximum acceptable intake of preservative.'' Stripped of the polite and cautious let's-not-offend-anyone language, this clearly conveys alarm at the amount of sulfur dioxide in the world's diet.

Modern fruit drying methods usually include the use of sulfur dioxide, which prevents browning, acts as a preservative, and makes the end product more attractive. While the amount used is enough to bother those who are sulfite-sensitive, it is limited, because an ''excess'' amount creates an unpleasant taste and odor in the food. It has been used since the time of the Romans and Egyptians as a preservative in wine and because of its long use had been considered harmless until we learned otherwise in the early twentieth century. Until July 8, 1984, the FDA included sulfur dioxide on its GRAS list, along with other additives whose use had been considered safe because they had been in use for so long without apparent harm to humans, but—like many other GRAS list additives—has now been banned from many foods (See Limited Sulfite Ban, pages 65–68).

In spite of this limited ban, the continued use of sulfites in wines and dried fruits (the fruit slices are dipped in it and kept standing for about two hours until the sulfur dioxide has completely penetrated the slice), imitation jelly, corn syrup, pickles, beverages, dehydrated potatoes (instant mashed potatoes, for instance), soups, and brined fruits and vegetables still presents a hazard to many consumers. Now that we are aware of its dangers, perhaps one day it will not be used at all in food; meanwhile look for it on the label and, when possible, buy the brand that does not use it. Chapter 9 describes the symptoms of sulfite reaction; if you suspect sulfite-sensitivity, familiarize yourself with them and avoid the foods that seem to trigger them.

Since dried fruit is not included under the present restrictions on sulfite use, the consumer wishing to avoid sulfited-dried fruit will have to buy it in a reliable health food store. It is impossible to be absolutely sure that dried fruit is unsulfured, although a brown, darkened appearance—unlike, for instance, the attractively moist and deep orange of sulfured apricots in the supermarket—is a fairly good indication of untreated fruit.

Dried fruit is very nutritious, even more so than fresh fruit. Some sulfured fruit may have even more vitamin C and carotene than untreated fruit, but the B vitamins may have been destroyed, and most consumers find the flavor inferior. Unfortunately, no attention seems to have been paid to the fact that whatever pesticides and insecticides have been used on the fresh fruit are probably incorporated, and possibly even concentrated, in the dried version. So the consumer needs to be concerned not only with the method of drying but also with the origin of the fresh fruit. This is clearly beyond the ability of the consumer, and the task should really be undertaken by experts. What consumers can do is raise questions concerning the safety of dried fruit from this standpoint. The fact that the problem is a complicated one to solve is no reason to jeopardize the nation's health by not tackling it.

Aside from sulfur dioxide, some dried fruits, such as pineapple, are heavily sugared; dried pineapple from Taiwan may contain as much as 80 percent added sugar. Banana chips, often sold in health food stores as a better snack than standard potato chips, are also heavily sugared. This information is easily available on the label or from your own taste buds; if you are avoiding excess sugar, snack on naturally sweet fruits like dates and unsulfured raisins.

C h a p t e r 2 0

Why Not Sugar?

There is no denying that Americans have a sweet tooth but they are not alone. Since prehistory man has considered natural sweets, such as dates, fruits, figs, and honey, a special treat. Even the Bible gives sweets its blessing when it describes the promised land as one that flows with milk and honey.

With the widespread use of sugar cane, probably about 325 B.C., when Alexander the Great's soldiers invaded India, refined sugar first became a possibility, though chewing on sugar cane was, and still is, one way of enjoying it. Today, when sugar is ubiquitous, it has gotten a bad name, both because it is considered fattening and because it is thought not to be "good for you." However, people are not willing to give up sweets, so artificial sweeteners keep being invented to fill the gap; aspartame is the latest example of an attempt to replace natural sugar.

What Is Sugar?

Sugar is a natural product, made from such plants as sugar cane and beets. It is a carbohydrate that, like all carbohydrates, is converted into glucose by the digestive process. Before refining, sugar contains such nutrients as calcium, phosphorus, iron, potassium, vitamin E and the B vitamins, pantothenic acid, thiamin, riboflavin, and niacin, along with such minerals as copper, iron, manganese, and zinc. After refining and processing, all the natural good in sugar is destroyed so that the finished product totally lacks nutritional value—which is why it is said to provide only "empty calories."

167

Of course under certain circumstances, even empty calories may be useful; in time of a high energy demand, calories equate with energy. Mountain climbers and serious hikers always include chocolate bars among their food supplies as a quick, easy, and compact energy source. Generally speaking, however, since the body changes all carbohydrates into glucose, high-carbohydrate foods are now considered a better source of energy than sugar.

Sugar by Any Other Name

We have seen in earlier chapters that the more food is processed, the more sweeteners (and salt) are added to take the place of the natural flavors that are lost in manufacturing. This has become a matter of concern to consumers, who have taken to reading labels on cereal boxes, canned goods, and peanut butter in an effort to cut down on their families' sugar intake. Unfortunately, labels are not completely informative unless the consumer knows all the names under which sugar can masquerade in the list of ingredients. If, as more and more nutritionists and consumers are asking, the total sugar content were to be identified on the label as a percentage of the total contents, we would all have a much easier time of it. Until that happens the best you can do is learn to recognize sugar, no matter what form it takes.

It is not only in recent years that sugar has come to be considered harmful. In the early 1900s Dr. Harvey W. Wiley, head of the Bureau of Chemistry, the pre-FDA agency that watched over the nation's food, took a dim view of giving sticky or hard candies to children. Sugar has long been indicted as the primary cause of tooth decay—although there is now some evidence that carbohydrates may be a more frequent cause—and has been accused by one or another scientist of causing heart disease, obesity, diabetes, and hypoglycemia.

However, eaten in normal amounts, sugar is not thought to be associated with any serious disease, nor need you avoid it because of specific conditions, unless you're diabetic. Tooth decay can be reduced considerably by proper dental hygiene, following such simple measures as brushing the teeth after breakfast and before retiring, rinsing the mouth after eating or snacking, and avoiding foods such as hard or chewy candies and chewing gum that keep sugar in the mouth. Obesity can be helped by reducing sugar intake, which automatically reduces caloric intake; this means cutting down on fats as well as sugar. There is no agreement among the experts that sugar actually does cause any other disease, but since they do agree that sugar in its refined form adds nothing to our general health, it is clearly a good idea to eat as little of it as possible.

Little Known Facts About Sugar

A 1980 conference in Savannah, Georgia, sponsored by the Institute of Food Technologists revealed some interesting new thinking on the relationship between sugar intake and tooth decay.

Dr. Michael C. Alfano, director of the Oral Health Research Center at Farleigh Dickinson University School of Dentistry, made the following points:

- Susceptibility to tooth decay may result from malnutrition in infancy, poor dental hygiene, and saliva deficient in minerals, fats, and organic agents that are protective agents.

- Eating high-fiber raw fruits and vegetables, such as apples, carrots, and celery, will not act as nature's toothbrush in humans as they do in other animals, because of the shape of human tooth surfaces.

- The frequency with which sugar is eaten during the day is more harmful than the amount of sugar eaten.

- Sugar eaten as part of a meal is less harmful than sugar eaten alone or as a snack between meals. Sugar eaten at bedtime without brushing the teeth is especially harmful.

- Eating peanuts or cheese right after sugar seems to adjust the chemical balance in the mouth and reduce the incidence of decay.

- In Scandinavia, where good tooth-brushing techniques are taught in schools, tooth decay among schoolchildren was reduced by 90 percent without any adjustment in diet.

- Sweets whose stickiness makes them difficult to remove from the surface of the tooth, such as honey, molasses, raisins, and figs, are more liable to cause decay.

Paradoxically, one of the easiest ways to reduce sugar intake is to increase the use of table sugar. The 16 calories in a teaspoon of table sugar is a better bet than the much larger quantity hidden in the presweetened cereals so heavily promoted (especially to children), and a teaspoon or two in homemade lemonade is obviously better than the 10 teaspoons in a 12-ounce soft drink. Unfortunately, the average consumer tends to feel guilty about the amount of table sugar added to a cup of coffee or a bowl of cereal, without realizing the far greater amount hidden in the processed foods that are eaten without a qualm.

There are more than a hundred substances that are sugary, but only a comparatively few of them are commonly used. Among them are sucrose, glucose, fructose, lactose, sorbitol, mannitol, xylitol, total invert sugar, brown sugar, turbinado sugar, raw sugar, and corn sweeteners. Even better, and more widely available without excessive processing, are honey, sorghum, maple syrup, and molasses.

Sucrose, also called table sugar, is the refined white stuff found in the sugar bowl. It is made up of two simple sugars, glucose and fructose, and is a basically pure product—99.9 percent. Three forms—granulated, tablet, or powdered (confectioner's)—are available to the consumer. The confectioner's sugar has cornstarch added to keep it from caking.

Glucose is also called *dextrose* or *corn sugar* (two more names to look for on labels). It may be straight glucose, or glucose blended with sucrose. It is, as we have seen, one of the simple sugars that make up sucrose, but commercially it is made from starch by the action of heat and acids or enzymes.

Fructose, also called *levulose,* occurs naturally in many fruits (as the name implies), but the fructose available to the consumer is not more "natural" than table sugar; *Nutrition Action* has said it is even more refined than table sugar. It can be much sweeter than table sugar but is not invariably so. It is available in food stores in liquid, powder, tablet, or granular form, but costs the consumer considerably more than table sugar.

Commercially, fructose is produced from sucrose by separating the glucose component; it is classified, therefore, as a nonglucose sweetener. It could be produced from honey (40 percent fructose) or from various fruits, but the cost involved makes these sources impractical.

Recently fructose has become popular, under the impression that it is more "natural," and it has been suggested as a substitute for table sugar for diabetics as well as a diet aid. Since claims of this nature come close to promoting it as a drug, the FDA has taken an interest and the agency's position, with which experts concur, is that there are no "clinical advantages" to diabetics in substituting fructose for table sugar. The possible long-term benefit for diabetics would have to be established by scientific studies, and so far, these have not been made.

The American Diabetic Association prefers to recommend a nutritionally adequate, controlled-calorie diet, but it agrees that fructose, along with sorbitol, mannitol, and xylitol, does not contain glucose (which in concentrated amounts could cause blood-sugar-level surges) and is metabolized in the same way as glucose. Because intestinal absorption is slower, insulin response is also slower, and this reaction is part of the basis for the claim that it is a more desirable sweetener for diabetics. Scientists are reluctant to put their stamp of approval on fructose for diabetics without more data. Dr. John Davidson, a diabetologist and professor of medicine at Emory University and director of the Diabetes Unit at Grady Hospital, Atlanta, says, "I'm a hard scientist, and I don't think you should compromise by saying: 'Well, maybe it's all right, and maybe it's not.' Nobody has done anything except short-term experiments, mostly on animals and a few humans."

To confuse the consumer further, it should be noted that the foregoing discussion does not apply to high-fructose corn syrups, which are mostly glucose or dextrose and are manufactured from cornstarch. Dr. Davidson sees little difference, however, between pure fructose and high-fructose corn syrups. His position is, "Neither one is preferable." Even if fructose were desirable, it would be difficult for the consumer to use it because high fructose syrups vary, from a 44 percent to a 50 percent fructose content. The remainder is made up of either glucose or dextrose, so the amount of pure fructose consumed could be only roughly estimated.

As to its advantages for dieters, fructose has the same number of calories as table sugar, so if used in the same quantity, it would be just as "fattening." The claim that fructose is better than sugar in reducing diets is based on the theory that a smaller quantity would be consumed, since under certain circumstances fructose may be from 15 percent to 70 percent sweeter than sucrose. You cannot depend on this, however, because temperature and acidity affect it. For instance, as the Fructose News Bureau puts it, it dissolves best and, therefore, is sweetest under certain specific conditions, "particularly in cold, slightly acidic applications." Unlike sugar, which dissolves best in hot liquids, fructose dissolves quickly and completely in cold water. Under less than ideal conditions, much more fructose might be needed to obtain the desired sweetness.

There is also the possibility that fructose is poorly absorbed by children. In a study of thirty-one children conducted in 1984 by researchers at the Department of Pediatrics in University Hospital, Groningen, the Netherlands, four suffered abdominal distress after consuming an oral dose of fructose; 71 percent of the group had increased breath hydrogen, indicative of poor absorption. The study concluded that children have a limited ability to absorb fructose; absorption was improved when glucose or galactose was added. This conclusion would apply equally to "natural" fructose-containing foods, such as apple juice.

In 1978 the Department of Nutrition and Food Sciences of Utah State University conducted a study that demonstrated how sweetness varied. Using sugar cookies, white cake, vanilla pudding, and lemonade, products whose sweetness and flavor would not be masked by other ingredients, the study found that fructose was not sweeter than sugar when used in cookies, cake, or pudding. Fructose lemonade was rated sweeter, however. Since the Utah State University study found fructose was not sweeter than sugar in cookies, cake, and pudding, it would appear to be of comparatively little help to dieters.

In promoting fructose to dieters, however, releases from the Fructose News Bureau no longer push the sweetness quotient of fructose. Instead they extrapolate from the theory that unlike table sugar, which raises blood insulin levels and causes excessive fluctuations in blood sugar, fructose does neither. Therefore, the argument goes, while "people who have pastry or doughnuts for breakfast often find themselves ravenous within a short time," this would not happen with fructose, which "does not cause a rapid rise in either blood sugar or insulin."

Advertising and promotion of fructose as a diet aid reached such proportions by 1979 that the Postal Service finally moved against mail order diet books that promised in their advertising fast and automatic weight loss through use of fructose. In the spring of 1980 the Center for Science in the Public Interest (CSPI) petitioned the FDA to halt such deceptive advertising and labeling of fructose and fructose-containing products. The CSPI objected primarily to the tablets, syrups, and crystal being sold as "natural" sweeteners, when they are actually less natural and more highly processed than table sugar. The CSPI also pointed out that "fructose is no sweeter than regular sugar" at room temperature.

A disadvantage of fructose that is not generally known is that it can have unpleasant side effects, due either to overconsumption or individual sensitivity. These range from diarrhea, the most common, to flatulence, and colic in babies. Since it is the sweetener most used in nondiet soft drinks, overconsumption is an ever-present possibility. According to the American Diabetics Association (ADA) and various reports prepared by the Federation of American Societies for Experimental Biology (FASEB) for the FDA, diarrhea may result from ingestion of 70 to 100 grams a day.

Sorbitol, mannitol, maltitol and *xylitol* are similar to fructose and are also sugar alcohols. Like fructose, they exist naturally in fruits but are produced commercially from cheaper sources, such as dextrose. Only xylitol equals sucrose in sweetness; the others are about half as sweet.

As with fructose, diarrhea may be an unpleasant side effect of overconsumption of any of these, but it is triggered in these nonglucose sweeteners by much smaller amounts. The ADA and FASEB say, for example, that this side effect may occur with daily consumption of 10 to 20 grams of mannitol, 20 to 30 grams of sorbitol, and 30 to 40 grams of xylitol.

Sugar Content of Some Common Foods

Food	Serving Size	Teaspoons of Sugar
cola drinks	12-ounce can	10
pudding mix	½ cup	10
bakery layer cake	1 slice	9
hard candy	1 ounce	7
commercial fruit yogurt	1 cup	7
vanilla yogurt	1 cup	3½

SOURCE: USDA.

Use of xylitol in the United States has been discontinued since FDA studies indicated it might cause tumors. It is periodically reviewed by the FDA because it appears to have a lower cavity-causing potential than other sweeteners and theoretically could be more desirable if further study determines that it is safe.

Lactose is milk sugar, commercially made from whey and skim milk; it occurs naturally in the milk of mammals, including humans. It is a common ingredient in pharmaceutical products.

An indication that babies may be born with a sweet tooth might be concluded by the fact that cow's milk is approximately only 5 percent lactose, while breast milk contains approximately 8 percent. In both cases, due to its lactose content, milk has been indicated as a prime cause of the decay of baby teeth, especially for infants who go to sleep sucking on a bedtime bottle.

Raw sugar is sucrose that is fully processed and is much coarser, ranging from tan to brown in color. Manufactured from the evaporation of sugar cane juice, it is liable to contain dirt, insect fragments, and other impurities, although FDA regulations require that these be removed before it is marketed. Blackstrap molasses, which is produced along with raw sugar in processing, contains many more nutrients; raw sugar itself is fairly rich in minerals but most of its vitamins have been lost. The term *raw* sugar is often used interchangeably with *turbinado* sugar.

Turbinado sugar may be different from raw sugar because it has had a further refining process, which removes most of the molasses, and is supposed to remove as well the impurities that make raw sugar often unacceptable. Unfortunately, the Sugar Association says this is not always the case and that contaminants have sometimes been found in turbinado sugar samples. It is not generally considered any more nutritious than brown or white sugar, though some health food experts think it is more natural, and less highly processed, when manufactured in certain ways. It is not worth the high price usually charged for it.

Brown sugar used to be sugar crystals in a molasses syrup, retaining some of the natural molasses flavor and color. Today, however, it is simply ordinary white table sugar that has had some molasses sprayed on it in a mixer or has been colored in some less desirable way. It is no improvement nutritionally over table sugar; in fact, it contains 91 to 96 percent sucrose.

Total invert sugar is a laboratory creation, a mixture of glucose and fructose. Available commercially, it is a liquid that is sweeter than sucrose but is used by manufacturers primarily to prolong the "freshness" of baked goods and candy and to prevent food shrinkage. Nevertheless, it is a sugar and needs to be counted as part of the consumer's total sugar consumption.

The Case for Sugar

If for some reason you do not like honey, molasses, or maple syrup, consider using table sugar instead of other forms of sugar and certainly instead of artificial sweeteners (unless you have a medical problem and your physician says no to real sugar).

The possible and/or proved dangers of serious side effects from the use of any of the artificial sweeteners make them a potential life-threatening hazard. No one knows for sure how much—or little—causes cancer, convulsions, genetic mutations, or any of the other suspected effects of ingesting these strange chemicals, but even those who advocate their use are becoming concerned over the widespread use of them in almost all consumer products, with the enormous increase in the amount to which consumers are exposing themselves in their foods. With the manufacturers of artificial sweeteners claiming, apparently correctly, that the public wants their products, it is up to the consumer to decide whether the easily avoided disadvantages of sugar—dental decay and obesity—can really match the risk of even "a little" cancer.

As a consumer, you need to educate yourself to resist the pressure of the extensive advertising that promotes these exceptionally lucrative artificial sweeteners. The use of table sugar—combined with a demand by consumers that better labeling make it possible for them to identify and avoid over-sugared processed foods—would put control of sweeteners back where it belongs: on the family dinner table.

CHAPTER 21

Salt—Keeping Your Perspective

An old Latin proverb states, Nothing is more useful than the sun and salt. Modern scientists might dispute that; some now tell us that exposure to too much sun may give us skin cancer and that salt can kill us by causing high blood pressure and strokes. At least that is the impression most people have been given, which only goes to prove the truth of another proverb, A little knowledge is a dangerous thing. We still need our fifteen minutes or so of sun a day in order to maintain an adequate supply of vitamin D; and we still need salt to maintain life, let alone interest in life. Before we blindly make drastic changes in our diet, let us examine the facts.

What Is Salt?

The salt we add to our food at the table or in cooking is sodium chloride; a combination of a metal (sodium) and a gas (chlorine). Sodium is the ingredient we try to avoid on a low-salt diet; it appears in many combinations, but sodium chloride is the most common.

How Do We Use Salt?

The Salt Institute estimates that there are about fourteen thousand uses for salt, including: to season food; cure meat and fish; pickle olives, cucumbers, and other vegetables; make sauerkraut; enhance the leavening of bread;

control fermentation of cheese; and inhibit harmful bacterial growth in pork products, such as bacon and sausage. Processed food relies heavily on salt to take the place of the natural food flavors lost in manufacturing; potato chips can lack all flavor except salt and still be popular.

Table salt comes in many forms; sea salt, kosher salt, large salt crystals for the salt grinder, and two kinds of shaker salt. The kinds of shaker salt are, of course, regular and iodized.

Iodized salt has been effective in practically eradicating goiter by supplying iodine to those areas of the country far from the sea. Due to the discovery that potassium iodate would make bread dough more manageable and make the finished product lighter, bread is also a source of dietary iodine. There is even some concern today that we may be getting too much iodine, due to improved transportation methods that deliver fresh seafood to inland populations; the amount of seafood consumed in these areas is much greater than it used to be, and as seafood in general becomes more familiar, frozen seafoods are also finding a wider market.

What Function Does Salt Perform in the Body?

Although sodium has many uses outside the body, its role within the body is even more impressive; without salt, we would die.

In a sense we run on electricity, and sodium, in conjunction with potassium, keeps the system functioning by maintaining an electrolyte balance. If our electrolytes are off, nothing in our body functions properly and even the strongest drugs cannot remedy the situation. The health of every cell depends partly on sodium in the body fluids outside the cell walls (only a little sodium is within the cell) and the potassium within the cell itself (with a small amount outside the cell wall).

Through osmosis, substances pass into the cells as nutrients and out of the cells as waste material, with the electrolytes acting as traffic cops. Too little sodium waterlogs the cells; too much drains the cells of necessary water. Maintaining the proper pH—the balance between acid and alkali— of the blood is also a function of the sodium/potassium connection, in conjunction with proteins, phosphates, and carbonates. Without this balance, nerves could not be effectively stimulated and muscles would not receive the nerve impulses necessary to activate them. Since the heart is one of the body's muscles, it is easy to see how life threatening a disturbance of the electrolytes could be.

The body has a built-in regulator that usually keeps sodium and potassium, among other nutrients, in balance. When the body gets low in either one, less is excreted in the urine. The reverse happens in the event of an excess, when more is then excreted. Certain events can interfere with this orderly process, such as excessive sweating, severe diarrhea, and vomiting. In all these cases the critical losses would be water and sodium, and both are fairly easily replaced. Salt tablets to replace the sodium are not recommended as freely as they used to be, but your doctor may still prescribe them under certain circumstances.

Nature has taken care that we normally receive adequate amounts of sodium; it is ubiquitous—present in almost everything edible, both plant and animal. All animals seem to require it, and those that do not get enough of it in their diet, such as deer and rabbits, respond quickly to the farmer who puts out "salt licks" for them.

What Foods Contain the Most Sodium?

Unprocessed foods that contain sodium include milk and milk products, meat, poultry, and fish, and most vegetables and fruits. Processed foods are frequently too high in sodium, but it is a necessary ingredient in making some foods, such as bread. The way food is prepared can affect the percentage of sodium, so it is important to read labels if you wish to avoid consuming excessive amounts.

It is estimated that Americans eat about 10 to 12 grams, or two to two and a half teaspoons, of salt a day. Salt is about 40 percent sodium, so that means an average daily intake of about 4 to 5 grams of sodium per person.

How Much Is Too Much?

Although recommendations have been made at various times as to how much of certain nutrients should be included in the ideal diet, sodium has presented a problem. Unlike most other nutrients, the need for it fluctuates. A person playing vigorous tennis, jogging extra miles, or sweating excessively on an August weekend would need more sodium than the same person watching a football game on television or sleeping in on a cold Saturday in December.

In 1979 the National Research Council of the National Academy of Sciences determined an "adequate and safe" sodium intake for adults to be 1,100 to 3,300 milligrams a day (1,000 mg = 1 gram). This was within the range that had been suggested by the McGovern Committee in 1977, which in its "Dietary Goals for the United States," suggested about 8 grams of salt a day (or 3.2 grams of sodium).

Finding the Sodium on the Label

Sodium, like sugar, is sometimes overlooked because the consumer doesn't recognize all its names. Any of the following names on a label indicates sodium; labeling that listed total sodium content would help the consumer keep track of sodium intake.

sodium ascorbate
sodium benzoate
sodium chloride
sodium caseinate
sodium citrate
sodium acid pyrophosphate
sodium phosphate
sodium bisulfite
disodium phosphate
calcium disodium
EDTA
monosodium glutamate
sodium preservatives
trisodium citrate
sodium aluminosilicate
sodium stearoyl-2-lactylate
sodium propionate
sodium saccharin
sodium tripolyphosphate
sodium alginate
disodium inosinate
disodium guanylate
sodium trisulfate
disodium dihydrogen pyrophosphate
sodium hexametaphosphate
sodium gluconate
sodium nitrate
anhydrous disodium phosphate
sodium biphosphate
dioctyl sodium sulfocuccinate
sodium hydroxide
sodium metaphosphate
sodium thiosulfate
salt

As we have seen, Americans on the average eat more sodium than that; hence the general recommendation at the present time is that we all cut down our salt intake. There are some scientists who are concerned that consumer education on the subject has been so vociferously one-sided that some people will cut down too far and do themselves harm through the consumption of an inadequate amount of sodium. We can see why this could be serious but how can we know—not how much is too much, but how little is too little?

Unless we are exceptionally disciplined, it is unlikely that we are going to get too little salt. We would have to throw away the salt shaker, eat no processed foods, and even, perhaps, watch our intake of natural foods which are high in sodium such as celery. Well water, also, is sometimes high in sodium (testing is the only way to tell), and a water softener adds sodium, though usually far less than that in all forms of milk. In any case, it certainly won't hurt most of us to cut our salt intake back to a more reasonable level.

What About Salt and Hypertension?

A connection between salt and hypertension has been suspected for some time. In 1920 twenty hypertensive patients were put on a low-sodium diet, with some success. Further studies seemed to corroborate these findings, and an interesting geographic correlation was found through the study of population groups. Although varying ethnically, geographically, and in size of the groups, researchers found a low sodium intake/low incidence of hypertension pattern among Sea Islanders, Brazilian Indians, Alaskan Eskimos, and others, while a high sodium intake/high incidence of hypertension pattern was found among groups such as the northern Japanese, whose diet includes large amounts of pickled vegetables. While they are interesting, these statistics could not be considered at all definitive since there were too many variables.

In 1953 an experiment with rats showed a positive correlation between increased salt and increased blood pressure. But in 1960 a more refined study, with two groups of rats—one genetically predisposed to hypertension and the other strain resistant to the disease—reported a somewhat different result. Neither group of rats showed increased hypertension on a normal diet, and only the genetically predisposed group developed the disease on a high-sodium diet.

In 1979 the *Harvard Medical School Health Letter,* taking note of more and more experiments reporting results similar to the 1960 study, said:

"Few experts claim that salt (sodium chloride) is the sole cause of hypertension; rather, they describe salt as an important contributing factor in the 10 to 20 percent of Americans who are genetically susceptible to high blood pressure. And for such persons, the hidden salt in processed food of the typical American diet is a real hazard."

The fact that the processed foods were singled out for special mention showed how much more important a part such foods were now playing in the American diet. In contrast, the USDA Yearbook of Agriculture for 1959 had written, "An oversupply of sodium comes from the excess salt we add to our food rather than from the sodium that is present in our foods as they are grown or produced," and assured us, "One can have a moderate intake of sodium if he does not add extra salt to foods after they are prepared and if he eats salted, pickled, and cured foods sparingly." In the 1980s it is no longer that simple, although eliminating salt in cooking and keeping the salt shaker off the table are usually two of the first things your doctor will advise.

Actually salt is no longer automatically ruled out of diets, except that it is wise to avoid excesses of everything. Two factors are usually taken into account in advising people as to sodium intake: (1) if you have a family history of high blood pressure; (2) if you already have the disease or signs of a tendency toward it. In both cases you would be wise to limit your salt intake somewhat more sharply until more is known about the connection between sodium and hypertension. (Ask your doctor; he will be monitoring your situation.)

Making the Best of a Low-Salt Diet

An unknown homespun philosopher, of perhaps tender years, put the dilemma succinctly, Salt is what makes things taste bad when it isn't in them. Thousands of Americans suffering from high blood pressure couldn't agree more. Told, however, that the choice is between tasteless victuals and an early demise, most people will reluctantly opt for the boringly bland no- or low-salt food. It really needn't be so bad as all that.

Tips for a Lower Salt Intake

Avoid Processed Foods As Much As Possible

A single serving of canned chicken noodle soup may contain over a gram (1000 mg) of sodium. So might turkey noodle, tomato, chunky beef, vegetable beef, cream of mushroom, and other soups. You're better off buying only low-sodium soups or making your own.

Nothing is easier to make than soup; you don't even have to know how to cook. If you're having fish for dinner, keep a raw piece for soup. Just boil it for 5 minutes in 2 to 3 cups of water. Remove and save. Add sliced onions and any other vegetables you want—a wedge of cabbage and a couple of small potatoes, peeled and cut up, will do—to the liquid. If you prefer not to peel the potatoes, scrub them and remove the eyes. Trim the tough edge off the cabbage wedge. Boil the vegetables in the liquid for 10 minutes. Add parsley, dill, or whatever other spices and herbs appeal to you, plus a little black pepper. Put the fish back for a minute to heat it up. Take off the burner and serve in a bowl.

This makes delicious soup in fifteen minutes; about the same length of time it takes to find a can of soup in the cupboard, open it, and heat it up. And this soup will start to cleanse your palate and get you back to appreciating the subtly delicious flavors of real food. If you don't eat it all, refrigerate what's left for another time.

Chicken soup and all the good soups you can make with chicken stock take a little longer, but are just as easy. Buy a 3-pound or larger frying chicken. Cut it up and save the chicken breasts; they are versatile and great for any kind of diet or company meal. Freeze the breasts individually wrapped.

Put the remaining chicken parts in enough cold water to cover. Add a sliced onion, diced carrot, chopped stick of celery, and a couple of slices of ginger root (or 2 tablespoons of ground ginger instead). Add a pinch of red pepper until you have found how much you like. Simmer for about 30 minutes or until the meat starts to fall off the bones. Strain the liquid and save separately from solids.

A bowlful of chicken broth, plus some chicken, together with a green salad and some good bread, will keep you busy while the rest of the broth simmers on the stove. (Refrigerate the chicken before you sit down to eat.) Simmer the broth for about 30 minutes, then cool by setting the pot in cold water. Cooled broth can be poured into ice cube trays and frozen. Store cubes in a plastic freezer bag.

Now you have a freezer full of chicken broth cubes, a base for all kinds of the best-tasting vegetable soups you ever ate; a good portion of boiled chicken that you can use in all sorts of salads, sandwiches or casseroles; and two chicken breasts (which would cost a lot more if you had bought them separately). And you haven't reached for the salt shaker once.

Ask Your Doctor About Salt Substitutes

Salt substitutes may help in adjusting to a low-salt diet, but be sure your physician approves of them. They contain potassium instead of sodium,

Foods High in Sodium

Since everyone agrees that Americans generally ingest too much sodium, the National Research Council advises limiting daily intake to from 1,100 mg to 3,000 mg. Not salting food at the table will help but can be more than offset by the high sodium content of many processed and packaged foods. Avoiding fresh raw celery (50 mg a stalk) and then eating a fast-food ham 'n' cheese sandwich (1,220 mg of sodium) doesn't make much sense, but unless the consumer has some idea of the sodium content of the two foods, it is hard to make an intelligent decision.

Here is the sodium content of some common foods.

Food	Quantity	Sodium (mg)
apple	1 medium	less than 1
Apple Jacks cereal	1 cup	125
apple strudel, frozen	3 ounce	215
asparagus	1 spear	less than 1
asparagus, canned	1 cup	896
asparagus, frozen	⅓ package	4
bacon	2 slices	228
imitation bacon bits	1 teaspoon	229
real bacon bits	1 teaspoon	54
banana	1 medium	6
baked beans with pork and tomato sauce	1 cup	1,181
bean and frankfurter TV dinner, frozen	10¼ ounce	886–1,995
green beans, fresh	½ cup	4
canned	½ cup	461
frozen	⅓ package	3
frozen, with butter sauce	⅓ package	297
beef, ground	3 ounce	39
Big Mac	1	1,010

and excessive potassium is nothing to fool around with; they also contain various other substances that may not be recommended for you. Taking time to learn the use of herbs and spices is a better idea than depending on the crutch of salt substitutes. And anyway, if you give your palate a little time, you will find that normally salted foods soon are distasteful to your awakened taste buds.

Foods High in Sodium (continued)

butter, regular	1 tablespoon	95
unsalted	1 tablespoon	less than 1
margarine	1 tablespoon	116
imitation margarine	1 tablespoon	130
stuffed pepper,		
homemade	1	581
frozen	7 ounce	851
pizza	1 slice	569–1,350
halibut,		
home broiled	4 ounce	168
frozen, fried	4 ounce	618
peanut butter, natural	1 tablespoon	4
smooth	1 tablespoon	94
soup, chicken,		
canned	1 can	1,290
turkey, roast	1 slice	21
canned	6¾ ounce	1,128

NOTE: These sodium contents have been adapted from USDA, HHS (Health and Human Services) Department and similar government sources. Obviously the sodium content will vary from brand to brand and the increase in low-sodium foods will help make even processed food choices healthier. Even allowing for variation in actual sodium content among brands, a clear pattern is revealed: foods prepared from scratch at home are lower in sodium (unless intentionally oversalted by the cook) than are processed and prepared foods. Plain frozen vegetables are as low or almost as low as home-prepared vegetables; canned vegetables are generally higher (low-sodium packs show considerable improvement). You can use these facts as a guideline without knowing the sodium content of a given brand. The more ingredients that have been added—butter or other sauces, for instance—the higher you can assume the sodium content to be. Even margarine is higher when it is "imitation" margarine. If you would like to know the sodium content of specific brands, write to the Center for Science in the Public Interest for their sodium poster.

Check Your Medications

Drugs—both over the counter and prescription—are often laced with sodium; you can't necessarily tell from the label. According to the USDA publication *The Sodium Content of Your Food,* those drugs most liable to contain sodium are antacids and analgesics. This useful little book is free for the asking.

Just write to The Food and Drug Administration, Rockville, Maryland 20857. It contains a table put together by the American Medical Association that shows the sodium content of a large number of selected nonprescription drugs by brand name.

Among the brands analyzed are Sal Hepatica, Rolaids Soda Mint, Alka-Seltzer antacid (gold box) and Alka-Seltzer antacid (blue box), Sleep-aids, Miles Nervine Effervescent, Metamucil Instant Mix, Milk of Magnesia, and Brioschi. It even lists a nondrug, Fleet Enema, because it contains sodium that is absorbed by the intestine. Some drug manufacturers are very helpful. The Alka-Seltzer blue box warns, "Do not use . . . if you are on a sodium restricted diet. Each tablet contains 55 mg of sodium." Gaviscon, Brioschi, Rolaids, and Bromo Seltzer also go out of their way to volunteer helpful information.

Ask Questions

Always check with your doctor to see whether he knows of or has any helpful literature to guide you, and don't hesitate to write to the manufacturer with your questions. Many manufacturers say right on the package, or in their advertising, that they will be glad to furnish information to anyone writing in.

Get a Good Low-Salt Cookbook

You may not have done much cooking up until now, but if you get desperate enough to try, you'll find it's easier than you think. And you can eat well for a comparatively small investment in time. Also, of course, you can eat at home like a king for a small part of what even a junk-food meal would cost you outside. Cookbooks will teach you shortcuts, and you will soon invent some of your own. Best of all, you will no longer be dependent on processed food.

This will work only if you cook from scratch. If you use processed foods as shortcuts—gussied-up rice, all sorts of mixes, TV dinners, frozen vegetables in sauces—you'll be right back in the salt cellar. Put your TV in the kitchen, if it helps you get started, and cook for health and longer life.

Take Advantage of Low-Salt Foods

Not so long ago it was impossible to get low-salt foods, except for a few cans of this and that in a health food store. Tomato paste was made without

Can a Low-Salt Diet Cause Hypertension?

A study conducted by Dr. David A. McCarron, Cynthia D. Morris, and Holly J. Henry from the Oregon Health Sciences University in Portland, Oregon, and John L. Stanton of Temple University in Philadelphia, of epidemiological data collected by the National Center for Health Statistics during the early 1970s led to a startling conclusion—that high blood pressure is associated with eating too little sodium or salt rather than too much.

The data was gathered in interviews and medical examinations of over ten thousand representative persons over eighteen years of age. It did not include anyone with a known history of hypertension or on low-salt diets. The number of persons in the study is impressive compared to the many studies conducted with twenty or thirty subjects.

Dr. McCarron, director of the Oregon Hypertension Program, was the senior author of the study. "We've always thought of heart disease in terms of excesses, especially excesses of sodium and cholesterol," he commented. "But these patterns are patterns of deficiency." The deficiencies indicated by the study were calcium and potassium, possibly caused by the attempt by the consumer to avoid high-cholesterol foods, such as dairy products, which are main sources of calcium and potassium.

The study's findings met with considerable negative reaction from many experts. Dr. William T. Friedewald, director of the division of epidemiological and clinical applications at the National Heart, Lung and Blood Institute, speculated that the findings might be the result of a statistical fluke or something wrong with the analysis. He did agree, however, that some previous studies had found that deficiencies in calcium and potassium were related to high blood pressure, so Dr. McCarron's study was "not surprising . . . rather confirming." He was bothered by the fact that the new findings conflict with hundreds of previous studies that found either a positive relationship between salt and hypertension or no relationship at all.

Dr. McCarron was understanding about the "most jarring" effect his group's findings had on many experts and the "remarkable contrast" they present to the conventional recommendation to cut back on salt intake. "I would not say that everyone should go out and buy two salt shakers. But this should serve as a very strong warning that we must reevaluate this long-standing, almost mythical commitment that if we just get sodium out of the American diet, our blood pressure profile would go down." He recommended, also, making sure the daily intake of both calcium and potassium at least meets the U.S. RDA recommendations.

salt, but almost no one knew it. Everything else tended to be loaded with sodium in one form or another.

Today, thanks to consumer demand, more and more foods are bragging about their low salt content and even advertising that they are "unsalted." Beware, though: *unsalted* and *no salt added* do not mean the products are salt-free, only that the manufacturer has not put any more in.

Tomato juice, previously a high-sodium product, can now be bought as low-sodium; seafood is available water-packed without added salt. Plain crackers come in a wide variety, from Melba toast to rice cakes. There's even a low-sodium spaghetti sauce. Del Monte offers about fourteen canned vegetables without salt, and Adolph's makes its meat tenderizer unsalted and natural. Salt-free seltzers, instead of club soda, are widely available— even flavored with real lemon, lime, or orange—and you can get low-sodium salad dressings (although it's better to make your own), cheeses, cereals, and breads. Even potato chips come unsalted.

The trick is not to give up on the first try; some products work, and some don't. Experiment, and throw out the ones you don't like; you'll soon find the ones that suit you. Manufacturers now know there is a big market for good-tasting, low- or no-salt items and will keep working until they suit you. Just make sure the product hasn't developed its pleasing taste by the addition of chemical additives that may be even worse than a little salt.

CHAPTER 22

Fiber—Why Bran Is Not Enough

Most consumers have heard about the importance of a high-fiber diet. As a result, many have switched to bran cereals or wood-cellulose-added breads and similar products, all of which are advertised as being healthful because they are high in fiber. Much of this advertising provides an excellent argument against putting the nutrition education of the consumer in the hands of the manufacturers (as has recently been suggested). Many of the practices that have long made the consumer suspicious of advertising claims are found in this area, including half-truths, untruths, deceptive nomenclature, and exaggerated health claims. Sugar and sodium content are often not mentioned; fiber sources are not always clearly revealed, as when they are wood or cotton lint; claims that high fiber will cure constipation or help prevent various diseases do not say that the particular type of fiber contained in the product may be useless for that purpose. The consumer, who has neither the time nor the desire to take a course in nutrition, must nevertheless in self-defense know more about fiber than is revealed on a cereal box.

Dietary Versus Crude Fiber

Fiber is an indigestible complex carbohydrate; it goes through the digestive system virtually unchanged. Our grandparents called it roughage. There are two basic kinds, crude and dietary, and the dietary is the only kind that is meaningful to the human body.

Crude fiber is extracted from plants and plant products through a process used by the textile industry. It consists of boiling them in sulfuric acid for half an hour, then rinsing the filtered residue several times with water, boiling the residue again with sodium hydroxide for another half-hour, rinsing, and drying.

At first crude fiber was thought to be the same as dietary fiber, the portion of undigested food found in the intestine, but new analytical techniques have found that crude fiber contains comparatively little of the important values of dietary fiber—hemicellulose, pectin, and lignin—compared to a high percentage of cellulose. Dr. Bandaru Reddy of the American Health Foundation puts down crude fiber in no uncertain terms: "Crude fiber has no meaning to human nutrition."

Most crude fiber is made from wood pulp and/or cotton lint; some is alpha cellulose derived from soy, bran, and wood pulp. The Center for Science in the Public Interest (CSPI) said in an October 1985 press release that eight breads, including Roman Lite, Lite Loaf, Lite's Up, Merita Lite, Tasty Lite, Sunbeam Lite, Vim, and 40, used wood pulp as a source; only one, Less, was named as using alpha cellulose from soy, bran, and wood pulp. In all cases the fiber replaced some of the flour that would normally have been used. Such breads are positioned to appeal to dieters and those seeking high-fiber food; they claim to have 30 percent fewer calories than regular white bread and 400 percent more fiber than whole wheat bread. Wood pulp fiber is not known to be harmful, but neither is it thought to be as healthful as dietary fiber. It is identified on the label as "powdered cellulose," with no mention of wood as its source.

The FDA does not propose to move against these companies, since it feels that under the present laws their labeling is technically in compliance, and the manufacturers of Roman Lite had actually worked with the FDA to make sure they used the proper terms in their labeling. The FDA proposed a regulation as recently as 1984 that would have required the use of dietary instead of crude fiber as the measurement in food. If this had passed, a claim of 400 percent more fiber could not have been made, inasmuch as crude fiber content is no longer considered a scientific measurement; dietary fiber is now generally accepted as a more meaningful basis for comparison.

As a matter of fact, ITT–Continental Baking Company was charged, in 1979 with false and misleading advertising simply because it had not disclosed that the cellulose in its Fresh Horizons bread was derived from wood pulp. The company was required to say in all its advertising, where applicable, that "the source of [this] fiber is wood." At the time the Federal Trade Commission, which brought the charge, said that "consumers would not expect to find fiber derived from wood as an ingredient in bread.'' It would seem that would be equally true today, but apparently Fresh Horizons was simply ahead of its time.

Dietary Fiber

Dietary fiber is much more complex than crude fiber. It includes hemicelluloses, pectic substances, gums, mucilages, lignin, and cellulose. Different foods contain dietary fiber elements in different combinations. This is important for the consumer to know, because each kind of fiber has its own characteristics and provides specific health benefits. To get the full benefit of fiber, the daily diet should include foods rich in the various kinds.

Pectins and Gums. These dietary fibers may lower blood cholesterol, thus possibly help to prevent high blood pressure, heart disease, and related illnesses. They are also helpful to diabetics because they prevent blood sugar levels from rising and falling rapidly, thus reducing the sometimes considerable increases and decreases that can lead to diabetic coma and other problems. Foods high in these dietary fibers include oat bran (not wheat bran), legumes, fruits, and vegetables. They are all water soluble so do not increase the bulk of stools, and since they slow rather than speed up intestinal digestion, are generally not thought to be helpful against constipation. Oat bran and pectin, however, are thought possibly to reduce the risk of colon cancer.

Celluloses, hemicelluloses, and lignin are water insoluble and, in contrast to the gums and pectins, do increase bulk, and therefore, decrease transit time of food in the intestinal tract. These may help with constipation, diverticulosis, and other digestive illnesses. From some of the current theories as to the cause of colon cancer, it would seem that these fibers would be helpful in preventing that disease, but so far a number of studies with wheat bran have not been able to duplicate some of the apparently positive benefits of oat bran. Research results are not clear cut; for example, pectin, one of the water-soluble fibers, seems also to play a part in reducing the incidence of colon cancer. Grains and grain products are good sources of the water-insoluble fibers, and they can be found as well in some vegetables and beans.

Bran

Bran, a comparatively inexpensive source of fiber, has been promoted to the public in a way that some nutritionists think is misleading; for example, the advertising for some cereals seems to imply that a diet sufficiently high in bran with confer all the benefits of rounded dietary fiber intake. The one thing definitely known is that bran contains the type of fiber that absorbs water as it passes through the intestinal system, thus creating bulk and speeding the passage of digested food, so any increase in bran intake will tend to have the obvious benefit of clearing up constipation.

The present American diet, low in fiber and high in processed foods, sweeteners, and fats, has made constipation a common ailment, and laxative manufacturers have benefited accordingly. So have cereal manufacturers, because bran really will help regularize the system. What is not so widely advertised is that many fresh fruits, vegetables, and other foods will do the job even better.

Wheat bran is the source of only one kind of fiber primarily, and it is not considered the best source of all fibers. Taken out of context (bran is only part of whole wheat), it has limited benefits. As we have seen, it is not thought to lower blood cholesterol. Fiber ingested directly from a variety of fiber-rich whole foods, rather than as an additive, appears to be more useful. In addition, wheat bran is said to be higher in phytates, which some authorities say can cause a deficiency in calcium, iron, and zinc—three minerals in which the majority of Americans are already thought to be deficient. (Other authorities claim that the mineral deficiencies caused in this way are only temporary and correct themselves over the long term.) There is nothing wrong with including wheat bran in your diet. Dr. Reddy himself has given it his seal of approval; but it is wise not to do so to the exclusion of other dietary fiber sources.

Incidentally, a good source of oat bran is rolled oats, as in that old-fashioned breakfast cereal, oatmeal.

Sources of Dietary Fiber

All whole grains are rich in fiber, as are flour and flour products (whole grain breads, rolls), fresh fruits (strawberries, mangoes, oranges, blueberries, bananas, pears), nuts and nut butters, fresh vegetables (though some, like carrots, should be eaten both cooked and raw to get the maximum benefit of all the nutrients available), including leafy vegetables, celery, tomatoes, cabbage, and legumes. All beans are a good source of fiber but are sometimes avoided by those who find they create too much gas. Soaking the beans overnight in cold water, which is drained before cooking the next day, will mitigate this problem. An even better solution might be to eat the beans in the form of sprouts. Most beans are easily sprouted in a jar in the kitchen. (See Sprouting Beans, following.) They will not satisfy a craving for baked beans but will help make a good salad even more nutritious.

Contrary to what you may think, foods rich in dietary fiber are not necessarily crunchy, stringy, or chewy; peas, for instance, are a very rich source. It would be hard to eat a diet deficient in fiber if you ate fresh fruits and vegetables and whole grains daily. Why then is our diet low in fiber?

Low-Fiber Foods

Americans could immediately switch to a high-fiber diet without having to think twice about what to eat when if they eliminated all processed foods. In our modern world, where almost everyone has a job or is busy with family and no one has time to cook, this is probably never going to happen. The fact remains that most take-out food, TV dinners, many instant foods, mixes, and fabricated foods tend to be low-fiber foods. An orange provides dietary fiber; an artificial powdered orange drink does not. White bread provides little if any dietary fiber, except possibly as an additive; whole grain bread is naturally rich in fiber. Our traditional American diet—high in meat, eggs, milk, white flour, and sweeteners—is low in fiber.

Dietary Fiber and Disease

There is no clear proof that a high-fiber diet will definitely prevent any disease except constipation (and that's enough of a boon to many people), but there are indications that it may. Researchers are presently working in a number of areas and have already exploded some old ideas about treatments for intestinal ailments.

Constipation

Among the problems created by a low-fiber diet are the small, hard, pebbly stools associated with constipation, together with inefficient peristaltic action. Peristalsis is the muscular contraction that moves the feces through the intestine. When it is not efficient, the feces stay in the intestinal tract too long and become increasingly difficult to evacuate.

A low-fiber diet is, of course, not the only cause of constipation. Other causes may be disease, insufficient intake of fluids, insufficient fat in the diet, poor muscle tone, too sedentary a life-style, and inattention to nature's

Sprouting Beans

Almost all beans and other seeds can be sprouted. Radish seeds, for example, make delicious sprouts. It is an easy process that can be done right in your kitchen or, if you don't have a kitchen, on any flat surface.

The only equipment needed is a Mason jar, a package of cheesecloth, and a rubber band.

There are many kinds of sprouts, each with its own distinctive flavor and texture. The dried beans from the supermarket will often sprout, or you can get beans for sprouting from many markets, health food stores, and garden centers. Mung beans (from garden centers or places where garden seeds are sold) are among the original seeds for sprouting, but soybeans and alfalfa seeds are also popular and not quite so expensive. If you buy the seeds from a seed catalog or rack, buy only those sold for sprouting, not the ones sold for planting. The seeds sold for planting may have been treated with fungicide.

To Sprout:

All you need is moisture—no soil, no fertilizer.

Soak beans—start with about half a cup—in warm water overnight. Drain and put on the bottom of the Mason jar.

Cover the top of the jar with two or three layers of damp cheesecloth, secured with a rubber band. It is important for air to circulate freely within the growing area.

Rinse with fresh water and drain (through the cheesecloth) by filling from the faucet, then turning the jar upside down over the sink. Do this

---

signs that you need to move your bowels. Regular habits, including sitting on the toilet at the same time each day, are a big help.

Once the problem is identified as constipation, many people may make it worse by resorting to laxatives, cathartics, and enemas; these temporary expedients can become a habit. Habitual use of any outside source of regularity defeats its own purpose and, even worse, can lead to serious illnesses of the digestive tract. Defecating is as normal as eating and is best, safest, pleasantest, and healthiest when performed in the manner nature intended.

The next time you have a problem with constipation, ask your doctor about trying a high-fiber diet. Going the added-bran cold cereal route is all right but comparatively expensive for what you get—compared to old-fashioned oatmeal or whole bran—and not nutritionally efficient. Instead, you might switch to true whole-grain cereals and breads, try prune juice

---

Sprouting Beans (continued)

twice a day for two to five days. The length of time will vary according to the sprouts and how you like them. Since you can see them growing, it will not be difficult to determine when they are ready to eat.

Do not put the sprouting jar in the sun. The seeds do not require much light, but the more light they get (short of direct sunlight), the greener they will be and the richer in nutrients (except for vitamin C). You will soon find whether you prefer greener or whiter sprouts and can adjust the light accordingly.

Once they have grown to your taste, rinse one last time, drain, and refrigerate. (Although some books will tell you to, do not remove the tan outer husks of the seeds.) And start on another batch.

To Use:

Sprouts can be used as is in salads, instead of lettuce on sandwiches, as stir-fry ingredients, or added to soup a minute before serving. A bowlful makes a good snack to eat while watching TV.

Caution: Once you become sprout-conscious, you will find that some vegetables sprout. Onions and garlic, for instance, will sprout in the spring, right in your vegetable bin. These sprouts make good eating, though usually their presence means the rest of the vegetable needs to be discarded. Potatoes sprout, too, but these sprouts should not be eaten under any circumstances; they are poisonous.

---

or a dish of prunes instead of orange juice, add wheat germ and bean sprouts to your sandwiches, cottage cheese, or salads. Eat more fresh raw fruits and vegetables and drink at least eight glasses of fluid a day, in the form of water, 100 percent fruit juices or vegetable juices, milk, skim milk, or buttermilk; soft drinks, fruit "drinks" or "punches," and coffee and tea are fluids but are not as desirable.

Colon Cancer

Among cancer victims, only lung cancer kills more people than colon cancer; colon cancer now strikes over 100,000 persons a year. President Reagan's own bout with this disease has brought it to the attention of many Americans who were not particularly aware of it before. Researchers have found that high fiber is a possible colon cancer preventative, and advertisers have jumped on the bandwagon, touting the benefits of their high-fiber products.

One of the most visible campaigns was conducted by the Kellogg Company, which quickly realized it had a natural with their All-Bran cereal, which is very high in fiber. Although it was approved by both the FDA and the National Cancer Institute, the campaign created a great deal of controversy because it linked consumption of All-Bran with the possible prevention of cancer. The National Cancer Institute received over 2,500 letters requesting dietary information on a cancer connection, and many concerned consumers actually phoned the institute (both its address and phone number were in the Kellogg advertisements). Although the FDA has not been going out of its way to chastise advertisers, it was impossible to ignore the concern aroused by the Kellogg campaign, and the agency has not only undertaken a study of how far advertisers can go in making health claims, but it is even considering using food packages to disseminate nutrition claims. According to the Food and Drug Act, health claims cannot be made for a food product—only for drugs, which are much more strictly regulated.

The FDA, in its Code of Federal Regulations, states, "It is the intended use which determines whether an article is a drug: thus foods and cosmetics may also be subject to the drug requirements of the law if therapeutic claims are made for them." (Requirements of Laws and Regulations Enforced by the U.S. Food and Drug Administration. HHS Publication No. [FDA] 85–1115.) In the 1970s the FDA took a strong stand against fats and oils but today the position of the compliance branch of the FDA, as explained to me in the course of a phone interview on the subject, is that applying the Act depends on how it is interpreted; which in turn depends on present "policy" as to whether a health claim will be deemed false and misleading, and "each claim and each product is considered separately, without regard to past precedents or rulings on any other product."

A discussion of the Kellogg's All Bran situation in Tufts University's *Diet and Nutrition Letter,* June 1986, predicted that new guidelines would probably be issued soon, but that they would require that labels "emphasize the importance of a healthy total diet and that any health claims . . . must be accompanied by nutrient information."

The newsletter further states, "The issue has direct implications for Kellogg's bran-and-cancer advertisement. It is based on recommendations from the National Cancer Institute, a reputable institution and a division of the prestigious National Institutes of Health, but it does not let the viewer know that the scientific community at large is far from united on the link between fiber and the prevention of cancer. In fact, the NCI itself recently found 'no conclusive evidence' that fiber could protect against colorectal cancer. And evidence from ongoing studies won't be available for three to six years. Package labels should be required to disclose such uncertainty.''

The first theory that linked high fiber to cancer prevention was expounded in 1969 by Dr. Denis Burkitt, one of a group of English physicians who had worked in East Africa among rural Africans and had observed that the natives on a high-fiber diet of unrefined cereal rarely had colon cancer—the incidence was one-fifteenth the rate among Americans—nor were they particularly subject to any of a number of other Western diseases, such as heart disease, gallstones, hypertension, hemorrhoids, varicose veins, or diverticulosis. Dr. Burkitt became convinced that the problem with Westerners was their low-fiber diet.

The pattern appeared clear as he examined his records. Diverticulitis, present in over one-third of middle-aged Westerners, had not been found by him among the natives in over twenty years of observation; appendicitis was almost equally rare. Dr. Burkitt's observations were especially important because he was a specialist in cancer; he was the discoverer of Burkitt's lymphoma, a cancer that occurs only among children.

The connection between disease and low- or high-fiber diets was further strengthened as more and more native Africans moved from their rural environment to cities, where they embraced the low-fiber foods of Western culture. Between 1952 and 1969 the incidence of appendectomies among the Ugandans increased twentyfold; in 1956 the first coronary heart disease victim in all of East Africa was a judge who had been living on the typical low-fiber Western diet for twenty of his forty-eight years.

Dr. Burkitt ascribed the beneficial effect of fiber to its ability to reduce the transit time of intestinal waste. He felt that feces contained carcinogens, which could attack the colon wall, and that fiber speeded up the digestive process so much that the carcinogens did not have enough time to do any damage. This was apparently confirmed by a study of the stools of the Africans and Westerners; the stools of the former weigh up to four times as much as the latter, and the transit time—the time between ingestion and excretion—is, on the average, about 35 hours for the former, as compared with 90 hours for the latter.

Dr. Burkitt's theories were widely discussed and generally accepted by the public, who reacted by eating more bran. The impetus toward high fiber was slowed somewhat when the Federation of American Societies for Experimental Biology in their 1980 report to the FDA, ''The Role of Dietary Fiber in Diverticular Disease and Colon Cancer,'' wrote that ''definitive proof of a casual relationship between low fiber intake and cancer of the colon is lacking.'' The National Academy of Sciences Committee on Diet, Nutrition and Cancer took the same position in 1982, but in 1984 the Department of Health and Human Services, the FDA's overseer, officially announced that if consumers increased their intake of fiber and reduced their fat intake, they could expect, according to cancer experts, to reduce the incidence of colon cancer by 30 percent.

Linking fat with fiber as part of a cancer-preventative diet is in line with current thinking that fat is often a villain in modern diseases. It follows naturally, in this instance, from the theories of Dr. Ernst Wynder of the American Health Foundation, who noted in a 1969 issue of the publication *Cancer* that colon cancer was common in countries with high-fat diets but not in countries with low-fat diets.

Dr. Wynder's theories led to the idea that bile acids might be turned into carcinogens by the effect of fatty foods on bacteria in the intestine. In an article in *Lancet* in 1971, he reported the finding that a high level of bile acids had been found in the feces of populations with high levels of colon cancer.

The connection between high-fat diets and colon cancer seemed to check out, but the role of a high-fiber diet proved more elusive. And as research continued all over the world, among both animals and humans, epidemiologically, geographically, and in the laboratory, even the fat connection seemed to be unprovable. The transit-time theory failed to hold up when in 1974 a research team tried to apply it to two groups of Japanese and Caucasian Hawaiians.

Gradually, however, more and more research began to implicate high-fat diets as a possible cause of cancer. The bile acids again appeared to be the agent. The rationale was that since their function in the intestine is to help digest fat, it was understandable that people on a high-fat diet had more bile acids in their feces than did low-fat eaters, such as Seventh Day Adventists. Further research determined that switching from a low-fat to a high-fat diet would increase the rate of bile acids that were excreted. The theory was that bile acids might irritate the colon wall and that, therefore, a high concentration of them would cause more irritation, making the colon vulnerable to carcinogens.

This theory fitted in with the results of a 1978 study by Dr. Bandaru Reddy of the American Health Foundation, a cancer researcher who had been responsible for much of the work up to that time. Dr. Reddy had been interested in the fact that the residents of Kuopio, Finland, had a lower incidence of colon cancer than did the residents of Copenhagen, Denmark, even though they had identical transit times. One difference in diet was that the Finns ate about twice as much fiber as the Danes. The result was that while both excreted about the same amount of bile acids, the Finns had about three times as much feces; thus the concentration of bile acids in the feces was more widely distributed—less concentrated.

Following this clue, Dr. Reddy identified another group, the residents of Malmo in Sweden, who followed a similar high-fat, low-fiber diet with high concentrations of bile acids, and compared them to those in Umeå, Sweden, who ate intermediate amounts of fiber and had intermediate concentrations of bile acids. As expected, he found the Umeå Swedes were at intermediate risk for colon cancer. This brought fiber back into the picture, since no other factor could increase stool bulk so effectively.

More recent studies appear to confirm fiber's role as a possible preventative of colon cancer. Dr. Sheila Bingham, a nutritionist with the MRC Dunn Clinical Nutrition Centre in Cambridge, England, was one of the researchers on the original Internal Agency for Research on Cancer (IARC) study in 1977. It demonstrates, she says, "that if you measure fiber accurately, you can show it has a protective effect."

With so direct a connection, why was it so hard to prove? One of the reasons appears to be that epidemiological studies tended to use "crude fiber" as the measurement of a population's fiber consumption. As we have seen earlier, crude fiber cannot be related to human nutrition; it is purely a laboratory product. It is interesting to speculate whether this lesson has been applied to other studies of human nutrients and ingested ingredients. These studies would seem to indicate that transit time in itself is no longer of any significance, but not all scientists agree on that. If it is natural to speed feces through the digestive system, then a quick evacuation would seem to be more beneficial than a slower evacuation time.

One point that should be made is that individuals react differently to fiber; a high-fiber diet for one person may be low for another. As Dr. Bingham put it, "If you feed a group of individuals a standard American diet, you find a two- to threefold difference in fecal weight." You can easily determine your own needs; if your diet is maintaining a regular schedule of excretion, and if your stools are bulky, soft, and easy to pass, you are probably getting enough fiber. If not, you might consider increasing the amount until you achieve the desired result, unless you have a digestive disorder.

Meanwhile, until all the facts are in—if they ever are—a high-fiber, low-fat diet seems to be desirable.

Other Diseases

A high-fiber diet is also thought to be beneficial for other diseases: possibly to help control diabetes mellitus, by slowing intestinal absorption of carbohydrates; to prevent diverticulosis, by speeding the smooth passage of bulky

Sources of Dietary Fiber

Food Item	# of Grams
All-Bran, ½ cup	7.9
whole wheat bread, 2 slices	5.4
rye bread, 2 slices	5.4
peas, cooked, ½ cup	5.2
baked potato with skin, 1 medium	5.2
orange, 1	3.8
Shredded Wheat, ⅔ cup	2.7
bartlett pear, 1	2.5
zucchini, cooked, ½ cup	2.5
strawberries, ½ cup	2.4
green pepper, raw, 1	2.4
kidney beans, ¼ cup	2.3
rye wafers, 3	2.3
spinach, 1 cup	2.2
brown rice, ¾ cup	2.0
plums, 2	1.7
grapefruit, ½	1.3
peach, 1	1.1
lettuce, 1 cup	1.0
orange juice, 6 ounces	0.6
celery, ½ stalk	0.6
apple juice, 6 ounces	0.3
Special K	0.1

material through the intestine, without straining; to reduce the incidence of hemorrhoids, by forming soft, bulky stools that pass naturally without discomfort or straining; to protect against duodenal ulcers (studies have shown that only about half as many duodenal patients on a high-fiber diet had a recurrent ulcer as those on a low-fiber diet).

How Much Fiber Do You Need a Day?

You will see all kinds of amounts given, but scientists haven't been able to determine yet just what the average American probably needs. It is estimated that the average intake of dietary fiber is in the neighborhood of 15 grams a day. Since our diet is considered low in fiber, the question is how much more should be recommended? The National Cancer Institute recommendation, in the fall of 1985, was 25 to 35 grams a day.

Dietary Fiber in Some Wheat Flour and Bread (g/100 g)

	Total Dietary Fiber	Non-cellulosic Polysac-charides*	Cellulose†	Lignin
flour				
white				
(bread-making)	3.15	2.52	0.60	0.03
brown	7.87	5.70	1.42	0.75
whole-meal	9.51	6.25	2.46	0.80
bran	44.0	32.7	8.05	3.23
bread				
white	2.72	2.01	0.71	Tr
brown	5.11	3.63	1.33	0.15
whole-meal	8.50	5.95	1.31	1.24

* Expressed as the sum of the component monosaccharides.
† Expressed as glucose.

SOURCE: The University of Connecticut, U.S. Department of Agriculture, and the County Extension Councils cooperating.

Dietary Fiber in Some Breakfast Cereals (g/100 g)

	Total Dietary Fiber	Non-cellulosic Polysac-charides*	Cellulose†	Lignin‡
All-Bran	26.7	17.82	6.01	2.88
Cornflakes	11.0	7.26	2.42	1.32
Grapenuts	7.00	5.14	1.28	0.58
Rice Krispies	4.47	3.47	0.78	0.22
Puffed Wheat	15.41	10.35	2.59	2.47
Sugar Puffs	6.08	4.00	0.99	1.09
Shredded Wheat	12.26	8.79	2.63	0.84
Special K	5.45	3.68	0.72	1.05

* Expressed as the sum of the component monosaccharides.
† Expressed as glucose.
‡ This value may include heat-induced artifacts analyzing as lignin.

SOURCE: The University of Connecticut, U.S. Department of Agriculture, and the County Extension Councils cooperating.

Dietary Fiber in Some Vegetables (g/100 g Edible Portion)

	Total Dietary Fiber	Non-cellulosic Polysac-charides	Cellulose	Lignin
Leafy vegetables				
Broccoli tops (boiled)	4.10	2.92	1.15	0.03
Brussels sprouts (boiled)	2.86	1.99	0.80	0.07
Cabbage (boiled)	2.83	1.76	0.69	0.38
Cauliflower (boiled)	1.80	0.67	1.13	Tr
Lettuce (raw)	1.53	0.47	1.06	Tr
Onions (raw)	2.10	1.55	0.55	Tr
Legumes				
Beans, baked (canned)	7.27	5.67	1.41	0.19
Beans, runner (boiled)	3.35	1.85	1.29	0.21
Peas, frozen (raw)	7.75	5.48	2.09	0.18
processed (canned)*	7.85	5.20	2.30	0.35
Root vegetables				
Carrots, young (boiled)	3.70	2.22	1.48	Tr
Parsnips (raw)	4.90	3.77	1.13	Tr
Rutabagas (raw)	2.40	1.61	0.79	Tr
Turnips (raw)	2.20	1.50	0.70	Tr
Potatoes				
Main crop (raw)	3.51	2.49	1.02	Tr
French fries	3.20	2.05	1.12	0.03
Potato chips	11.9	10.6	1.07	.032
Canned*	2.51	2.23	0.28	Tr
Peppers (cooked)	0.93	0.59	0.34	Tr
Tomato (fresh)	1.40	0.65	0.45	0.30
(canned)*	0.85	0.45	0.37	0.03
Sweet corn				
(cooked)	4.74	4.31	0.31	0.12
(canned)*	5.69	4.97	0.64	0.08

* Drained.

SOURCE: The University of Connecticut, U.S. Department of Agriculture and the County Extension Councils cooperating.

Dietary Fiber in Some Fruit and Nuts (g/100 g Edible Portion)

	Total Dietary Fiber	Non-cellulosic Polysac-charides	Cellulose	Lignin
Fruits				
Apples				
(flesh only)	1.42	0.94	0.48	0.01
(peel only)	3.71	2.21	1.01	0.49
Bananas	1.75	1.12	.037	0.26
Cherries				
(flesh and skin)	1.24	0.92	0.25	0.07
Grapefruit				
(canned)*	0.44	0.34	0.04	0.06
Guavas				
(canned)*	3.64	1.67	1.17	0.80
Mandarin				
oranges				
(canned)*	0.29	0.22	0.04	0.03
Peaches				
(flesh and skin)	2.28	1.46	0.20	0.62
Pears				
(flesh only)	2.44	1.32	0.67	0.45
(peel only)	8.59	3.72	2.18	2.67
Plums (flesh				
and skin)	1.52	0.99	0.23	0.30
Rhubarb (raw)	1.78	0.93	0.70	0.15
Strawberries (raw)	2.12	0.98	0.33	0.81
Preserves				
Strawberry jam	1.12	0.85	0.11	0.15
Marmalade	0.71	0.64	0.05	0.01
Mincemeat	3.19	2.09	0.60	0.50
Nuts				
Brazils	7.73	3.60	2.17	1.96
Peanuts	9.30	6.40	1.69	1.21
Peanut butter	7.55	5.64	1.91	Tr

* Fruit and syrup.

SOURCE: The University of Connecticut, U.S. Department of Agriculture and the County Extension Councils cooperating.

Until labeling laws require the listing of dietary, rather than crude, fiber content, the consumer may find it difficult to keep count or to make comparisons, as examination of the following packages shows:

Nabisco Shredded Wheat says "A Good Source of Natural Bran Fiber" in fairly large type under "100% NATURAL WHOLE WHEAT," on the front, but on the side it says "provides 2% non-nutritive crude fiber (0.5 g. per 1 biscuit)." No dietary fiber content is given.

Grape Nuts Flakes on the front says, "Natural Whole Wheat Cereal . . . fortified with 8 vitamins & iron," and the side panel, "Carbohydrate Information," for one ounce (⅞ cup) of cereal includes, "Dietary fiber 2 g."

Since both are given for a supposed single serving (but specified so that you could adjust for your usual quantity), almost anyone would recognize that 2 grams is more than 0.5 grams, but only a very knowledgeable consumer would realize that these figures were not comparable and that a meaningful comparison could be made only if both were given as dietary fiber.

What we come back to is that given the difficulty of determining our individual dietary fiber needs, the only way we can be sure of getting enough is to minimize our intake of the foods we know are low in fiber and replace them with the natural foods we know are high. Since these are also the foods we should be eating more of for a variety of health reasons, we cannot lose. If, due to an extended period of constipation, we wish to temporarily increase our fiber over and above what we normally eat, we should also be sure to increase our fluid intake and perhaps ingest—either in food or in supplements—more calcium and iron than usual. This can probably be worked out with your doctor or nutritionist, who can monitor your own personal needs.

CHAPTER 23

What We Really Know About Fats and Cholesterol

Anyone concerned about nutrition and health is concerned about fat, especially how much to eat, what kind to eat, and which high-fat foods to avoid or minimize. For some reason fat has become a subject that seems to arouse strong emotions, both pro and con, and some of the most dogmatic and least substantiated statements in the health field are made about fat and its sometime companion, cholesterol.

The Difference Between Saturated and Unsaturated Fat

All fats are insoluble in water but will form emulsions with liquids to form such foods as mayonnaise. There are many types of fats: hard, such as beef suet; soft, such as butter; and oily, such as safflower, sunflower, corn, and olive oil.

Fats are similar in composition to carbohydrates but contain less oxygen in proportion to carbon and hydrogen; all three types combine to form glycerol (glycerin), which is not a fat but an alcohol, and fatty acids. So fats are composed of glycerin and fatty acids, and it is the fatty acids that we classify as saturated or unsaturated, according to how much hydrogen they contain.

Saturated fatty acids are saturated with hydrogen; that is, their molecules are constructed with single bonds between carbon and hydrogen atoms and contain the maximum number of hydrogen atoms possible. Like most fat, unsaturated fatty acids include the "essential fatty acids (EFA)"—linoleic, linolenic, and arachidonic—and, depending on the number of double bonds they contain, are either monounsaturated—containing one double bond— or polyunsaturated—containing two or more double bonds—with both missing some hydrogen atoms. What the consumer really needs to know for practical purposes is that unsaturated fat, whether mono- or polyunsaturated, is always liquid, while saturated fat is always solid, and that unsaturated fat can be turned into saturated fat by the addition of hydrogen through the process known as hydrogenation. Generally, vegetable and fish oils are unsaturated, except for coconut and palm oils, which are very highly saturated, and olive and peanut oils, which are neutral and in a class by themselves. Animal fats are primarily saturated.

Using these facts, it is possible for the consumer to look at food and determine that some fat is saturated and some unsaturated without knowing beforehand which is which. The fat on meat, for instance, is solid; therefore, it is saturated. (What you can't tell by looking is that meat fat is more saturated today than it used to be due to the confined methods of raising beef; range-fed beef is generally considered to have been more healthful.) Salad and cooking oils are liquid; they pour out of the bottle and are, therefore, unsaturated (unless they are coconut or palm oil). Which brings us to margarine, which many consumers eat because it is low in cholesterol and made from unsaturated fat. That is true as far as it goes: it is mostly "made from" unsaturated fat, but when you eat it, it is solid so it must be saturated. How can this be?

Hydrogenated "Unsaturated" Fats

The answer to how a liquid fat can be turned into a solid, saturated one lies in the processing. The unsaturated fat in margarine, as the label clearly states, is either "hydrogenated" or "partially hydrogenated." The missing hydrogen atoms have been added, and a fat that started out unsaturated has, by the modern technology of the food processor, been turned into saturated fat. If it hadn't been, you'd have to pour it on bread or on baked potatoes. It may still be low in cholesterol, however, because fats of vegetable origin do not contain cholesterol.

As you will see when you read labels, most of the fat used in processed foods is all or partially hydrogenated; few contain only fats that are still unsaturated. Fats can be hydrogenated in various degrees but, apparently, the more they are hydrogenated, and thus the harder they are, the more they raise the level of serum cholesterol. So not only can unsaturated fat become saturated; it loses its serum-cholesterol-lowering properties the more it is hydrogenated.

In his book *Chemicals in Food and in Farm Produce* (Faber and Faber, 1960), Dr. Franklin Bicknell says that hydrogenation destroys the oils' natural vitamins and minerals, and either destroys or changes the essential fatty acids (EFAs) into abnormal fatty acids that are both toxic and antagonistic to normal EFAs. He describes how the body fat is fooled into accepting these new EFAs as if they were the real thing, with the result that they block the use of the true EFAs because the body thinks it has already accepted its quota. Since the body synthesizes EFAs only to a limited extent, if at all, and since they are essential (as the name indicates) to numerous body functions, this could have a serious and deleterious effect on health. The result, of course, is a deficiency of EFAs, since the abnormal ones cannot be utilized by the human system. A number of other scientists agree with these findings and think that hydrogenation of unsaturates has an adverse effect on the human system.

Studies show that consumers take the fat problem seriously, but most of them are familiar only with the extremely negative view of cholesterol and are unaware there is another side. In a true-or-false test most readers would probably mark the following statements true.

1. All vegetable oils are unsaturated fat.
2. All the fat in margarine is unsaturated.
3. Polyunsaturated fats are good for you.
4. Saturated fats are bad for you and you should eat as little as possible.
5. Thrifty cooks are smart to save polyunsaturated fats and reuse them, straining them when necessary.
6. Polyunsaturated fats are better for you than olive oil.
7. Eating polyunsaturated fats will keep you younger longer.
8. Everyone should eat as few eggs as possible.
9. Cholesterol is bad for you.
10. It's a proved fact that eating cholesterol will clog your arteries and cause heart and artery disease.

As you have probably guessed by now, many experts would say that all these statements are false. If this comes as a surprise, take a look at a food label. Many foods that are low in cholesterol are now allowed to list this information on the label along with other nutrient information. But the government also requires that the label also include the statement: "Information on cholesterol content is provided for individuals who, on the advice of a physician, are modifying their total dietary intake of cholesterol." Obviously if cholesterol were the harmful stuff most consumers have been led to believe, no such statement would be necessary. After all, isn't a low-cholesterol diet necessary for everyone?

Well, no . . . not according to the latest scientific thinking on the subject. What is now thought to be good for you is a "low-fat diet"; in other words, eating less of all kinds of fat, both saturated and unsaturated. Many experts think that both saturated and unsaturated fats are necessary to good health and that it is very unhealthful to lean heavily to unsaturated fats at the expense of saturated fats.

Let's take a look at some of the facts.

Will Eating Cholesterol Clog Arteries and Cause Heart and Artery Disease?

Research on fats has not so far led to conclusive results, and scientific evidence as to the role cholesterol and the various kinds of fat play in human nutrition and disease is still not all in. Unfortunately for the American consumer, the anticholesterol fad has proved a bonanza for part of the food industry, which publicizes every study that says cholesterol is bad and ignores every study that says maybe it's not only not bad but actually necessary and good.

As long ago as the spring of 1973, the Federal Trade Commission, acting on a complaint against the makers of Fleischmann's Margarine, decided to "allow the company to make certain claims that are not scientifically established." Fleischmann's had been running ads that claimed use of their margarine would prevent or alleviate heart and artery disease. The advertising urged parents to feed children margarine so as to spare them heart attacks in middle age, implying that continuing to feed them butter was to run the risk of giving them heart attacks.

Dr. Edward R. Pinckney, an internist from California, had contended that some of the claims the commission was allowing had not been established by competent and reliable scientific evidence. He also pointed out that the advertising neglected to mention an important point: any detectable reductions in blood cholesterol would be only temporary and would require "an inordinate amount of margarine" to accomplish even that. For example, Dr. Pinckney said, ingesting an 8-ounce steak (17 percent saturated fat) would necessitate eating at least 6 ounces of safflower oil margarine or 11 ounces of corn oil margarine for the countereffect (the margarines being made only partially of pure polyunsaturated fats) and would provide 240 calories.

The commission agreed with Dr. Pinckney but said: "atherosclerotic disease is one of the principle public health problems confronting the nation today," and added, in effect, that educating the public about this disease, even if the information was somewhat inaccurate, was still a good thing to do. Morton Mintz, a *Washington Post* investigative reporter, wrote at the time:

> On the basis of evidence it admits is inconclusive, the FTC is telling the margarine and oil makers that they are free to go on conducting advertising campaigns that can terrify parts of the public, despite the fact that leading scientists—a task force of the National Heart and Lung Institute, the Council on Food and Nutrition of the American Medical Association, and the chairman of the Food and Nutrition Board of the National Academy of Sciences—all have said that the general public, without proper warnings, explanations, or medical advice, should not modify diets to stress polyunsaturated fats. In many individual cases, certainly, a physician may have sound reasons for telling patients to do precisely that. But the FTC is licensing margarine companies and their advertising agencies, whose eyes are more often on their own financial health than on the public health, to encourage people to follow particular diets without evidence of efficacy and without notice to the public that lowering cholesterol, even if that is accomplished, could be either detrimental or beneficial.

This had long been the government's position also. The FDA, in its Code of Federal Regulations, states:

> . . . A number of common food fats and oils and some other forms of fatty substances are being offered to the general public as being of value in the control or reduction of blood cholesterol levels and for the prevention or treatment of diseases of the heart or arteries.
>
> The role of cholesterol in heart and artery diseases has not been established. A causal relationship between blood cholesterol levels and these diseases has not been proved. The advisability of making extensive changes in the nature of dietary fat intake of the people of this country has not been demonstrated.
>
> It is, therefore, the opinion of the Food and Drug Administration that any claim, direct or implied, in the labeling of fats and oils or other fatty substances offered to the general public that they will prevent, mitigate, or cure diseases of the heart or arteries is false and misleading, and constitutes misbranding. . . .

The FDA left no doubt what industry it had in mind; it stated further that it would "proceed against such health claims made for vegetable oil products" and that "terms such as 'polyunsaturated,' 'unsaturated,' 'low in cholesterol,' and similar statements mislead many people to believe that these foods will reduce blood cholesterol and thus be effective in treating or preventing heart and artery disease.'' Further, it said that a claim such as ''made from 100% golden corn oil'' is misleading because it implies there is a dietary benefit to be derived from ingesting this kind of oil and there is no proof that such a claim is true.

By 1982 things still had not changed for the better; the public was still being presented with the possible as if it were a proved fact. In its January 5, 1982, issue *The New York Times* ran an item headlined ''Life-Saving Benefits of Low-Cholesterol Diet Affirmed in Rigorous Study.'' The lead paragraph read: ''A major, well-designed study has shown more persuasively than any previous experiment that eating less fats and cholesterol can reduce the chances of suffering a heart attack or of dying suddenly from heart disease. The study also showed a smaller benefit from stopping smoking or reducing the number of cigarettes smoked.'' And the item continued: ''The study, conducted in Oslo among more than 1,200 healthy men who had high levels of cholesterol in their blood, is considered by experts in the United States to be the best evidence to date of the life-saving value of changing dietary habits. . . .'' In later paragraphs it was explained why this study was being hailed so warmly: ''Previous studies were mostly conducted with smaller groups, among men living in institutions or among those who had already suffered one heart attack. In 1980, the Food and Nutrition Board of the National Academy of Sciences concluded that no study had yet convincingly shown a life-saving benefit of dietary changes designed to reduce cholesterol levels in the blood.''

In other words, from early 1970 to ten years later, while the consumer was being told repeatedly in advertising and on packages that butter was bad and margarine was good, and that they would die of heart attacks if they ate natural foods like butter instead of chemical foods like margarine, *''no study had yet convincingly shown a life-saving benefit of dietary changes designed to reduce cholesterol levels in the blood.''* But more and more consumers—and not a few physicians—believed, as the ads kept telling them, that the case against cholesterol had long ago been proved.

A few days later the same paper carried a large advertisement, reprinting the entire news item with the addition of a banner headline, ''Fleischmann's Margarine wants you to know . . .'' At the bottom of the ad was the payoff: ''Fleischmann's Margarine. 0% Cholesterol.''

The day the news item appeared, I happened to have had a public lecture scheduled, and I brought the clipping along. When I stated that there was no proof that dietary cholesterol caused heart attacks, hands went up all over the audience, and as I had expected, a number of people called my attention to this latest "proof." I asked them if they had read the article all the way through and everyone said they had. So I read them the next-to-last paragraph:

> The researchers conceded that "if this had been a diet trial only, the difference in MI [myocardial infarction, or heart attack] incidence in the two groups would probably not have reached statistical significance." However, they added, the combination of diet and smoking examines "two important life-style factors" and is "more relevant to usual medical practice."

In other words, the evidence concerning the beneficial effect of a low-cholesterol diet "would not have been meaningful" (i.e., "reached statistical significance"), or, to put it in other words, would not have shown any results. As it stands, there was no way of determining whether the beneficial results were due to a low-cholesterol diet, or to not smoking, or to a combination of the two. All the study actually showed was that the combination of not smoking and eating a low-cholesterol diet appeared to be good for your health.

For some reason this methodology is typical of low-cholesterol studies; they keep being made in tandem with other variables. A recent National Institutes of Health study, conducted for over ten years, also claimed to show the importance of reduced cholesterol intake in reducing the risk of heart disease, but it, too, was not a pure diet study; it included the use of a cholesterol-lowering drug.

What Harm Can a Low-Cholesterol Diet Do?

At this point the consumer may well ask why not just switch to low-cholesterol foods; wouldn't such a diet be harmless? Unfortunately there are several ways in which this apparently easy solution may be detrimental to your health. (See also Chapter 24, A Surprising View of Polyunsaturated Fats.)

For one thing, many high-cholesterol foods are very good for you and are inexpensive sources of important (and otherwise expensive) nutrients. Among these foods are eggs and whole milk. A glass of orange juice, a glass of milk, and a couple of boiled eggs, with two slices of whole wheat toast, and maybe butter and honey, used to be considered a good way to start the day. Now it is often replaced by a glass of imitation orange juice, a dish of sugar disguised as cold cereal, skim milk or decaffeinated coffee, and white toast with margarine and an artificially sweetened jam. The only real food left in the picture is the skim milk. The consumer has been scared away from all the wonderful nutrients in the old-fashioned breakfast by fear of cholesterol and calories. And fear of food is only one harmful effect.

The fact is that not only do scientists not yet understand the connection between serum cholesterol and heart attacks—or even whether there is a connection—they are still finding out that the metabolism of fats is far more complicated than they had previously thought. Recent examples of this are the new discoveries about fish oils.

Fish Oils and Fatty Acids

Many consumers who had switched to a high-fish diet in an effort to cut down on cholesterol-rich meats were dismayed to be told a few years ago that many kinds of fish were high in equally undesirable fatty acids. The consumer was specifically warned to keep to a low intake of salmon, tuna, whitefish, bluefish, and other fatty fish, and all shellfish, which were thought to be high in cholesterol. A communal groan went up as adjustments were made in menus and people tried to comply with these new restrictions.

All this changed when in its May 9, 1985, issue *The New England Journal of Medicine* published three studies that "support the possibility that the consumption of fish may be of special benefit to human health." The studies showed that not only was fish not a cholesterol-raising food but that, on the contrary, it was a cholesterol-lowering food. This kind of turn around in nutrition knowledge and nutrition advice is normal as research studies in this area proliferate, but it makes it increasingly important that the consumer not be pushed into taking extreme dietary positions or into making severe modifications in diet.

The First Study The first study, which took place in Zutphen, the Netherlands, grew out of the observation that the Greenland Eskimos, who eat a high-fat (blubber) diet, have a low incidence of coronary heart disease (CHD), presumably because of their high intake of fish. This seemed also to confirm a previous theory that the low death rates from CHD found in Japan are due to the high fish intake of the Japanese, especially since the lowest death rate is found in Okinawa, where the highest fish consumption exists. In addition, another study in Japan, which compared a fish-eating fishing village with a farming village, found that the fishing village, with higher fish consumption, had significantly lower rates of heart disease than did the farming village. Fish began to look better and better; but the problem was that Americans were unlikely ever to modify their diet so as to include fish three times a day seven days a week (the Eskimo diet) or even 400 grams a day (the Japanese diet).

The Zutphen study had started in 1960, with the gathering of dietary information, particularly fish consumption, from 852 middle-aged men without coronary heart disease and their wives. The study group was followed up regularly for twenty years. The result was that the mortality rate from heart disease (78 of the participants died during the period of the study) was more than 50 percent lower among those who consumed at least 30 grams of fish per day than among those who did not eat fish. The study concluded, therefore, "that the consumption of as little as one or two fish dishes per week may be of preventive value in relation to coronary heart disease." This was good news to all the Americans, who might balk at a large fish intake but have no problem with a diet that calls for only one or two fish dishes a week.

Incidentally, the study reported that "the relation between fish consumption and death from CHD seemed to be *independent of other risk factors, such as age, blood pressure, and serum cholesterol levels.*" Whether it was important to avoid fatty fishes and shellfish was still unclear, however, and it was exactly this question that was addressed by the other two studies.

The Second Study The second study, conducted in the United States, attempted to identify the constituents in fish that protected against coronary vascular disease. As it turned out, it appears that the polyunsaturated fatty acids of all fish are the constituents that have the protective effect. In addition, the metabolic effects of fish fatty acids appear to differ substantially from the fatty acids in vegetable oils—the polyunsaturated fats the consumer had been urged to eat in a 1-to-4 ratio with saturated fats. Specifically, the highly polyunsaturated fish fatty acids proved much more effective than vegetable oil fatty acids in reducing "triglyceride-rich lipoproteins in the plasma [and] plasma cholesterol. . . ." Very low density (VLD) fatty acids were also reduced "markedly." This is apparently due to the unusual types of the fatty acids; their cholesterol has such low bioavailability that the body is unable to utilize it.

The Third Study The third study dealt further with the effects of the polyunsaturated fatty acids in fish. Both studies identify the beneficial fatty acid as "omega-3." Since "different types of polyunsaturated fatty acid can have vastly different metabolic effects," there is the possibility that omega-3 is much more effective at preventing the conditions that cause atherosclerosis than are other polyunsaturated fatty acids. Whether it is effective enough to offset other risk factors still needs to be determined through further studies.

What These Studies Mean to You

The immediate practical effect of these studies had been anticipated by some nutrition writers during the previous year. "Ironically, the very same fatty fish and shellfish that in the past you've been urged to avoid for the sake of your heart now seem to be the most helpful. For fish oils have been found to contain fatty acids that can lower harmful fats and cholesterol in your blood and can reduce the tendency of blood cells to form artery-blocking clots. The net result may be a diminished risk of heart disease and stroke" (Jane E. Brody, *The New York Times,* June 13, 1984).

Dr. William E. Connor, professor of medicine and director of clinical nutrition and lipid metabolism at the University of Oregon Health Sciences Center, who conducted the second and third studies, warns that even if eating fish has this beneficial effect, it doesn't mean that you are free to go on a high-cholesterol diet. His position is that the fish dishes should be eaten instead of some of the cholesterol-rich foods. The good news is that all the fishes especially rich in omega-3 fatty acids turn out to be precisely the ones we had been told not to eat. Newer studies have shown that most shellfish are not high in cholesterol (as was previously thought) and that some, such as scallops, oysters, and mussels, are actually very low. Even those such as lobster and shrimp, which do contain more cholesterol, are low in calories because they are low in fat (which is why organizations like the Diet Center allow them). In Dr. Connor's opinion, you could safely eat shrimp once in a while even on a low-cholesterol diet.

If you don't care for fish, you may be tempted to take cod liver oil or fish oil pills instead. You would be better advised to cultivate a liking for fish; it's quick and easy to cook and there are a wide variety of ways to prepare it. And it's the only way you can be sure of getting what appear to be the beneficial results of these studies. Next year we may find that the extracted oils are missing some essential ingredient found only in the whole fish; you will have spent a lot of time and money taking still another pill, and all to no effect. In addition, there is also the danger that in your enthusiasm you may ingest an excess of the potentially toxic, oil-soluble vitamins, A and D.

Is Cholesterol Bad for You?

Cholesterol is a substance manufactured by the body itself; if your diet doesn't provide all that is needed, the body makes up the difference. It is found in every cell in the body and is involved in a number of important functions. It is a constituent of breast milk; a building block for hormones;

necessary for healthy skin, liver, and many other organs; needed to help your nerves transmit impulses to activate your muscles; and normally found in high concentration in the brain. It is obviously essential to human health; without it, sex hormones wouldn't exist, corticosteroids could not be made by the adrenal gland, and digestion of fat would be impossible because there would be no bile acids. If this is not the image you had of cholesterol, you may begin to feel that perhaps the totally negative image that has been projected was not as balanced as it might be.

How Did Cholesterol Get Its Monster Image?

The idea of cholesterol as a harmful ingredient in the diet arose originally from the discovery that the fatty material that causes atherosclerosis (by accumulating on the walls of the arteries) consists of 30 to 40 percent cholesterol, with the remainder divided among triglycerides, fibrous tissue, and red blood cells. The next step was to determine where the cholesterol came from; serum cholesterol—the amount in the blood—was indicted as the culprit. Logically enough, further studies indicated that an increase in dietary cholesterol—how much you ate—caused an increase in serum cholesterol. So the fat (although cholesterol is technically an alcohol) was in the fire, and low-fat, low-cholesterol diets were recommended by many nutritionists and other experts.

One of the side effects of these recommended diets was the suggestion that saturated fats (which contain cholesterol if they are from animal sources) were "more dangeous" than unsaturated fats. As a result, it was sometimes suggested that polyunsaturated fats be substituted for saturated fats whenever possible. Some experts took a rather extreme position against cholesterol; Dr. Mark D. Altschule, professor of medicine at Harvard University Medical School, publicly stated that mother's milk was bad for babies because it contained "too much" cholesterol. Personally, I would rather trust Mother Nature to create the best possible balance of nutrients in what is meant to be an infant's first food.

This anticholesterol bandwagon was not as universally joined as the American public was led to believe. Even the American Medical Association (AMA) took the position that "there is no evidence that a low-cholesterol diet reduces blood cholesterol levels, or even that it would be desirable that it did." Dr. Philip L. White, then secretary of the AMA's Council on Foods and Nutrition, firmly stated that the relationship of heart disease to diet had not been established. In a strong statement he added, "We are all tired by now of the unending advertisements for oils and margarines that

Another Plus for Soybeans

In 1980 a study was undertaken involving 127 participants with hereditary high cholesterol levels (type II hyperlipoproteinemia) at nine European medical clinics to determine whether ingesting soybean foods has been part of the reason for the low serum cholesterol found among vegetarians and natives of China and Japan. Animal protein foods were replaced by textured vegetable protein on an eight-week diet regimen.

The results were all that the researchers had hoped. Serum cholesterol levels dropped dramatically: 23 percent in men, 25 percent in women. Even when the diet was supplemented with 500 milligrams of cholesterol (the average daily American consumption), the soybean diet markedly reduced cholesterol levels. The study appeared to indicate that this type of diet had similar effects to those produced by cholesterol-lowering drugs.

The researchers used a soy product, cholsoy, made by Pro-Gen of Bologna, Italy, which the study's participants found easy to use and pleasant tasting, and recommend that those who do not respond to the usual low-fat, low-cholesterol diets might like to try cholsoy. If so, consult your physician.

promise to clear out our arteries in much the same way a drain cleaner works.'' Even the American Heart Association issued a policy statement a few years ago: "It is not proven that dietary modifications can prevent arteriosclerotic heart disease in man.'' (It has since changed its mind.) The AHA did, however, suggest that a low-cholesterol diet might be a good idea. Finally, in 1980, as already noted, the Food and Nutrition Board of the National Academy of Sciences officially reported their findings of a survey of the latest studies, stating that no study had yet convincingly shown a lifesaving benefit of dietary changes designed to reduce cholesterol levels in the blood.

As we have seen from the studies reported in the 1985 *New England Journal of Medicine,* not only is the cholesterol story much more complicated than a mere reduction in dietary cholesterol, but it is even possible we have been led up the wrong scientific alley.

Is Cholesterol Good for You?

The body needs cholesterol; it is essential to many body functions. And we had better be very certain that we are doing so for sound scientific reasons before we try to eliminate it from our diet or to substitute some other substance. So far those reasons do not appear to exist.

Feeling Better with Oats and Beans

A study reported by J. Anderson, L. Story, B. Sieling, et al., in the *American Journal of Clinical Nutrition* (1984; 40: 1146–155) further suggested the beneficial effects of ingesting oats and beans, with their guar gum, pectin, and other water-soluble dietary fibers.

In the study, which was conducted at the College of Medicine, University of Kentucky, three groups of men with high serum cholesterol were fed: (1) a diet high in oat bran; (2) a diet high in beans; (3) a diet with half the total fiber and one-third the soluble fiber of groups 1 and 2. All diets were otherwise equivalent in energy, fat, and cholesterol content.

As might have been expected, diets 1 and 2 had different beneficial effects, except that both reduced serum cholesterol levels by 19 percent. The oat bran, however, reduced LDLs (low-density lipoproteins) by 19 percent, whereas the bean diet reduced it by 24 percent. Oat bran increased fecal weight by 43 percent, whereas beans had no effect on weight. Oat bran caused an increase in bile acid secretion; beans, a decrease.

The researchers concluded that both oat bran and beans lower serum lipid levels: oat bran by removing excess cholesterol along with bile acids; beans by an as yet undiscovered mechanism.

Are Polyunsaturated Fats Good for You?

In an effort to lower serum cholesterol (although, as we have seen, even when this can be done it is not necessarily a good thing to do), recommendations were made to substitute polyunsaturated fats for saturated fats whenever possible. Predictably, food manufacturers loved the idea; meat, egg, and dairy producers hated it. What the public was sadly lacking was a balanced presentation of all the facts. The resulting confusion of claims, counter-claims, and general brouhaha made it impossible for the public to determine the facts; many simply gave up and switched to margarine, corn and safflower oil, skim milk, and a reduced egg intake; they tried to avoid saturated fats and cholesterol as far as they could and sharply increased their intake of polyunsaturated fats—or what they thought were polyunsaturated fats. What no one bothered to tell the consumer was that an excess of polyunsaturated vegetable oils was not universally thought to be at all desirable.

CHAPTER 24

A Surprising View of Polyunsaturated Fats

Much of what the consumer "knows" about polyunsaturated fats has been "learned" from the advertising of manufacturers who have something to gain by increasing the sales of their products through badmouthing saturated fats. Understandably, this is not the best source for an unbiased presentation of the facts. Yet much of the advertising is not untruthful; rather it is often a collection of half-truths presented as the whole truth. The result is misinformation, and the government, which is supposed to police this sort of thing in the public interests, has been notably lax in doing so.

But What About Cholesterol?

Cholesterol, which is contained only in foods of animal origin and not in plant foods, seems sometime to be increased in the blood by the intake of saturated fats. Conversely, blood cholesterol appears to be lowered sometimes by intake of unsaturated fats, unless, as we have noted, they have been hydrogenated. It is from this observation that saturated fats have been thought to be harmful.

Further studies have indicated, however, that fat chemistry and the metabolism of fatty acids by the body is much more complicated than was originally thought. For instance, contrary to the popular view, a direct correlation between serum cholesterol and heart attacks or atherosclerosis has so far eluded researchers. On May 22, 1984, two members of the advisory committee reviewing the federal government's official dietary Guideline Three, "Avoid Too Much Fat, Saturated Fat and Cholesterol," objected to the wording of this heading and the accompanying text. They wanted, among other changes, to add, "Studies of several American populations have shown no correlation between blood cholesterol levels and cholesterol intake." (See also Chapter 30, The RDAs—What They Really Mean.) In addition, studies have now shown that overemphasis on polyunsaturated fats can have detrimental effects on health.

Polyunsaturated Fats, Cancer, and Other Diseases

Polyunsaturated fats speed the process of oxidation. Oxidation causes metals to rust and the deterioration of many other things; its action within the body is also detrimental.

Dr. Denham Harman, professor of medicine and biochemistry at the University of Nebraska College of Medicine and originator of the free-radical theory of aging, feels that the increased use of polyunsaturated fats in the American diet is partially responsible for many of our health problems, especially heart disease. In a lengthy interview he described how he has found in animal studies that the more polyunsaturates he feeds the animals, the sooner they die. He is of the opinion that concentrated use of polyunsaturates can shorten your life by as much as fifteen years. "The more you increase polyunsaturates," Dr. Harman says, "the more you increase chemical reactions in your body, including the chemical irritation of the arterial walls, which leads to hardening of the arteries; I think they are more liable to cause heart disease than to prevent it. At this present state of our knowledge, from my point of view, polyunsaturates are not the way to go."

Although Dr. Harman was the first to set forth the free-radical theory of aging, it is now widely accepted by gerontologists throughout the world. The aging process is still not understood, but free radicals—the elements in the oxidative process that turn fats rancid (unsaturated fats are unstable and spoil more quickly than saturated fats, unless treated), make leather hard and brittle and, as we have noted, rust metals—do seem to play an important part. Free radicals are produced by the body's cells during the normal process of oxidation; in excess, they have been shown to produce premature aging. Nature apparently is well aware of the action of free radicals in polyunsaturated fats because in their natural state the fats contain vitamin E, an antioxidant, which helps counteract the effect of oxidation and the damage it causes.

Manufacturers, having discovered this source of vitamin E, often remove it to sell as a vitamin supplement. Even when not removed deliberately, it is often lost through the long processing of the oil (which may include being treated with alkalis, steamed, bleached, dissolved by a petroleum solvent, degummed, filtered, and/or deodorized). There is no way at present that the consumer can tell whether the polyunsaturated oil used in home cooking still contains its vitamin E. This puts the consumer in an awkward position, since ingestion of polyunsaturated oils should be accompanied by an antioxidant (such as vitamin E or C) or it is liable to deplete the body's stored supply and result in a subclinical deficiency.

Also, from a health standpoint, it is better to get the vitamin E from the foods in which it occurs, so that its natural antioxidant qualities are present exactly at the time when they are most needed. This is especially important with polyunsaturates, which produce free radicals, may damage the molecular genetic process, and in doing so may cause cancer and increase the clogging of arteries.

As long ago as 1978, *Lancet* (Volume 2, November 25, 1978) and the *New England Journal of Medicine* (December 14, 1978) both ran editorials commenting on reports of increased cancer in people with high polyunsaturated diets. The thrust of both editorials was a strong suggestion that perhaps a better way should be found to lower serum cholesterol. The *Lancet* editorial had reference to a previous article by Dr. Mike Oliver, who had conducted an eight-year study of the diet of Europeans and their intake of polyunsaturates.

This research confirmed a previous study made in 1973 by Dr. E. R. Pinckney, who reported in the *American Heart Journal* (1973, 85: 723) that skin cancer was more common in humans on diets high in polyunsaturated fats. In the *New England Journal of Medicine* (September 6, 1976), Dr. Mackie observed that "subjects eating polyunsaturates have a higher incidence of malignant melanoma and squamous cell carcinoma." This study is particularly interesting in view of the fact that today Americans are eating much more polyunsaturated fats at the same time that melanoma is one of the fastest growing types of cancer in the United States.

By 1979 evidence of the harmful effects of polyunsaturates had been increasingly documented, and an article by Saul Kent in the January issue of *Geriatrics* reported on studies by Kenneth K. Carrol and associates at the University of Western Ontario in Canada that indicated, "Rats on diets high in unsaturated fats such as cottonseed oil, corn oil, soybean oil, and sunflower seed oil developed somewhat more tumors than rats on a similar diet containing saturated fats such as butter, tallow, and coconut oil."

Further evidence cited in the article came from the laboratory of Garry J. Hopkins and Clive E. West of the Australian National University in Canberra City, who found, "When rats were fed a polyunsaturated-fat diet, they developed significantly more DMBA-induced mammary and skin tumors than rats fed a saturated fat diet.'' The study confirmed these results by reversing the diets in the two groups; significantly fewer tumors were found in the new group on the saturated fat diet.

Polyunsaturated Fats and Aging

In addition to Dr. Harman's theory of the free-radicals' role in aging, there have been a number of studies that seem to point to excessive use of polyunsaturates as an aging factor. One particularly interesting one, because of its visibility, has been conducted by Dr. Edward R. Pinckney in cooperation with the Research Foundation for Plastic Surgery in Los Angeles. For over ten years Dr. Pinckney has been conducting a study on the effects that polyunsaturates have on the visible signs of aging, particularly on wrinkled skin.

What this study shows is premature aging; at least 78 percent of those in the study who ate an excess of polyunsaturates "showed marked signs of premature aging of the skin of the face, some actually appearing more than twenty years older than they were.'' The difference was profound when compared to those who made no special effort to eat polyunsaturated fats but simply consumed a normal diet, consisting of both kinds of fat. Only 18 percent of the latter group had outward physical signs of premature aging. Four times as many of the former group looked markedly older than they really were.

The Problem with Cooking with Polyunsaturates

In addition to the possibly adverse effects of increased intake of polyunsaturates, there are the problems that arise when they are used in cooking. Heating polyunsaturated oils, as in frying, actually changes them. As Dr. Pinckney states in his book *The Cholesterol Controversy*,

> The longer a polyunsaturated fat or oil is heated, the more dangerous it becomes. Think of this the next time you visit a commercial establishment that deep-fries its foods. Almost all of these food suppliers re-use their cooking oil. They . . . add new oil to the vat to maintain the proper cooking level, as the old oil is withdrawn on foods that have been cooked. In Germany, the re-use of cooking oil in a commercial establishment for more than three days resulted in the imprisonment and harsh fine of the restaurant owner.

In one experiment performed by Dr. Daniel Melnick and his colleagues at CPC International, the heating of corn oil raised the amount of a component (DNUA fraction) of that oil three times the amount that was present before the oil was heated. After his heated oil was fed to animals, the female animals had a 127 percent increase in breast cancer. In the same experiment, when a saturated fat was subjected to the same heat treatment and then fed to similar animals, the amount of breast cancer was not increased at all, and these animals lived much longer.

David Kritchevesky of the Wistar Institute in Philadelphia, says using polyunsaturated oils for deep-fat frying promotes atheroma formation in the arteries; the hotter the oil, the greater the danger. Thrifty housewives who have been following advice on how to reuse cooking oils (traditionally the method was to strain oil after use and not reuse if fish or other foods with strong odors had been cooked in it) might want to consider using fresh oil each time they deep-fry to minimize the formation of toxins. Or, better yet, they might decide to bake, broil, steam, or sauté, instead of frying. Olive oil and butter would appear to be more healthful for sautéeing.

Lipoproteins—HDLs and LDLs

The difficulty researchers had been having in proving a correlation between high serum cholesterol and added risk of heart disease was thought to be partly explained with the discovery that the quantity of total serum cholesterol was apparently not the critical factor. Physicians knew that some of their patients had healthy, completely clean arteries in spite of extremely high serum cholesterol levels. The puzzle was what protected these patients from arterial disease.

One of the first clues came from the Framingham, Massachusetts, study, which, starting in 1948, had followed more than 5,000 residents to see what their health record could tell the researchers. Records were kept of habits, life-styles, diet, and the effect of these on health. For many years the Framingham study found an apparent correlation between such factors as high blood pressure and high serum cholesterol, with increased risk of atherosclerosis. But as the study went on, much to the surprise of the study's director, Dr. William P. Castelli, this correlation failed to lead to the expected conclusion. In fact, according to Dr. Castelli's findings, "Even if your cholesterol level is relatively low—such as 200—you could . . . get into trouble." Since three-fourths of the heart attacks in the United States occur among people with cholesterol levels between 150 and 300 and half occur in men with levels below 250, it was clear even to dedicated cholesterol watchers that there must be another factor.

The factor was, as almost everyone now knows, the difference between what are called high-density lipoproteins (HDLs) and low-density lipoproteins (LDLs). These are two major kinds of lipoproteins, or cholesterol-carrying proteins, which can dissolve in the blood. The LDLs are associated with the risk of atherosclerosis; the HDLs appear to protect against the adverse effects of cholesterol (even to the extent of removing it from areas where there is too much of it). Evidence was provided by the Framingham study in 1977, when researchers found a correlation between low HDL levels and a higher incidence of heart disease among the participants. Dr. Castelli summarized the results up to that time: "The most surprising finding of our study was the observation that the cholesterol contained in the HDLs was inversely related to the incidence of coronary heart disease. As the HDL went up, the rate of coronary events went down."

By 1985 Dr. Castelli was expressing the risk of getting heart disease in terms not of total cholesterol but of the ratio of HDL to total cholesterol. He recommends that the ratio of total cholesterol to HDL cholesterol should be no higher than 4.5 to 1. The importance of HDL is presently so widely accepted that blood test analysis commonly include total cholesterol, HDL and LDL cholesterol, and the percentage of HDL cholesterol. If you are curious about yours, ask your doctor to tell you what it was last time he did a blood test.

Now that attention has been focused on HDL, other statistics have been gathered. Fifty percent of the total cholesterol of newborn infants is in HDL lipoproteins. Women (who have lower heart attack rates than men until after menopause) have higher HDL levels than men. And high HDL levels seem to run in families, just as does a tendency to high serum cholesterol.

How to Increase HDLs

If you are genetically inclined to low serum cholesterol or high HDLs, you needn't pay any particular attention to that element in your diet. If you want to hedge your bets and increase your HDL ratio, researchers say there are some things you can try:

1. If you smoke, stop. Smoking lowers HDL levels.
2. Lose excess weight. Thin people seem to have higher HDL levels than fat or obese people.

3. Drink moderately—but no more than two or three drinks daily. Moderate alcohol intake raises HDL levels more than abstinence.

4. Exercise regularly. Although evidence is mixed as to the effect of exercise on total cholesterol, it definitely seems to increase HDLs.

5. Eat a low-fat (both saturated and unsaturated) diet. What this does is not clear, but it apparently reduces both LDL and HDL levels, so you can hope for the best.

Cholesterol and Estrogens

By now it should be evident that we still have much to learn about fat metabolism and the role of cholesterol before we undertake making drastic changes in our diet. Numerous studies are going on all over the world to determine the role of cholesterol in health and disease (although the bias is still on disease) and further findings about LDL and HDL will undoubtedly be made. Other factors (exercise, life-style, heredity, etc.) are also being correlated, and as our technology becomes increasingly sophisticated, we are able to delve even more deeply into the mystery of metabolism, aging, and other processes.

But there is still the human element, and the personal mind-sets of researchers are bound to affect the way they interpret the results of their studies and even what they study. An example is the fact, now known for several decades, that women are less prone to heart disease than men, especially before menopause. Although this has puzzled scientists, it was not until 1983 that this area attracted intense study.

In that year Columbia University and the Framingham Heart Study found that men who had had heart attacks had more of the hormone estradiol than did men who were free of heart disease. Estradiol is one of the female sex hormones known as estrogens. Since there was no correlation between those who had heart disease and those who did not in the usual risk factors of smoking, high blood pressure, HDLs, and cholesterol, the evidence seems to suggest the possibility that heart disease is a hormonal disorder primarily. For example, of the fifteen patients with the highest estradiol levels, thirteen had coronary heart disease, but of the fifteen with the highest cholesterol levels, only three did.

As Dr. Castelli, Framingham Heart Study director, said of the new research, "It excites many more questions than it answers, but it will encourage us to start looking in other directions." It may be that in years to come we will look back in wonder at our present preoccupation with cholesterol;

New Role for Olive and Peanut Oils

Olive and peanut oils are monounsaturated oils and until recently were not thought to have the "good" characteristics of the polyunsaturates. On the other hand, they weren't considered to have the characteristics of saturated fats, either; they were "neutral," neither good nor bad, but at least harmless.

Recent research now indicates that they lower serum cholesterol and, unlike polyunsaturates, do not lower HDL levels in the process. Since, as we have seen, high HDL levels appear to be more important than the serum cholesterol level, this makes them much more beneficial in that regard than polyunsaturates.

Also, olive oil is usually much less processed, although U.S. laws required that it be pasteurized. To get the best quality and least "refined" olive oil, buy the brands that are packed abroad. They may be somewhat more expensive than the repacked kinds but the extra nutrients are worth it, and if you use it instead of the polyunsaturates, you may be able to buy larger, more economical quantities.

In addition, olive oil, in particular, has a pleasant flavor—in contrast to the tastelessness of the typical polyunsaturated oils—and can enhance the dishes in which it is used.

already Dr. Gerald B. Phillips, of St. Luke's–Roosevelt Hospital Center and Columbia and director of the study for Columbia University, is theorizing that regarding causative factors in heart disease, cholesterol may be of secondary importance or even incidental.

PART FOUR

Real Food
at Risk

CHAPTER 25

The Antibiotic Steak

On February 18, 1983, Michael Osterholm of the Minnesota Health Department put in a call for help to the Centers for Disease Control in Atlanta, Georgia. What had alarmed him was the fact that ten people in the Minneapolis–St. Paul area had become ill within the past four-week period with salmonellosis. Furthermore, the cause was a particular strain of the salmonella bacteria, *Salmonella newport,* which normally accounts for only about a dozen cases of salmonellosis a year in Minnesota. Six of the ten people stricken with the diarrhea, vomiting, stomach cramps, and high fever that are symptomatic of this illness were so ill as to require hospitalization.

Since seven of the ten victims had taken antibiotics before becoming ill, investigators thought at first that the antibiotics themselves might have been contaminated. This quickly proved not to be the case, and the search for the source of the bacteria went into high gear.

The "smoking gun" was discovered by the detective work of Dr. Scott Holmberg and his associates at the Centers for Disease Control. The breakthrough came when Kenneth Senger, state epidemiologist in neighboring South Dakota, revealed that his state had had four cases of *S. newport* in three months. The important similarity between the South Dakota cases and the those in Minnesota was that in all instances the bacteria, which is usually easily controlled with antibiotics, were antibiotic resistant. And they were antibiotic resistant specifically to ampicillin, carbenicillin, and tetracycline, antibiotics of choice for human beings.

Dr. Holmberg's investigation revealed that the South Dakota four lived near one another, on farms only six miles apart. They had gotten beef from a single source, a nearby feed lot where the cattle were raised on

227

feed that routinely included chlortetracycline among its additives. It also turned out that meat had been shipped from this same feed lot to eight supermarkets, which were in Minnesota and which the Minnesota ten said they all shopped at. The beef was targeted as the source of the contamination, since the victims said they had eaten it in the form of hamburgers during the week before they came down with the symptoms of salmonellosis.

What had happened seemed clear once the detective work had been done. The cattle, routinely fed antibiotics, had developed within their systems antibiotic-resistant strains of the bacteria. These bacteria had continued to live and increase in the processed beef that was sold to the consumers. If the beef had been thoroughly cooked before being eaten, it might not have caused a problem, but due to the tendency of housewives to taste the raw hamburger while preparing it and to the preference of many consumers for rare beef, the bacteria had been ingested along with the meal.

In addition, the "good" bacteria contained in the human intestinal tract had already been immobilized, along with the "bad" resident bacteria, by the antibiotics some of the consumers had been taking. So when the antibiotic-resistant bacteria arrived on the scene, there were no friendly bacteria to fight it. And if and when a physician, confronted with symptoms of salmonellosis, properly prescribed tetracycline, the resistant strain ignored it, while all other bacteria were knocked out of the fight. This left the host human being defenseless, sicker, and sometimes fatally stricken.

The Minnesota incident provided scientists, who had for many years protested the use of antibiotics in animal feed, with what they felt was clear evidence that antibiotics routinely fed to animals were creating resistant strains of bacteria. It also provided evidence that these same bacteria, when introduced into people's bodies through eating, could infect human beings and create serious health problems.

Although this connection had been suspected for many years, proof had been a long time in coming. As long ago as the early 1960s, England was encountering instances of resistant salmonella bacteria in cattle. Because of resultant serious illnesses due to this bacteria, the Swann Committee was established by the English government to study the matter. The committee's subsequent report, attributing the increase in resistant bacteria to the subtherapeutic (when no illness is present) use of antibiotics in feed animals, resulted in the banning of antibiotics for subtherapeutic use throughout England in 1971. By 1973 other European countries had passed similar laws, but America had lagged behind to this day.

To give credit where it is due, the USDA and the FDA, which has jurisdiction in this area, have tried. Since 1977 it has regularly surfaced with a proposal to ban subtherapeutic use of at least penicillin and tetracycline in animals, since these drugs are so important to humans. As recently as January 25, 1985, the FDA held hearings on this subject, which continued to hear arguments from both sides for over twelve hours. In almost every hearing the result has been a decision, by the USDA or the FDA, to refer the matter for "further study."

What the consumer may ask at this juncture is why antibiotics are fed to healthy animals in the first place. When animals were range fed and roamed and foraged at will, many of the diseases they are now liable to acquire were not a problem. When, however, cattle were more commonly raised in confined and crowded pens, disease became a potentially serious problem. Nor is this true only of cattle. Pigs and poultry—particularly poultry—are raised in what many would consider unnatural conditions.

When diseases occurred, it was important to catch them before they spread and wiped out an entire feed lot. Antibiotics were as effective against animal diseases as against those of humans, so the farmers used them to treat their sick animals. A side effect of the antibiotics was accelerated growth, which meant it was possible to get meat to market in a much shorter time. The price of feed being what it is, this saved the farmer much of the money he had had to spend to raise the animal, and some of that savings was passed on to the consumer in the form of cheaper meat prices.

Subtherapeutic quantities of broad-spectrum antibiotics have been routinely added to animal feeds since about 1955. And while the meat industry may protest that it is necessary to prevent disease, scientists generally agree its purpose is primarily to promote much rapid growth. Under pressure to discontinue the practice after the Minnesota incident, the industry protested that not only would such action reduce meat production but that it would raise meat prices to the consumer. However, the danger to the consumer in the current practice may more than offset the hardship of a price increase. Given a choice, the consumer may prefer to pay a higher price, even if it means eating less meat, than to suffer ill health, even possible death, due to increased antibiotic resistance among hostile bacteria.

Unfortunately, antibiotics are big business, and large profits are at stake. In 1983 alone $270.9 million worth of antibiotics—over 35 million pounds—was supplied for use in animal feed. Approximately half of all antibiotics sold are fed to animals. The other half is fed to humans, and the meat industry contends that overprescription by physicians and abuse by patients is the real cause of the growth of resistant bacteria. Certainly it would be wise to encourage doctors not to prescribe antibiotics inappropriately and to resist the demands of their patients for what is sometimes looked upon as a quick fix. Also, people have to be educated against taking antibiotics whenever they feel so inclined. But closing one door is not enough. If we are being invaded by resistant organisms at our own dinner table, we need to take every possible measure to reduce the risk—including limiting animal treatment with antibiotics to those sick animals that truly need them.

Part of the opposition's position is that the case has not really been proved. Drug manufacturers accurately contend, for instance, that no salmonella was found in the suspected beef herd and, therefore, that Dr. Holmberg's conclusions were based on circumstantial evidence. The fact is that the whole herd had been slaughtered—and presumably processed into such items as hamburger—and was no longer available on the hoof for testing.

Dr. Holmberg did, however, examine a dead cow he found in an adjacent field, and that animal contained not only salmonella but even the identical strain that had been the cause of the illnesses in Minnesota and South Dakota. So the evidence, while admittedly circumstantial, was strong. So strong, in fact, that it made it possible for the National Resources Defense Council to file a petition for an "imminent hazard" ban. If concurred with by the Department of Health and Human Services (HHS), the ban on subtherapeutic use of antibiotics could take effect immediately. If, on the other hand, HHS forces the FDA to go through usual procedures, it could take up to three years to adopt the ban.

For a long time meat producers argued that while it was true that resistant bacteria were to be found in animals, they were not able to cross over to people. Animal guts and human guts, the argument went, were not comparable. Unfortunately, by 1977 we no longer could hope that this was the case. Plasmids, which are extrachromosomal DNA molecules, can transfer acquired resistance from one kind of bacteria to another. Studies indicate that antibiotic use has increased the number of resistance plasmids—those that have acquired resistance determinants. Since most resistance determinants are carried on tiny bits of DNA that can transpose or jump from one plasmid or chromosome to another, resistance to more than one antibiotic can thus be created, destroying the effectiveness of a large group of (perhaps even all presently known) antibiotics and returning us to the dark ages before the discovery of penicillin. Once introduced into our bodies, these multiply resistant plasmids can in turn jump onto resident plasmids—not yet resistant—in, say, the human intestine. What this means is that resistant salmonella bacteria that finds its way into the human intestine by way of a medium-rare hamburger can turn other bacteria—for instance, those that cause gonorrhea or influenza—into equally antibiotic-resistant bacteria, or, to put it another way, from controllable to uncontrollable harmful bacteria. And where bacteria resistance ends is now anybody's guess. The vista thus opened up—of a world full of virulent, resistant bacteria against which we have no drugs left to defend us—is like a science-fiction nightmare.

If you think this picture is an exaggeration, consider the picture painted by Dr. Stuart B. Levy of the Tufts University School of Medicine, New England Medical Center. Writing in the *New England Journal of Medicine,* September 6, 1984, he said:

Every animal or person taking an antibiotic (therapeutically or subtherapeutically) becomes a factory producing resistant strains through selection of existing and newly emerging resistant organisms. Since there are two to three times more livestock than people in the United States, the number of animals fed antibiotics at subtherapeutic levels (almost all poultry, pigs and calves) is enormously greater than the number of people taking antibiotics in therapeutic amounts ($<1\%$). Depending on the animal's size, its daily fecal excretion can be five to four hundred times greater than the 100 to 200 grams excreted daily by adult human beings, and dispersal of animal feces is not well controlled. Therefore, one can understand why many consider the use of antibiotics in animals to be a more important contributor to the environmental pool of resistant strains than their use in human beings.

The uproar that has been created over the dangers posed by the proliferation of drug-resistant bacteria has had some effect on the meat industry. *The New York Times* reported in its February 6, 1985, issue that "a number of cattle raisers have stopped using the antibiotics. Kenneth Monford, president of Monford of Colorado, Inc., in Greeley, said his feed lot, which sends 500,000 head of cattle to market annually, stopped routine use of tetracycline about five years ago. 'I decided it wasn't a good practice,' he said. He said he had continued using an antibiotic developed specifically for cattle, until a few months ago, 'and then I decided that wasn't cost-effective either.' "

His company owns two meat-packing plants that process 1.1 million head of cattle annually, and he said an informal survey of packing plant customers indicated "only about 25 to 30 percent were using these drugs." When told of that figure, Roger Berglund, communications director of the National Cattlemen's Association in Denver, said, "I'd estimate the use is much less than that."

In addition, Cactus Feeders Inc., the country's largest cattle feeder, has said it will voluntarily eliminate tetracycline from its feed from now on. And the National Cattlemen's Association has now advised its members to discontinue antibiotic feeding until the FDA has determined the extent of the hazards it poses for the consumer.

Milk—A Beef "Product"

As meat consumption has decreased in the United States, the consumption of milk products such as cheese and yogurt has increased. In addition, milk and ice cream are popular and are often fed especially to the vulnerable young. Unfortunately, contaminated beef can lead to contaminated milk and milk products and can, therefore theoretically, pose a danger even to ovo-lacto vegetarians who never eat meat.

The CDC recently reported the death of a seventy-two-year-old woman who had drunk raw milk. The milk contained antibiotic-resistant salmonella bacteria, and she came down with an especially severe infection. She was given chloramphenicol, an antibiotic similar to penicillin and tetracycline but one that could be effective against salmonella bacteria resistant to them. Unfortunately, the bacteria had already developed resistance to chloramphenicol as well.

Another instance of resistant bacteria in milk occurred in 1985 in Illinois, where more than sixteen thousand people became ill from salmonella bacteria. The source was thought to be contaminated raw milk found at a single large dairy plant. A CDC scientist said the resistant strain possibly had come from antibiotic-feed-fed animals, but the matter was not pursued and this conclusion remains speculative. To date, this is the largest outbreak of salmonella food contamination ever recorded.

The speed with which death can occur is illustrated by the case of Thomas Levins, a Rockford postal clerk who was a victim of the Illinois incident. He became ill and was dead the next day. Winnebago County Coroner P. John Seward said "he had salmonella everywhere." While no one could say for certain what had happened, Mr. Levins had been taking penicillin for treating an abscessed tooth, which could have destroyed his disease-fighting bacteria and left his body defenseless against the invading resistant bacteria, which were able to flourish uncontrolled.

It is encouraging that the industry feels under pressure to discontinue, or at least cut down on, therapeutic antibiotic use, but the only way the consumer can be sure this is really being done throughout the industry is if the United States can follow the lead of England and other European countries and officially ban antibiotics as a routine feed additive and if the law provides for enforcement of such a ban. Banned pesticides, insectides, and other harmful chemicals are all too often found by FDA inspectors still in use long after the laws are passed, and merely putting a law on the books is no guarantee that it will be obeyed.

CHAPTER 26

Antibiotics and the Bottom Line

If you've read the previous chapter, you may now be asking why the FDA and the USDA continue to allow the use of subtherapeutic antibiotics for feed animals, given the proved health hazards and dangerous proliferation of drug-resistant bacteria. One reason is a firm conviction on the part of meat manufacturers that it is more profitable to raise beef with antibiotics, accompanied by a refusal to accept that the procedure has been shown to be truly hazardous.

The reluctance of the industry is only to be expected, but it is not so easy to understand the actions of the government—which should be looking out for and protecting the interests of its citizen consumers, and is instead going along with the excuses that industry presents. This is especially baffling in light of the government's own findings, an example of which occurs in one of its own reports: that the industry would not suffer any economic loss through discontinuing the use of antibiotics.

Agricultural Economic Report No. 414 is entitled "Economic Effects of a Prohibition on the Use of Selected Animal Drugs." It bears the imprint of the USDA's Economics, Statistics and Cooperative Service, and runs sixty-eight solid pages. The material it contains deserves close examination. Written in 1978, seven years after England had already banned the use of antibiotics in feed animals, the report starts mildly, "The subtherapeutic uses of some animal drugs are being questioned, because of evidence linking resistant strains of certain organisms to the chronic intake of antibiotics. For example, the Food and Drug Administration (FDA) has demonstrated that strains of *Pasteurella multocida* and *Pasteurella haemolytica* have developed a resistance to penicillin, streptomycin, sulfonamides, and tetracyclines. The development of such resistance is a serious concern, because it makes the use of these antibiotics potentially less effective in dealing with health problems.''

Other drugs considered were the nitrofurans (''these antibacterials produce tumors in laboratory animals. . . . Since manufacturers have been unable to produce adequate methods of analysis to assure the absence of residues in human food, there continues to be doubts whether their use in animals feeds poses a threat to human health''), and sulfamethazine in hogs (''a potential proposal to restrict the use stems from the continued high levels of sulfa residue being detected in pork tissue''). The fact that all these potentially dangerous additives were being used purely to increase profits is revealed in the next paragraph: ''Farmers have used drugs at subtherapeutic levels in raising animals for approximately twenty-five years. Over the years, they have come to believe that such use (a) reduces the risk of animal disease outbreaks, (b) improves feed efficiency, and (c) reduces condemnation of the final product. In short, while limited scientific evidence is available to either support or refute the notion, the subtherapeutic use of animal drugs is not believed responsible for reducing the unit costs of animal production.''

To translate this into consumerese, for the past twenty-five years consumers have unwittingly been consuming meat laced with drugs of various sorts, fed to or injected into the live animals so that they would grow faster on less food (feed efficiency) and not get sick in spite of the crowded and unhealthful conditions under which they are raised, ''finished,'' slaughtered, and delivered to the corner butcher store. And the result of all this is that it reduces the cost of ''animal production.'' Noticeably missing in this description is any benefit to the consumer. But actually, when pressed, the industry has always insisted—and still does—that without the use of all available drugs, less meat would be produced and what was available would cost more. The question of ''less meat'' is addressed in the report: ''Advancements in production, harvesting, processing and storage technology, plant and animal genetics, nutrition, and management (including the use and availability of chemicals and drugs) were the factors that contributed to the agricultural revolution. Today, largely as a result of these advances, our society is more concerned about managing a food surplus and protecting the safety and quality of food than it is about food shortages and the consequences of not having enough to eat.'' There is a certain irony in this statement, since the society's concerns about safety and quality are clearly not the priorities of meat manufacturers, who are using potentially harmful chemicals and drugs to produce meat that is lower in quality—if by that we mean flavor, texture, and healthfulness—than at any time in our history. And further, in respect to the industry's concern for safety, as the study says, "The huge and increasingly widespread use of antibiotics has to be regarded as a significant factor in explaining any possible increases in health risks associated with their use."

One of the objectives of this study, as the title states, was to determine what effect "restrictions" might have on consumer prices of meat; in other words, whether the industry's expressed concern for consumer prices was justified. The report's summary contradicts the industry's position. It says in a succinct paragraph:

> While the results of this study must be considered as merely suggestive, they do indicate that the economic system would generally be quite resilient to a more restrictive policy on animal drug use. Costs of production, and, therefore, consumer prices would increase initially. However, farm prices would increase more proportionally, because the farm-level demand for most livestock products is inelastic. As a result, total net revenue to farmers would initially be enhanced. The increased profitability would encourage farmers to expand output in subsequent years; by the fifth year following the restrictions on animal drug use, production and prices of most affected species would recover to approximately their baseline levels.

Farmers would also benefit because meat production would become less capital-intensive, and the smaller farmer would once again have a place in what is now considered agribusiness, suitable only for wealthy, oversized producers. As the report describes the present conditions situation, "Large-scale-confinement animal production systems require large investments of capital . . ." And, a little later in the text, "Improved sanitation and pasture rotation could reduce the magnitude of even the first-year effects as they are shown."

In other words, our meat could easily be made more wholesome, not only by freeing it of drugs but also by improving the conditions (sanitation and pasture rotation) under which it is manufactured. The flavor of beef, pork, sheep, and poultry might even return to the good meat our great-grandparents enjoyed, and the twin dangers of a worldwide explosion of drug-resistant bacteria and the loss of the help of all the miracle-drug discoveries (penicillin, tetracyline, and so on) that have done so much to control disease among us would perhaps be arrested.

And all without any cost to the meat producers. The animals might grow a little more slowly—and more naturally—but they would be range fed, so the rancher would save on expensive feed. Since the British government, acting on the report of the Swann Committee, banned subtherapeutic use

---

Effect of Cost of Meat if Drugs Banned

From Report No. 414:

Consumers would spend $32 more for the market basket items in the first year. By the fifth year, costs would be $5 more than the base estimate. In no instance is the change in food costs greater than 5 percent; by the fifth year, the percent increase is less than one percent.

---

of antibiotics in feed animals, it has found that ''use of drugs has been more selective and effectively monitored without a sacrifice in food production.'' In addition, all the elaborate testing apparatus that the state and local governments have had to put in place in order to monitor drug residues in carcasses, milk, and milk products could be put to other uses, and the FDA could spend more of its time in other areas and less in prosecuting ranchers who violate even the present mild drug restrictions.

If that sounds too utopian to be true, it is. Nine years later the use of drugs in American meat production is still widespread and, as we have seen in the previous chapter, serious health problems directly related to this type of antibiotic use are now being identified. What is even more incredible is that the use of subtherapeutic drugs the meat manufacturers are fighting so hard to retain has not even been proved to confer any benefit to the industry itself. Not only has it not been proved, but lack of information makes any chance of evaluation difficult. As the report puts it: ''Basic science data are essential to a study such as this. Without good data on the effect of subtherapeutic drug use on feed efficiency, growth rates, mortality, and product condemnation rates, it is impossible to develop precise estimates of the economic effects resulting from a ban. . . . Most of the data were from tests conducted when the additives were first introduced in the 1950's and 1960's. In many instances there were wide variations in test results, making estimates of the changes in production coefficients subject to error.'' With all our modern technology and highly trained food scientists, determination of this crucial problem is resting on the shaky data that was gathered thirty years ago!

The question of human health was not the primary thrust of this study, although the report does mention it in the introduction: ''Public health and safety impacts are identified where possible. The assessment focuses on the incidence rates, trends, and costs for cancer, food-borne bacterial diseases, and allergy problems associated with drug residues. Due to the broad recognition of the importance of the problem of chemical and drug usage in food product and insufficient knowledge about their side effects, a list of research projects and associated data needs to be developed.''

In other words, approximately twenty to thirty years after drugs began to be used as additives in feed animals, our government still didn't know what side effects they had or whether they were making us ill. This lack of knowledge was practically presented as a plus, with the consumers constituting a nation of guinea pigs. Of course, that is not quite the way the report put it:

"Numerous scientific advancements in the fields of epidemiology, toxicology, and pharmacology now provide evidence that health hazards may have evolved from the continuous use of chemicals once considered safe. As future advancements are made to more specifically identify the causes of human and animal diseases, it is likely that other, now commonly used animals drugs will be the subject of regulations further restricting their use.''

And further:

> The health hazards posed by the widespread and indiscriminate use of antibiotics at subtherapeutic levels in animal feeds and for human and animal therapy are potentially dangerous. The most serious hazard to human health is represented by the large reservoir of plasmids carrying genes for antibiotic resistance existing in humans, animals, and in the environment. The hazard is not the resistance carried by the pathogens, but the therapy problems created by the resistance patterns. Once the disease is diagnosed and the treatment of choice is realized to be ineffective, considerable time may be required to find a substitute therapy to combat the disease. Practitioners would have recourse only to less effective, more expensive, and possibly more toxic antibiotics. In the meantime, the disease could spread and reach epidemic proportions. This would result in greater human suffering and greater economic losses in the form of higher medical costs and lost production of goods and services.

So much for the bottom line—reduced profits for pharmaceutical companies, as compared to the just-described result.

When the report talks about out-of-control diseases, it is not speaking about salmonella poisoning and similar food-borne diseases but about the horrors of the Middle Ages.

> More recently, a number of epidemics among human populations have been characterized by the emergence of R-plasmid-mediated pathogens. These include resistance to chloramphenicol in a Mexican typhoid epidemic. There is considerable anxiety about the possibility of development

---

The Shape of Things to Come?

Atlanta, Sept. 19, 1985 (Associated Press news item)—Government medical researchers today reported the first cases of gonorrhea that cannot be treated with tetracycline, a drug often prescribed for patients allergic to penicillin.

Twelve cases of tetracycline-resistant gonorrhea have been identified since February, according to the national Centers for Disease Control. Nine were in the Atlanta area and three were in Philadelphia.

"We don't know yet what the prevalence is nationwide," said Dr. John Zenilman of the center's Sexually Transmitted Diseases Division.

---

of tetracycline-resistant forms of psittacosis, ornithosis, and Q-fever. There is also considerable apprehension about the recent emergence of ampicillin-resistant strains of *Haemophilus influenzae* and penicillin-resistant strains of *Neisseria gonorrheae.*

So far these are mostly fears of what might happen as antibiotics become useless as human medicine, but the writing is on the wall, and many scientists feel we ignore it at our, and our children's, peril.

The report clearly puts the responsibility for action on the consumer. "The extent of regulatory decisions to restrict the use of possibly hazardous additives and drugs will depend upon society's knowledge, anxieties, and willingness to make tradeoffs and amend the law. On the one hand, extreme concern about the possible adverse impact of chemicals used by the food system on one's health could lead to restrictions on their use, and ultimately to higher costs to produce food, and a reduction in the variety of foods on the market." (The report itself shoots down this argument, and properly should not even be repeating it since the summary in the first few pages established that a ban would not increase food costs.) "On the other hand, little expressed concern by society could be associated with further cost reductions in food production and greater food variety." (Here again this statement is puzzling, since the report establishes that this would not happen.)

But how can society respond to a danger of which it is not aware? How many consumers even know this report exists, or the facts it presents:

Of the three major types of animal drugs addressed in this report, the nitrofuran class has caused tumors or cancer in laboratory animals, and, therefore, is suspected of being carcinogenic for humans. Of further concern, the widespread use of antibiotics such as penicillin and tetracycline as animal growth stimulants is suspected of causing the development of organisms resistant to one or more antibiotics. These organisms, now known to be capable of transferring newly acquired resistance patterns to pathogens, could become the causative agents of epidemics among human or animal populations.

Finally, some researchers suggest that the sulfa drugs, especially sulfamethazine residue or sulfa metabolites in animal (pork) tissue, can cause allergic reactions to susceptible humans. The widespread use of sulfa has also been connected with development of antibacterial-resistant organisms and pathogens. In addition, administration of large doses of sulfa to laboratory animals results in enlargement (hyperplasia) of the thyroid gland, an indication of possible cancerous growths.

These are the drugs, more or less, that have been added to meat since before 1950 to increase production and reduce cost. The price we are paying in human health is unknown, which would seem to be a good reason for not allowing their use until we have a greater knowledge of the effect on our families and ourselves ingesting them along with our steaks, barbecued ribs, and chicken nuggets. Instead the attitude is that since we do not have "scientific proof" that they are harming us, let's keep on using them for now.

What about the cases cited in the previous chapter? What about the CDC survey of salmonellosis outbreaks occurring between 1971 and 1983, which the February 1985 issue of *Acute Care Medicine* said "dramatically illustrates how resistance [of bacteria to inappropriately used antibiotics] affects mortality. In nineteen of the outbreaks the organisms were identified as antibiotic-sensitive, and the case fatality rate was 0.2 percent. The death rate was 4.2 percent—twenty-one times higher—in the seventeen outbreaks that were caused by antibiotic-resistant salmonellae." The article, written for physicians, quoted Dr. Scott Holmberg of the CDC (see Chapter 25) as recommending, under "Clinical Implications," that the physician who sees a severe Salmonella, Campylobacter, or other bacterial infection soon after starting antibiotic treatment should suspect he's dealing with a bacterium that is resistant to the drugs he's been using." In other words, the value of all our most commonly used antibiotics, which have so improved and simplified the treatment of many serious and intractable bacterial diseases, has been seriously compromised. Not only will they be useless to us when we need them, they may make us even more ill if our physician isn't aware of this problem. And meanwhile we may be at risk in areas about which we know nothing.

The final irony may be breeding back at the ranch. The use of antibiotics for farm animals was originally developed to prevent diseases in the animals.

USDA Inspection System as Described in Report No. 414

The meat inspection system was developed and implemented long before the modern era of strict regulation of substances such as food and color additives, and before the development of increasingly sophisticated technology to detect the residues of such substances. While visual inspection during slaughter and processing is effective in locating signs of disease and other forms of adulteration, which may be apparent to trained USDA personnel, residues of various additives which may also render the product adulterated are not so readily detectable. Inasmuch as the USDA inspector does not see the meat and poultry until it is brought to slaughter in a federally inspected establishment and has no jurisdiction over articles such as animal feed, his ability to control or monitor residue problems at their source—the farm or the feedlot—is limited.

Use was stepped up as it was found that with these drugs, animals could be raised successfully under what are unnatural and unhealthful conditions. This led to the use of antibiotics not only in sick animals but in well animals. The discovery that antibiotics appeared to make animals grow faster and, therefore, consume less food led to even greater use. The problems that this is creating for human health now present a danger to the animals themselves. The CDC report recognizes this.

Livestock and poultry producers are finding themselves in the midst of a serious dilemma. Proposed restrictions on animal drug use at low levels is expected to result in less efficient feed conversion and growth rates, higher incidence of diseases and mortality, and higher costs. However, continued use may also reduce the therapy value of these animal drugs in preventing or curing some potentially serious animal diseases. FDA has recently demonstrated that strains of *Pasteurella multocida* and *Pasteurella haemolytica* have developed plasmid mediated resistance to penicillin, streptomycin, sulfonamides, and tetracyclines. Consequently, production efficiency may be impaired regardless of the regulatory decisions.

The industry that denies their drug practices are dangerous to human health may respond differently when it finds its feed animals facing these same dangers.

CHAPTER 27

What You Need to Know About Additives and Pesticides

Additives

Pick up any processed food package and try to read the list of ingredients. I say "try to" because the package design often makes it difficult. Ingredients listings are generally in very small type (I carry a magnifying glass) and often printed in a way that makes them practically invisible—white type on a clear plastic or black type on a dark red background, for instance. It's almost as if the manufacturer is ashamed of what he is putting in his product and is doing everything in his power to prevent you from finding out. Granted space is sometimes limited; that may excuse the choice of small type, but there is no excuse for using color combinations that render reading matter illegible.

If you persevere, you may find most of the list practically meaningless unless you are a food chemist or have had a course in food science. There are over ten thousand chemicals that may be added to your food, not including vitamin and mineral supplements, and not one of them is a household word or has anything to do with nutrition.

Why Additives Are Used

Since these chemical additives do not add to the nutritional value of your food, why are they there? From the food processor's view, food additives make food attractive, palatable, cheaper to manufacture, longer-lasting, more uniform, and less dependent on natural or high-quality ingredients. The label often explains that sodium propionate is added "to retard spoilage," BHT is "an antioxidant," and sodium nitrite is "a preservative." Actually all these particular chemicals serve one purpose: to keep food from deteriorating naturally (see also Chapter 8, Forever Foods—The Food Processor's Dream) and having to be withdrawn from sale when they have lived their normal life span. This is presented as a consumer benefit, but it is debatable whether the consumer really wants to ingest foods that have been kept alive artificially.

Chemical additives are often used cosmetically to mask how processing has denatured food. As we have noted in previous chapters, artifical colors and flavors replace natural colors and flavors lost by processing and make possible the use of less expensive ingredients. They also make possible totally artificial "foods," manufactured foods that appear to be the real thing.

The argument for additives is that they are necessary if we are to continue to enjoy the variety of safe, palatable foods to which we have become accustomed year-round. After all, it is said, man has always sought ways to preserve food in times of plenty so that it would be available during lean periods. The trouble with this argument is that additives have simply gotten out of hand and are being used for more and more trivial reasons in larger and larger quantities. Unless the public resists this trend, fabricated food will take over and real food will disappear from the marketplace entirely. It is already estimated that a ban on all additives would eliminate supermarkets, since so many of the eight thousand "food" items they now carry could no longer exist.

A Checklist of Some Common Additives

Here are just a few of the additives commonly found in food, and their function:

stabilizers and thickeners To keep foods in suspension and from separating (as in salad dressings); to increase viscosity; to stabilize foam (as in beer); to improve "mouth feel"; to keep gels from "weeping"; to prevent graining (as in ice cream):

gum arabic, gum tragacanth, gum karaya, agar, alginate, carageenan, furcellaran, pectin, guar, corn hull and wheat gums, quince and locust bean gums, amylose, amylopectin, methyl and ethyl cellulose, sodium caseinate, sodium carboxymethylcellulose (CMC).

preservatives To keep food from spoiling:

benzoic acid, sodium benzoate, sulphites and bisulphites, sulphur dioxide, calcium (or sodium) propionate, potassium bromide, sodium nitrite, sodium nitrate.

bleaches To whiten or to render food colorless so that artificial color will "take" better, and to make dough rise more quickly. Vegetable oils, flour, fruits, maraschino cherries, and other foods are subjected to such bleaches as hydrogen peroxide, nitrogen peroxide, and chlorine dioxide. Nitrogen trichloride, known as agene, was a popular bleaching agent until 1949, when, after years of proved toxicity, it was finally banned. Many of its uses, such as to bleach flour, could be accomplished by natural processes, but they would take longer and, therefore, be more expensive.

antioxidants To prevent food deterioration, such as fats going rancid:

tocopherol (vitamin E), ascorbic acid (vitamin C), butylated hydroxyanisole (BHA), butylated hydroxytoluene (BHT), propyl, octyl, and dodecyl esters of gallic acid (propyl gallate, etc.), erythorbic acid.

chelating agents To remove minerals that might cause rancidity and other deterioration of foods, such as canned pears turning pink, shellfish turning blue-green, corn turning gray-green, and soft drinks clouding. EDTA (ethylenediamine tetracetic acid) is the leading one.

humefactants To keep food moist by absorbing and retaining water; polyphosphate solutions are injected, tumbled, or massaged into meat (such as ham and poultry):

glycerol (glycerine), mannitol, sorbitol, propylene glycol, pholyphosphate solutions.

enzymes To ferment milk, tenderize meat, alter starches, remove oxygen (to slow or prevent oxidation), clarify fruit juices, clean shellfish, remove diacetyle from beer, degrease bones, reduce lactose by hydrolzying it into monosaccharides, to hydrologize proteins, to remove bleaching agents (as hydrogen peroxide from cheese):

microbial enzymes.

acids and alkalis To aid coagulation (as in cheese); as a preservative; to reduce excessive acidity or alkalinity.

Nutrients are often specifically affected by a change of pH (acid or alkaline condition) different from their natural environment; vitamins A, B_{12}, and C; tryptophan; threonine; histidine; argenine; and thiamin are among the nutrients that may be altered or lost through the use of these additives.

The preceding list is by no means definitive and does not identify additives as being probably toxic, possibly toxic, or considered safe at present. It would take a book of its own to list all the most common additives, tell what they do, what foods they are most commonly used in, and how hard the consumer should try to avoid them. Such books exist in handy paperback form and are inexpensive and practical sources of this information for the consumer.

How to Become an Instant Additive Expert

While the consumer cannot expect to learn overnight which additives to avoid, there is an easy way to cut down on additive intake. Just compare the ingredients lists on labels on different brands of the same foods—soups, staples (such as cottage cheese and yogurt), bread, cookies, potato chips, mayonnaise. You will quickly find that some brands use many fewer additives than others. In some instances—cottage cheese and yogurt, for example—you will be able to purchase brands that are additive free.

The only homework you will need to do first is to learn or bring a list of the vitamins and minerals. Now that these nutrients are often listed along with other ingredients, the consumer can be confused by a long list that consists primarily of these vitamin supplements. If you don't have such a list, you can always check the ingredients list against the nutrient information, which will also list the nutrients.

The aim is not to eliminate all additives from the diet, which is clearly impossible, but to reduce the overload that is bound to result from eating too large a proportion of processed foods, restaurant food, and fast food. Each product may pride itself on being more or less harmless when considered in a vacuum, but as part of the day's food intake, it may add up to a much larger quantity of certain additives than the FDA ever intended.

Pesticides

Pesticides, insecticides, and similar chemicals are different from additives in a very important way: they were never meant to get into our food.

Approval of such chemicals always specifies certain conditions to ensure that this will be prevented; unfortunately, such is not always the case.

An instance of the difficulty in preventing an allowed substance from getting into the food chain is the chemicals allowed for use around food crops. Once these are sprayed on fields, they may leach into the soil, be carried by the wind to crops, or leach into waterways, where they poison fish and groundwater.

EDB (*Ethylene Dibromide*)

Even after EDB, a fumigant, had been described by scientists as an unusually potent carcinogen, it was allowed by the EPA to be used on citrus products and stored grain. Since it had been widely used for over twenty-five years, even this limited ban was a step in the right direction, but in view of its extreme toxicity, consumer groups were far from satisfied. When it was found, subsequently, as a residue in fruit and grain products, in Florida drinking water, and in produce from Texas and Mexico, public concern as to its safety was more strongly aroused.

In 1981 a proposal to ban EDB was successfully opposed by the citrus industry, concerned with control of the Mediterranean fruit fly. Consumer groups, upset by the failure of the government to act more decisively, accused the EPA of dragging its feet. Soon, however, the amount of residues found reinforced public concern. The issue received wide media coverage when Florida ordered seventy-seven types of packaged food products removed from store shelves because they were found to contain more than one part per billion of EDB.

According to government guidelines, safety levels had been set at a maximum of 900 parts per billion in raw grain; 150 parts per billion in flour and cake mixes, and 30 parts per billion in ready-to-eat products, such as bread and cold cereal.

By February 4, 1984, evidence of dangerous residues had mounted so alarmingly that the Environmental Protection Agency (EPA) finally took action and ordered the immediate suspension of any use of the chemical on grain products; the ban did not, however, apply to citrus fruit.

On February 6, 1984, New York State found traces of EDB in 50 percent of a variety of food products in random sampling throughout the state. Although the residue was lower than the "safe level" that had been set by the EPA, State Health Commissioner Dr. David Axelrod said he would recommend more stringent standards for food produce EDB residues. "The effect of the federal guidelines is very, very little," Dr. Axelrod said. "I think there is a need for a very large safety factor." Dr. Axelrod's concern stemmed not only from EDB's admitted carcinogenicity, but also because it had been shown to cause reproductive abnormalities in test animals and to alter DNA.

Three days later, on February 7, Governor Mario Cuomo said the state would order all grain products removed from grocery shelves throughout the state and would bar their replacement until the products met the state's standards. The speed and decisiveness with which the state acted to protect their constituents not only contrasts favorably with the slowness of the federal banning process but points up the serious flaws in the currently proposed law that would prevent the states' similar action regarding irradiated food. Federal laws of this sort have always been subject to state regulation, and the EDB story is a clear instance of the importance of retaining the states' right to set their own safety standards, when they are stricter than those of the federal government.

Fusilade

Another problem is that often these chemicals turn out to be so dangerous that they are subsequently banned. By then, however, produce or meat producers have found them so useful that they continue to apply them in spite of the ban. An example of this occurred in August of 1985, when Fusilade, an herbicide approved for limited use on certain crops such as soybeans, was illegally applied on some Maine potato farms. Although the farmers denied using it, investigation revealed that as much as 420 gallons of it had been sold so far that year. Potatoes were tested without revealing any Fusilade residue, but for some reason none of the samples had been taken from the area where most of the Fusilade had been sold. Sales of Maine potatoes fell off temporarily when the story surfaced in newspapers throughout the East, but the episode was soon forgotten by the public.

Captan

A fungicide that is used in paints, wallpaper paste, animal dusts, shampoos, textiles, and paper, captan is also used to treat corn and soybean seeds and on fruits, such as strawberries, apples, and peaches, and on some nuts. (Its use on seeds means the consumer must be especially careful not to use such seeds for sprouting. Captan-treated seeds are easily recognized and avoided because they are always colored a bright color, such as green or pink.)

In June 1985 the EPA proposed banning captan because it had been shown to produce cancer in mice and rats. A statement released by the agency explained the reason behind the proposed ban: "The potential risk from eating foods with captan are not immediate but are estimated from a lifetime exposure to the pesticide. We have indications that the risks of captan may be lower than our assumptions estimate, but the residue data currently available simply are not reliable enough."

An interesting comparison might be made between captan and cholesterol in that the exact same statement could apply to ingesting cholesterol ("potential risk . . . not immediate . . . but estimated from a lifetime exposure . . . may be lower than our assumptions estimate"). The consumer can make a point of buying only untreated seeds and can join groups working to ban or reduce the use of all pesticides in agriculture.

Waxes

Have you noticed lately how waxed produce is increasing in the market—or did you just think the shiny apples and cucumbers had been washed and polished? If so, take another look.

Commercial waxes, derived from petroleum and other sources, are usually a combination of shellac, carnauba, polyethylene and a paraffin-type wax. These are mixed with water and emulsifying and wetting agents so that a thin, continuous wax coat can be applied by foaming, brushing, fogging, or through immersing the produce in a tank of wax.

Commonly waxed produce includes all nuts in shells, avocados, beets, bananas, coconuts, eggplant, garlic, grapefruit, lemons, limes, oranges, tangerines, pineapples, plantains, pod peas, rutabagas and other squash, turnips, watermelons, and sweet potatoes. Many of these are always peeled before using but others are eaten without peeling, and some, such as the citrus fruits and watermelon, are often used rind and all.

Although the FDA considers the wax itself safe, it is often combined with artificial food colors (especially on citrus) that are not safe, and if any pesticide or other undesirable residue remains on the skin or peel, it is sealed in. Since washing, even with warm, soapy water, does not remove the wax, the consumer is bound to consume some of it.

As usual, the reason given for the use of wax is the consumer: waxing makes the food more attractive. The FDA condones the practice also on the ground of a consumer benefit: Waxing "adds a protective coating that helps retard moisture evaporation." Since, as the FDA explains, "During the growing period, produce accumulates dirt and residues from chemical spraying, many products are cleaned with solvent detergents by packings, which may remove the natural wax coating. This can reduce the market life of many perishables. Washing increases the rate of water loss through evaporation. . . ." The consumer may think a simpler method might be to eliminate the "chemical spraying" and the detergent washing to give us fruit and vegetables that can really be washed in the home kitchen. "Clean," shiny fruits and vegetables that have been exposed to chemical sprays, detergents, artificial coloring, waxes, and heaven only knows what else, which cannot be washed off at home even with warm, soapy water, is not exactly what the consumers think they are getting.

PART FIVE

When the Government Lends a Helping Hand

CHAPTER 28

What's in a Name? A Look at the Label

One of the good things about the good old days is that the consumer didn't have to be so well informed. Everyone knew what was in a jar of grandmother's preserves, pickles, or canned vegetables, home-baked bread, and the pork and bacon that came from the family pig raised on table scraps. Times have changed; today our food is "engineered," "manufactured," or "fabricated," and if you think that sounds more like ways of making television sets, clothing, or plastics, you aren't entirely wrong. Not only have we lost control of what is done to our food before we eat it, but worst of all, we often do not know, and neither can we find out, what exactly it is that we are eating. We cannot tell whether the cheese on the pizza, the eggs in our sandwich, or the shrimp in our salad is real or fabricated. At present we cannot even tell when the breakfast cereal we are feeding our children contains more that 50 percent sugar. Without laws that require the public to be told these things, we will continue to consume "foods" that may make us ill—especially if we have allergies, sensitivities, or special health problems, such as diabetes. And we are denied our right to chose the chemicals and additives we are putting into our bodies, because we are not told which of them are in what foods.

Part of the solution to this problem is better labeling.

Labeling Today

The good news is that labels are now more informative than ever. The bad news is that they still don't list many ingredients.

Responsibility for food labeling is divided between the Food and Drug Administration (FDA) and the United States Department of Agriculture

251

(USDA). The FDA is responsible for all foods except meat, poultry, and egg products, which come under the jurisdiction of the USDA. They, and the Federal Trade Commission (FTC), which theoretically oversees food advertising, have responded recently to consumer pressure and proposed improvements. Since 1978 these agencies have been gathering consumer opinions through five nationwide public hearings at which 450 consumers spoke up, and from approximately nine thousand letters written directly to the agencies. In addition, the FDA surveyed food store shoppers. The result was a decision to propose some of the following labeling changes:

1. List all ingredients in foods, even those previously hidden under the standards of identity provision.
2. Label ingredients by percentages, not by quantity.
3. Require more specific listing for colors, spices, and flavors.
4. Increase nutrition labeling.
5. List quantity of total sugars as part of nutrition labeling.
6. List quantity of sodium (salt) and potassium as part of nutrition labeling.

To understand exactly how these proposal would work, it is necessary to know something about the facts behind the present labels.

Standards of Identity

More consumers are reading labels more carefully than ever before, but what many do not know is that the ingredients list is far from complete. One of the regulations that can hide a multitude of ingredients is the mandatory ingredient labeling on foods for which the FDA has set "standards of identity."

The Department of Agriculture's Yearbook, *Protecting Our Food*, explains:

An example of standard-setting or rulemaking can be found in section 401 of the Federal Food, Drug and Cosmetic Act. . . . It provides for the establishment of reasonable standards of identity, quality, and fill of container for foods, with butter, fresh and dried fruits, and vegetables exempted.

Standards define what a particular food product shall consist of, setting minimum figures for valuable ingredients and in some instances maximum figures for less valuable ingredients.

Standards have been established for cocoa products, macaroni and noodle products, cheeses, dressings for foods, food flavors, tomato products, and many other foods. The standards may include enriched varieties of foods, ensuring that the amount of enrichment is a substantial one.

Most of the standards established thus far have been standards of identity, specifying permissible ingredients and quantities of ingredients to be present.

Among the specific foods subject to the standards of identity are: mayonnaise, catsup, certain canned fruits and vegetables, milk, certain cheeses, ice cream, certain breads, and margarine. The idea may have been a good one to begin with; for instance, in order to make mayonnaise one must combine oil, egg yolks, and vinegar or lemon juice; leave any one out and the result will not be mayonnaise. Salt and dry mustard are fairly standard additions, but nothing more is actually needed than the three original ingredients. The government's thinking was that as long as these three ingredients were used, the result could be called mayonnaise. If any one of the basic three was eliminated or substituted, the result could be called salad dressing or something else, but not mayonnaise. So rather than require the manufacture to take up precious label space listing the obvious, the standards of identity for mayonnaise simply specified what mayonnaise must contain in order to be labeled mayonnaise. Any additional ingredients had to be specified.

Theoretically, this protected the consumer, who then knew that if it was labeled mayonnaise, it came within his understanding of what mayonnaise was. A good idea in theory perhaps—but it has not worked out that way in practice.

The standards of identity have come a long way from allowing just the ingredients the consumer would associate with the product. For example, even the oil used in mayonnaise—traditionally, olive oil—may be any number of other oils (and today, is almost *never* olive oil). The standards of identity do not require that which oil has been used be disclosed on the label. As it happened, some manufacturers, proud of their pure ingredients, listed them anyway. And other manufacturers of similar products have followed suit. For instance, Cains Mayonnaise, which is not required to list any ingredients, has a complete list: soybean oil, egg yolks, distilled vinegar, sugar, salt, water, and spice. This makes it easy to compare one brand with another and to choose the one you think has the best ingredients.

In practice, I have found that most consumers assume they know what mayonnaise contains and never bother to read and compare labels. They buy what advertising has persuaded them is the best and are sometimes surprised, on comparing labels, to find they prefer a different brand.

Incidentally, many people have asked me why labels sometimes use the words *and/or* before listing a number of different oils. The USDA–FDA policy allows this when the fats or oils are not the primary ingredient. In other words, a bottle of oil must say exactly which oil—safflower, peanut, sunflower, olive—it contains; the kind of oil when it is as merely one ingredient among many need not be specified beyond listing the several possibilities. The reason for this is purely commercial and in no way related to a consumer benefit. As the FDA puts it, "It permits processors the flexibility to use different oils to take advantage of price fluctuations to produce a more economical product"—which is governmentese for saying it allows the manufacturer to use whatever oil was cheapest the day he bought it. It's thus a "more economical product" for the manufacturer, but the savings are not necessarily passed on to the consumer. Consumers have protested this lack of specificity, and the agencies have proposed amending these regulations to require foods with 10 percent or more fat content, on a dry weight basis, to list the specific fat or oil used. Foods containing less than 10 percent would be allowed to continue using *and/or*.

Ingredients by Percentages

At present ingredients are listed according to the amount of them in the food item: the largest quantity listed first, the rest listed accordingly until the last ingredient represents the least amount. While this is some help, it does not provide an accurate picture. *Meat* listed as the third ingredient in a product does not reveal whether the product contains, for example, 40 percent meat or 10 percent. This system makes it difficult to know what you are getting and impossible to compare different brands. Consumers have long asked that this system be replaced by actual percentages. The FDA has new proposals that would expand the use of percentage labeling for key ingredients. A can of peas, for instance, might specify "peas, 65 percent; water, 32 percent; sugar, 2 percent; salt, 1 percent." This would help determine whether a more expensive brand was delivering more peas or merely more water or sugar than a less expensive one. It would also enable the consumer on a low-salt or low-sugar diet to determine which brand to buy. If these proposals become law, the USDA has indicated it also would apply to the foods under USDA jurisdiction.

More Information on Colors, Spices, and Flavors

At one time food coloring was presumed safe and the consumer trusted in the generally recognized as safe (GRAS) list to contain only additives that were harmless when added to food. (See Chapter 11, Forever Beautiful—The Dubious Magic of Food Colors, for a more detailed discussion of GRAS.) As science advanced, it discovered that many substances that had been added to foods for many years were actually harmful or, at the very least, might be the cause of various illnesses and adverse reactions.

One of the groups discovered to be most harmful was some of the artificial colors, used to make food more attractive. Gradually these have been banned for use in food, but some food colors are still allowed because they are considered safe. Many consumers who were previously not aware of the widespread use of artificial colors in their food are now looking at labels for this information, but it isn't always there. Butter, cheese, and ice cream may contain artificial colors but the manufacturer is not required to say so on the label. Since the use of artificial colors is purely cosmetic—the manufacturer thinks the consumer prefers butter to be yellower than it sometimes is naturally, for example, and yellow coloring is sometimes added to foods to make them look as if they were made with egg yolks—there is no health reason for using them, so perhaps they could simply be eliminated altogether. If not, however, they should be listed on the label so the consumer can avoid foods that contain them. An alternative would be to use natural coloring ingredients. The manufacturer of Perdue chickens boast that their yellow color comes from natural sources, and specifies, in TV commercials, exactly what those sources are. There are many natural sources, such as marigolds, that will make foods yellow, and most cooks know to add turmeric, curry, or saffron to foods such as rice when they want a yellow color.

Spices are generally "natural," but flavors are largely imitation. Some artificial flavors, such as vanillin, are generally specified, but most of the time the ingredients list simply says "artificial flavors." The new proposal would require inclusion of specific names of all colors and spices but only of those flavors that are "known to cause health problems, such as allergies." It would seem the consumer would want to know the names of all the artificial flavors, if only to be able to compare the quality of one brand with another.

Increased Nutrition Labeling

The present law requires nutrition information only for foods that make nutritional claims. When it is given, nutrition information must be accurate; the FDA specifies the format, including serving size; number of servings; number of calories; amount of protein, carbohydrates, and fat per serving; and percentage of U.S. RDAs of seven vitamins and minerals. This sounds very complete, but it is not quite what it seems. The "per serving" requirement specifies the size of serving, whether in cups, ounces, or spoonfuls—but does not require unform sizes within a product class. As a result, a consumer doing a cursory reading of two labels may fail to note that the serving sizes vary. Always compare number of servings per equal-size containers when comparing two products; the more servings, the smaller the serving size will be.

If the manufacturer does not make nutritional claims for his product, nutrition listing is voluntary, although more and more manufacturers are doing it. The agencies would like to see more nutrition labeling, but public response to the question of whether to increase label information in this area has been mixed.

Listing Sugar As a Total

There are a few ingredients about which consumers have expressed a desire to be told more. One of them is sugar. Because so many forms of sweeteners are used—for example, sugar, corn syrup, fructose, corn sweeteners, glucose, dextrose, sorbitol, mannitol, xylitol, total invert sugar, and brown sugar—the consumer might not be aware that they all mean added sugar. And even if they are recognized for what they are, it is impossible to add the various listings to determine the total sugar in the product.

Total sugar content listing would simplify the consumer's task and make very clear which of a wide range of foods—soft drinks, cold cereals, salad dressings, and various processed items—contain startlingly large amounts of sugar.

List Salt (Sodium) and Potassium by Quantity

Sodium and potassium—a balance of which is essential for proper working of the body's electrolytes—are two more ingredients consumers have asked to have listed quantitatively. As with sugar, it is often difficult to recognize them under the various names by which they may be listed.

An estimated 60 million Americans have high blood pressure and they and other Americans may be on low-salt diets. Unfortunately, the manufacturers' description of salt content has not always been reliable. Foods labeled low-salt have been found to be higher in sodium than the regular version of a product, and "low salt" itself is a relative term that covers a quantitative range.

As of July 1, 1985, a new regulation required that the sodium content be listed "on all processed foods regulated by the FDA that carry nutrition labeling," which excludes meat and poultry products that are under the regulation of the USDA. Getting this regulation passed took three years and considerable consumer activity; the FDA considers it "one of the most successful public education campaigns in recent years, as well as one of the more outstanding examples of industry-government cooperation."

Due to this regulation, terms have been clearly defined so that the consumer need have no doubt what they mean. "Sodium free" means less than 5 milligrams per serving. "Very low sodium" means 35 milligrams or less per serving. "Low sodium" means 140 milligrams or less per serving. "Reduced sodium" means the product has been processed to reduce the level of sodium it usually contains by 75 percent. "Unsalted" does not mean it is salt free or even low in sodium, but that additional salt has not been added. (An example is unsalted potato chips, which may naturally contain salt, but which have not been salted by the manufacturer.)

The listing of potassium content is still voluntary and not affected by the sodium regulation.

Other Labeling Considerations

Fats, Cholesterol, Fatty Acids

Fats, cholesterol, and fatty acids are subjects of great interest to today's consumer. The agencies are in favor of defining terms such as "low cholesterol," "reduced cholesterol," and "cholesterol-free"—which presently are not defined by the government—so that their use on packaging is more meaningful. Until recently any use of these terms to indicate a more healthful product was prohibited by law. Obviously it is some time since this law has been enforced, and over the years the consumer has been led to believe that research linking cholesterol, saturated fats, and similar ingredients to disease was much more positive than in fact it was. (For a more detailed discussion of this issue, see Chapter 23 and Chapter 24.)

Open Date Labeling or Code Dating

These terms refer to the dates found on a number of perishable foods, such as milk, yogurt, and cottage cheese. Almost all of the approximately 45 percent of the consumers who expressed an opinion on open dating favored it. Although it is required by some state and local jurisdictions, it is voluntary elsewhere, under federal law.

Consistent dating policies would give consumers some guidance as to how fresh the food they propose to purchase might be. Consumers often do not realize that not all the dates mean the same thing. Some dates indicate when the item was packed, some the last date on which it should be sold (with the understanding that it may be kept in the home for a period after that and still be considered fresh); some dates indicate the probable date after which the item will spoil. The consumer is rightfully confused by this lack of uniformity, and there is usually nothing on the package to indicate which of these meanings applies to the date shown.

The proposed USDA regulations would require open dating for perishable and semiperishable foods under its control. At that time, perhaps, the meaning of the dates could be standardized.

Food Enrichment and Fortification

Most consumers are aware of nutrient additives in foods that say they are "enriched" or "fortified." Most frequently, processed foods have lost much of their nutrients and those specified have been put back; the manufacturer does not say which have been lost but does make a virtue of the fact that some have been returned in the form of supplements. A peculiar result is that advertising that focuses on fortification may confuse the consumer into thinking that the advertised food is more nutritious than the naturally nutritious food, which cannot advertise itself as being fortified or enriched, because it contains these nutrients naturally. Sometimes nutrients that were not present to begin with have been added, as in the case of iodine in table salt and vitamin D in milk. Usually fortification is a selling point, both on the package and in advertising, as "lemonade-flavored drink, rich in vitamin C."

It is possible for a manufacturer to overdo fortification in an effort to prove that one product is better than another; an excess of certain added nutrients or ingredients might be harmful. Getting all your nutrient requirements in one meal, when you will be eating several other nourishing meals, just might not be such a good idea, even if it were possible.

CHAPTER 29

How to Read a Label

The Format

Labels often contain information in which you are not interested, and do not tell you everything you want to know. Somewhere in between is the useful information that will help you get more for your money and your health. The trouble is no shopper has time to wade through all the fine print in a typical grocery cart—yet how else is one to winnow the wheat from the chaff and end up with the good stuff?

Here are some tips:

Bring a magnifying glass. The light in supermarkets is fine for shopping but not strong enough for reading dark blue print on a dark red ground. If the manufacturer really wants you to read something, he'll put it in big type, but that may not be what you want to know. Be prepared— go armed.

Learn typical label formats. Usually you are looking for two copy blocks, the one headed "Ingredients" and the one headed "Nutrition Information Per Serving." If you want to go deeper, continue on to the one headed "Percentage of U.S. Recommended Daily Requirements (U.S. RDA)." Cereal boxes are easy; the information is usually all on one panel. Other labels make you hunt for what you want to know. If you are especially interested in sugar (which would be included under "carbohydrates" in "Nutrition Per Serving") or salt (sodium), you will soon become familiar with its place in the nutrition grouping. Take your time and don't try to learn everything at once.

Start by picking a few foods to learn about and read those labels. For instance, compare a couple of highly advertised brands of cold cereal, or mayonnaise, or soup.

Resist the hype. The front of the package is for advertising the name, and all the special new features, such as "new easy opener," "natural," "no sugar (fat, cholesterol)," "fortified with," "enriched with," "the best," "provides X essential vitamins and iron." Never mind all that; the nutrient information is a better basis for comparison.

Watch for advertising "weasels," such as "no other (item) contains more (whatever)." Well, maybe not, but how about just as much as? Such wording doesn't say the product is the only one that contains that much, but it tries to give you that impression.

Don't rely too much on the labels. Although they tell more than they used to, labels leave out a lot of important information. Ice creams, for example, may legally contain—but not have to list—sixteen hundred different additives. Butter may contain color—natural or artificial—but doesn't have to say so.

Today over 2,800 substances are intentionally added to foods. In addition, ten thousand other compounds are added indirectly during processing, packaging, or storage, including pesticide residues, drugs fed to animals, and chemical substances that migrate from plastic packaging materials [from *Never Too Old,* by Geri Harrington and Ty Harrington].

Understand "imitation" foods. A food that is not what it purports to be need not say so, according to current policy, "unless it is nutritionally inferior to the original product." (And it can be made nutritionally equal by fortification, which may not make it truly equal, except for certain specified nutrients.) Consumers have expressed dissatisfaction with this policy, but so far it stands. The FDA's justification is: "This policy permits manufacturers flexibility in developing foods that may be substituted for a traditional or standardized food while maintaining the food's nutritional quality."

What this means in practice is that a new "food," so long as it is similar to and substitutes for an existing food, does not have to be labeled imitation. "New" foods are being created at an astounding rate. In 1928 the number of items offered in the typical supermarket was nine hundred. In 1981 that number exceeded twelve thousand.

The question is: are they really new foods or just shadows of the real thing? When the FDA requires them to be the nutritional equal of the foods they replace or for which they are substitues, it is relying on our limited knowledge of the nutrients in our food. We have not isolated all the nutrients, neither do we know all the trace minerals or

nutrients we ingest when we consume real food. Since nutritional deficiencies manifest themselves in unknown ways over sometimes long
periods of time, we may be ignorantly creating future health problems
for ourselves and our children. At the very least, the consumer ought
to be told clearly when foods are invented foods, not be denied the
"imitation" appellation that would allow an opportunity to avoid them,
if such is their desire.

The present policy, for example, allows a cheese that is "nutritionally
equivalent to and which conforms to the fat and moisture content requirement of the cheese it imitates"—but does not meet the standard
of identity for that cheese—to be called a cheese substitute. Some
consumers might prefer the imitation to the real thing—if, for instance,
they knew it contained vegetable fat and protein instead of cow's milk
and thus had lower cholesterol. Because the standards of identity presently mean that the "real" cheese (with some exceptions) doesn't have
to list its usual ingredients, the consumer has no way of comparing it
with the substitute and cannot make an informed choice. For example,
calcium chloride, which is added to many cheeses as an aid to curd
formation, must be listed as a nutrient if added to cheese substitutes
but not when added to real cheese. Obviously it would be better to
give the consumer *all* the information for *all* cheeses.

The informed consumer can pick up some clues from the name of
the product. For instance, "artificial vanilla ice cream" or "artificially
flavored vanilla ice cream" indicates the produce contains more artificial
than natural flavors, or even all artificial flavors. Whether a product
is labeled fruit juice or fruit drink tells you exactly how much fruit
juice and how much water you are getting for your money. Fruit juice
must be only the liquid squeezed from the fruit; fruit drink can be 90
percent water and usually has to have sweetener added to make it
palatable. Some products, such as Tang, contain zero percent of the
real thing, as the label makes clear to the careful reader.

Sometimes the information on labels appears to be complete when
it is not. An example is stuffed olives described as stuffed with minced
pimientos. As we saw in the section on real foods, this is not a very
forthright description of what is actually inside the olives. The old-
fashioned foods—when you can find them—still have the most comforting labels; Baker's Unsweetened Chocolate package says, "No ingredients other than chocolate," Domino Confectioners 10-X Powdered
Sugar says, "Ingredients 97 percent sugar, 3% cornstarch (added to
prevent caking")—a classic definition of powdered sugar. Baking from
scratch still has a lot going for it; you can convince yourself by reading
the ingredients list on baking mixes.

Learn some common additive terms. It doesn't do any good to read a list of ingredients if you don't know what the names mean. Most consumers don't have the time or the inclination to become food technologists, but in the interests of self-defense, they ought to learn at least the more common additives and be able to distinguish the good from the bad—not all additives are necessarily bad—or at least recognize the harmless against the less desirable.

Whey. I have had audiences ask what whey, is, and I am always surprised; I thought Mother Goose was known even to the new generation and that everyone would remember little Miss Muffet eating her "curds and whey." Whey is simply the liquid that milk products break down into during cheese making; curds are the solids. Whey is the liquid you see in yogurt and cottage cheese when you've taken out a spoonful. It is rich in vitamins, minerals, and lactose and should not be wasted. Add it to stews, soups, and casseroles; put it in a glass of milk. Just keep it in a jar in the refrigerator and use within a few days.

Alkali. Another listing that seems to bother people is alkali. The alkali used as a food ingredient is derived from plants (unlike the metal alkali) and is used in some chocolate manufacturing to darken the chocolate cocoa and give it its characteristic "Dutch" cocoa flavor. At some point I noticed that chocolate ingredients were changed and were broken down into listings like cocoa butter, chocolate liquor, and sugar (instead of just saying *chocolate*), or "Dutched cocoa (Processed with Alkali to enhance flavor, aroma and color)"—which is really overkill, since *Dutched* means "processed with alkali" and is the usual way of making this type of cocoa. This description doesn't do anything to reassure the consumer who wonders what alkali is doing in his chocolate bar.

Vanillin. This happens to be one of my pet peeves. I'm very fond of good chocolate and am not happy about how expensive it has become, but I really feel ripped off when chocolates that cost twenty dollars or more a pound use vanillin instead of real vanilla. The difference in taste is enormous; the savings in cost to the manufacturer is a few pennies. I would rather have the packaging a little less elaborate and the flavor truer to real chocolate than the other way around. If you think I am nit-picking, take a minute sometime to check the ingredients on your favorite box of chocolates or chocolate bar. Work up to the most expensive brands you can find; you will be amazed to discover how very few brands use real vanilla. By now most consumers have never tasted chocolate made with real vanilla, and I consider that true deprivation.

Vanillin is a crystalline phenolic aldehyde that is the chief fragrant component of the vanilla bean. Using that instead of vanilla is like spraying a fast-food restaurant with a baked ham aerosol (something that is actually done): it's satisfying only if you've never eaten home-baked ham or real chocolate.

Vitamins. Many consumers do not know all the names of vitamins. The manufacturer adds them to a product, carefully listing them as a plus; he would be surprised to find the number of consumers who wonder whether they should buy a product that contains thiamin (B_1), riboflavin (B_2), pyridoxine (B_6), and alpha tocopherol (vitamin E). I know, because these names constantly crop up when I am asked whether an additive is safe. Learn your vitamins so you can get on to other matters.

Some additives and preservatives are discussed more fully in another chapter; it is a big subject and deserves a book of its own. There are some excellent paperback books that list and describe additives and tell which ones to avoid. An especially good one is Michael Jacobson's *Eater's Digest,* which is inexpensive and small enough to fit in a pocket.

Don't try to memorize all the ingredients you come across; look up one or two every so often; you will remember quite a few after a while. You may even develop your own pet peeves, such as avoiding anything that contains monosodium glutamate or other "flavor enhancers," in favor of food that doesn't need its flavor enhanced. You might try buying fewer foods that contain preservatives; this will reduce your shopping list materially and automatically eliminate many of the more highly processed foods, pushing you closer to cooking from scratch. (If you think you don't have time, maybe you aren't using the right cookbook.)

Changing the Rules

Until the summer of 1985, the FDA in its Code of Federal Regulations had a strongly stated policy of forbidding manufacturers to make health claims about their products. In considering claims that manufacturers were trying to make about cholesterol and fats, for example, it said

A number of common food fats and oils and some other forms of fatty substances are being offered to the general public as being of value in the control or reduction of blood cholesterol levels and for the prevention or treatment of diseases of the heart or arteries.

The role of cholesterol in heart and artery diseases has not been established. A causal relationship between blood cholesterol levels and these diseases has not been proved. The advisability of making extensive changes in the nature of the dietary fat intake of the people of this country has not been demonstrated.

It is, therefore, the opinion of the Food and Drug Administration that any claim, direct or implied, in the labeling of fats and oils or other fatty substances offered to the general public that they will prevent, mitigate, or cure diseases of the heart or arteries is false and misleading and constitutes misbranding.

The FDA further stated that it would "proceed against such health claims made for vegetable oil products" and that "terms such as 'polyunsaturated,' 'unsaturated,' 'low in cholesterol,' and similar statements mislead many people to believe that these foods will reduce blood cholesterol and thus be effective in treating or preventing heart and artery disease."

Step into any supermarket and it will be obvious that this rule was never been enforced. Consumers are bombarded with claims that low or no cholesterol is a health benefit, even though that is still not established as a fact and even though the latest findings seem to indicate that a reduction in overall low fat intake is desirable but that ingesting a higher proportion of unsaturated (as compared with saturated) fat may not be healthful. The same sort of thing has been done with advertising and packaging of nonsugar sweeteners, which are always presented as being beneficial to the health— even when the package contains a warning to the contrary.

Now the FDA itself is planning to allow the dissemination of misinformation on labels through exactly this sort of health claim, and the consumer, believing that such claims could not be made if they were not substantiated, will be poorly served. For example, terms such as "low cholesterol" and "reduced cholesterol" will not only continue to be used but will now have the agency's blessing. The reason given is that "studies have repeatedly shown an association between dietary fat and cholesterol and the occurrence of coronary heart disease," which is like saying flying saucers are a fact. (They may be, but we certainly do not have proof, only an indication that something else is out there.)

The agency release continues, "Manufacturers should be permitted to use the food label to communicate" proper diet information regarding reducing the risk of cancer, heart disease, and other ailments. As we see elsewhere in this book, there are some dietary recommendations—such as eating more fiber—that may reduce the risk of, for example, colon cancer. But that is far from being able to say that if you eat enough fiber, you won't get colon cancer. If it were that simple, we could wipe out colon cancer tomorrow. But that simply isn't a known fact—and as we learn more about fiber, we find that bran, the most highly advertised fiber, is not the type that reduces the risk of colon cancer. With this new, relaxed regulation, however, there is a good chance that "eat bran, lick colon cancer" is the message the consumer will be getting from the advertising and the package.

With health information as complicated as it is, the simplistic approach required by advertising and label messages would not seem to be the best way to educate the consumer. If the government really wants to do the job, it should undertake the responsibility for getting the latest and best information on health matters to the consumer. Unfortunately, such information is actually becoming harder for the consumer to get from unbiased sources; even the Government Printing Office's own publications, which were mostly free or very inexpensive for years, have been whittled down to almost nothing, with those that are left often priced out of the average consumer's reach.

The FDA does realize that it may be inviting abuses in this critical area. Joseph P. Hile, associate commissioner of the Food and Drug Administration, comments, "Our problem is how to permit appropriate health claims without opening the door to outright fraudulent ones." Given the true state of our knowledge of nutrition, it would seem that the best way would have been to stay with the old regulation and enforce it. Since so clearcut a rule apparently proved impossible to enforce, one cannot help being dubious about any control under the new permissive climate.

An example of how claims may change under the new rule is the Kellogg Company's campaign, which started last October, promoting Kellogg's All-Bran cereal as a help in reducing the "risk of some kinds of cancer." Kellogg apparently consulted with the National Cancer Institute and got their blessing before committing this message to their packaging and television advertising. Not all manufacturers feel this freedom is necessarily a good thing. James. L. Ferguson, chairman of the General Foods Corporation, which makes the Post cereals, feels health claims by food manufacturers might be confusing: "Unless there is absolute proof that a specific food prevents a disease, health claims can mislead the consumer." Since there is not yet absolute proof in most instances that a specific food can prevent a disease, Mr. Ferguson would appear not to be in favor of such health claims at the present time.

The trouble with claims such as Kellogg's is that there is no room, either in advertising (TV commercials are notably brief) or on the package (already crowded with small print), for a complete, substantial, and accurate presentation of the facts behind any such claim, and anything less is automatically misleading. For instance, many experts feel that bran is not a solution to a "high fiber" diet because a combination of fibers is necessary to be really effective. According to this thinking, reliance on bran to the exclusion of other fibers could lull the consumer into a false sense of security and prevent the ingestion of a better diet.

The old problem of telling the truth, nothing but the truth—but not the whole truth—can be critical when health claims are made. A case in point, cited by Michael F. Jacobson, executive director of the Center for Science in the Public Interest, is the advertising for certain Campbell Soups, which promotes their high vitamin content by saying "Soup is Good Food" but does not point out their high sodium content, which has been linked to increased risk for people with high blood pressure and lessens their desirability to many consumers.

It is inevitable that a company will put its best foot forward in order to gain a competitive advantage, but it is questionable whether the government should allow health information to be used in this way—selectively disseminated to the trusting consumer. On the other hand, the label is an advertising medium for the product and is not meant to be purely informative. Somehow a balance must be achieved between the manufacturer's and the consumer's interests. A disinterested third party should be the one to see that both sides are dealt with fairly, but the government has not always shown itself to be disinterested. Until a better solution is found, consumers must look after their own interests and let the legislators know that knowing what is in food is of concern to the people who are going to eat it.

CHAPTER 30

The RDAs— What They Really Mean

Food packages that list nutritional information usually have a table showing also the percentage of U.S. RDAs (Recommended Daily Allowances) of selected nutrients that the contents provide. This information may be helpful in comparing different brands of the same item, but you may be reading into it more information than it really provides. Most consumers do not know that there are two RDAs: the U.S. Recommended Daily Allowances (U.S. RDAs) and the Recommended Dietary Allowances (RDAs). They differ appreciably and in some very basic ways.

Recommended Dietary Allowances (RDAs)

RDAs were first established by the Food and Nutrition Board, National Academy of Sciences Research Council, in 1941 and have been updated periodically ever since to incorporate the latest findings in the field of nutrition. The nutrient allowances are broken down into twenty-six groups, including age and sex, and are for "healthy people," whoever they may be. Since nutrient needs are strongly affected by these factors—for instance, a child under five has very different nutrient requirements from one sixteen years of age—these tables are a better guide than U.S. RDAs. The resultant tables, however, are somewhat lengthy, so, if for no other reason, they are not the ones listed on food packages.

U.S. Recommended Daily Allowances (U.S. RDAs)

Even if you consult the FDA tables, you will not be able to translate the U.S. RDA percentages easily. Lacking the detailed breakdowns, you can apply the percentages only very roughly; the U.S. RDAs are not an exact and precise guide to your nutrient needs. The U.S. RDAs, compiled by the FDA, are based on the highest values of RDA tables. The amounts given are what is usually considered the highest levels for a healthy diet. The tables are broken down not by age or sex but by four general population groups (compared to the National Academy's 26 groups), so the recommendations, at best, are very general and, at worst, may be seriously inappropriate. The four groups are: pregnant or lactating women; infants of up to one year; children under four years; adults and children over four years. Obviously the nutrient requirements of a five-year-old are very different from those of an eighteen-year-old or an eighty-five-year old. Sex also makes a difference in needs for certain specific nutrients, such as calcium and iron. Yet the majority of Americans are lumped together in the "adults and children over four years" group. A recommended amount may be too much for a girl of five and not nearly enough for a man of eighty-five.

The FDA revises the U.S. RDAs periodically as the nutrition data published by the Food and Nutrition Board of the National Academy of Sciences' National Research Council is updated. The latest change, issued in 1980, were not so incorporated, partly because they were so minor, and partly due to strong disagreement amoung the scientists.

The program requiring nutritional information on labels was initiated in 1972, and final regulations governing nutrient labeling of food products were published in 1973. According to the regulations, any food with added nutrients or for which a nutrition claim is made must list this information on the label. Obviously not all foods are required to list this data, but consumer interest has led more and more manufacturers to provide it.

The standard heading is 'Percentage of Recommended Daily Allowances (U.S. RDA).'' It then lists approximate percentages per serving (which are arbitrarily determined by the manufacturer) of various nutrients and, usually, the number of calories. The nutrients required to be listed are protein, vitamins A and C, thiamin, ribloflavin, niacin, calcium, and iron. Optional are vitamins D, E, B_6, folic acid, B_{12}, phosphorus, iodine, magnesium, zinc, copper, biotin, and pantothenic acid. If the optional list is used, the other must be also. Other nutrition information may include carbohydrates, fat, and sodium.

What the U.S. RDAs on the Label Mean

The percentage indicates the amount of the daily requirement, as established by the tables, that is in a serving. *Twenty-five percent* means a serving provides one-fourth of the recommended need for that day. This is only a rough guide, not only because your age, sex life-style, and various other individual factors may require more or less than the 100 percent working base, but also because you may already have an adequate supply of those the body itself accumulates. On the other hand, intake is not necessarily a reliable guide since, due to interactions with other foods or with drugs, or to a malfunctioning metabolism, you may be utilizing only a small part of your intake and thus may need much more than usual. There is also the question of the source of the nutrients; some sources may be more bioavailable (able to be utilized by the body) than others.

The FDA defends its limited breakdown by saying it was done "to make it simpler and easier for consumers to use the information on a label." As we have seen, what this limited grouping really does is make the information much less useful. Even this, however, is a step in the right direction; every little bit of information is helpful.

In 1985 an effort was made to revise the RDAs in view of new nutrition studies, especially those relating to fats and cholesterol, to carbohydrates, fiber, sugar, and minerals, such as calcium. For the first time in its history the advisory committee reviewing the guidelines were unable to agree, and the National Academy of Sciences, announcing "an irreconcilable conflict," said it would be unable to issue a new set of recommended dietary allowances "at this time." For a more detailed discussion, see Chapter 36, Fats Under Fire—When Scientists Disagree.

CHAPTER 31

GRAS—Are Food Additives Really Safe?

During the past fifty years the number of additives used in food has grown enormously; since 1958 over one million different organic molecules have been chemically created in the laboratory, and many of them end up as food additives. At the present time over 2,800 substances are intentionally added to food; as many as 10,000 compounds are used either directly in food or during processing, packaging, or storage; this does not count all the pesticides, insecticides, fungicides, detergents, and other indirect additives that may be found as residues in food.

Although poisonous residues in food had been regulated by the Pesticide Chemicals Amendment of 1954, the amendment hadn't been particularly effective because residues were often at such low levels that they couldn't be detected by methods then available, and it was thought that such low levels were "inconsequential." With the advanced chemical analytical methods of the 1980s, it became possible to detect residues of parts per billion, and with generally advanced technology, it became possible, also, to determine whether, far from being inconsequential, even these small amounts could be seriously toxic. As a result, some pesticides, such as endrin, when used on cauliflower, now have no permitted residue or tolerance levels. This has led to seizures of cauliflower crops by the FDA when endrin residues have been found.

The first Food and Drugs Act was passed in 1906, but it was not until the more comprehensive Food, Drug and Cosmetic Act of 1938 that the government was given the authority actually to remove adulterated and obviously poisonous foods from the market. The next amendments, the Food Additives Amendment in 1958 and the Color Additive Amendments in 1960, included laws that specifically regulated food additives. One of their most important stipulations was that the manufacturer was now required to prove the safety of his product; previously the burden had been on the government to prove it unsafe.

The Delaney Clause

One of the most important parts of the 1958 amendment is the so-called Delaney Clause, named after its sponsor, Representative James J. Delaney, Democrat, of New York. This section says that "no additive shall be deemed safe if it is found to induce cancer when ingested by man or animal, or if it is found, after tests which are appropriate for the evaluation of the safety of food additives, to induce cancer in man or animals."

Before the Delaney Clause, carcinogens were not regulated any differently from any other additive. Often tests that would have revealed that a substance was carcinogenic were simply not done, and when a substance was found to be carcinogenic, the FDA set use levels for it, just as for any other regulated substance, in spite of the fact that experts firmly state that our present knowledge of cancer does not allow us to determine how much of a cancer-causing substance is "safe."

The Delaney Amendment was loudly opposed, not only by industry but by some within the FDA itself. It was argued that banning carcinogenic substances would bring financial hardship to some manufacturers, and that we didn't absolutely, positively have proof that very many consumers would get cancer from foods that contained these substances. It would be easy to say that given a choice, consumers would vigorously object to being exposed to even a small amount of a carcinogen, especially when it is used primarily to increase a manufacturer's profits; it is hard to take that position, however, in light of the fact that even today, when the facts are generally known, and when warnings must be printed on the labels of foods that contain saccharin, many consumers go right on drinking beverages that contain saccharin (and are only discontinuing this practice in favor of an unknown and possibly even more harmful substance, aspartame), even though these beverages are nonfoods and in no way necessary to human health.

The Delaney Clause has been under fire ever since it was put into effect, and many efforts have been made to dilute or circumvent it. The word *appropriate* has been seized upon as a possible loophole, and some scientists have tried to challenge subcutaneous animal tests of suspected carcinogens, saying such tests are not "appropriate." Dr. Hueper, when he was chief of the Environmental Cancer Section of the National Cancer Institute, entered the fray in defense of subcutaneous tests, pointing out that no one questioned these tests until they became inconvenient for the additive and food industry. In a strongly worded statement he said that questioning the validity of such an excellent and particularly sensitive method of determining whether a substance is a carcinogen "has opened, intentionally or unintentionally . . . the door to a legalized inclusion of carcinogenic chemicals in common goods, especially foodstuffs, and thereby has become the pernicious instrument in perpetuating the avoidable and needless exposure of the general public to certain environmental chemical cancer hazards." Dr. Hueper continued to fight against this downgrading of tests for cancer, and many leading scientists joined him, but the result was a serious weakening of the protection intended by the amendment. Many food dyes, shown by subcutaneous injection tests to be carcinogens, were banned in Europe but were continued to be added to American food. Although most of them have now been taken off the GRAS list, a few suspected ones still remain or are allowed with restrictions (See Chapters 10 and 11.)

The 1960 amendments required rigorous premarket testing for colors used in food, drugs, and cosmetics. Those colors already permitted or already commonly used received automatic provisional approval pending investigation and confirmation of safety. This particular list has at one time or another included as many as two hundred colors, but over time it has been reduced to a handful. As we note in the section on artificial colors, over the years more and more have proved toxic, including Red No. 2, which was in its time the most widely used red coloring agent. Artificial colors, like artificial sweeteners, have a higher record of toxicity than most classes of additives and are consumed in great quantities because they are used in such a wide variety of foods. Even today there are both colors and sweeteners in use whose safety is suspect and under investigation.

The GRAS List

GRAS, short for "generally recognized as safe," is the official government list of additives that may be used in food, drugs, and cosmetics without testing because the government says they are safe and will not cause illness. Among the additives included are artificial colors and flavors, pesticides, and chemicals. For regulatory purposes GRAS substances are not considered food additives. If they were legally classified as such, they would be more strictly regulated than GRAS substances. This distinction is not a real one, and both groups have always been called "food additives" in this book.

"Prior sanctioned" substances are those that had been permitted under previous laws, such as the FD&C Act, the Meat Inspection Act, or the Poultry Products Act. This group is also presumed to be safe.

In allowing an additive to appear on the GRAS list, a distinction is made as to whether it is safe for use in food and/or drugs and cosmetics. For instance, some substances are GRAS for food but not for cosmetics, while some may be used in cosmetics but not in food and drugs.

The GRAS list was established in 1958 in an amendment to the Food, Drug and Cosmetic (FD&C) Act. At that time it included only substances that were generally recognized by experts as having been "adequately shown" to be safe for their intended use in food. The primary way they had been shown to be safe was by obtaining the opinion of a group of scientists, and by choosing those substances that had been in general usage for some time. Extensive testing prior to inclusion on the list was not required at that time, inasmuch as the whole point of the GRAS list, as the FDA has repeatedly explained, was "to avoid the huge burden of proving the safety of substances already regarded as 'safe,' thus diverting FDA resources from the more pressing task of checking the safety of new additives." The public tends to consider that a substance being on the GRAS list is an assurance of its safety, but until recently there was little scientific basis for such an assurance.

The law differentiated between *intentional* and *indirect* additives. Intentional, or direct, additives are substances that are purposely added to food. These include all the substances the consumer usually thinks of as additives. Indirect additives are substances that were never meant to become part of the food; an example of this is some of the preservatives that are incorporated into food packaging and that sometimes "migrate" into the actual food. Concern has been expressed about the dangers of ingesting some of these indirect additives, but since it is only recently that their ability to migrate into food has been discovered, they are not presently banned on that account. In one way these additives are similar to substances like DES (diethylstilbestrol), which was never approved as a direct food additive but only for use in live animals. It finally had to be completely banned for any use when dangerous residues of it kept showing up in the food supply.

When the GRAS list was first published in the Federal Register on December 9, 1958, interested persons were invited to present their views to the FDA, and approximately 900 qualified experts outside the FDA were sent copies of the list with a request for comments; 355 responded. The GRAS list was then put into place, and manufacturers and food processors felt these substances could be used without fear of consumer lawsuits or government interference, since they took the position that the government had assumed the responsibility for their safety. Growers, manufacturers, packers, and distributors who had incurred financial losses when cyclamate was finally banned clearly set forth this position in congressional hearings in September and October of 1971.

Changes may be made in the list three ways: the removal of approved items; the ban of approved items, and the acceptance of new items. In 1971 a procedure was established whereby a chemical or food additive on the list could be removed and put under "interim regulation." It could also become a "regulated additive" if there was scientific evidence that would indicate that its use should be restricted. A substance in either of those categories may still be used in food.

Food Additives Not on the GRAS List

The FDA calls a food additive "any substance the intended use of which may be expected to result in its becoming a component of food." Substances not classified as GRAS or having prior sanction are subject to "pre-marketing approval"; the manufacturer is required to produce results of a variety of tests to determine the composition and purity of the ingredients and to measure the strength of all toxic effects the substance can produce in feeding experiments in at least two animal species. Food additives have never been required to be on the GRAS list; many substances are not on the GRAS list partly because they have never applied to be on. The list has been primarily a convenience for the FDA to cut down on the number of additives that needed to go through the regulatory process.

In 1971 the GRAS list consisted of six hundred substances that ran the safety gamut from salt (sodium chloride) to cyclamate. The FDA made no attempt, however, to create a complete list and admitted that "you will find some of the common things that you think about as food additives not on the list not because they would not be considered generally recognized as safe, but because they were just not put on." Sugar, for example, is not on the list. The agency hopes, however, eventually to have an all-inclusive list.

If a proposed new additive passes the required tests, the maximum amount of the substance that does not produce undesirable effects, known as the "no effect level," is determined. This amount is divided by 100, and this $\frac{1}{100}$ amount is the amount the FDA ordinarily sets as the permitted amount of the additive that may be used for human consumption. This does not mean that the additive is not toxic; it means that the FDA has decided that the amount permitted to be added to food allows a sufficiently large margin between toxic and nontoxic amounts so that it is safe for humans. In the event that the amount that would be permitted to be used by this formula is more than the food processor needs to achieve the desired result, only the lesser amount is permitted. The rub is that future tests may show that even that amount is toxic and that humans have therefore been exposed to deleterious substances in their food with the consent by their own government. This has happened repeatedly in the past; it will undoubtedly happen in the future.

If a food additive is not on the GRAS list, it may still be used, if approved, but it is then regulated as to what it may be used in and how much of it may be used. Saccharin is an example of an additive that is no longer on the GRAS list but is not banned; it is a regulated additive. (According to the Delaney amendment, if animal studies show it produces cancer in animals, it technically must automatically be banned.) At present it has "interim regulation" and the amount that may legally be added to food has been set by the formula just described.

The GRAS List Reviewed—1971

In 1971–72 a group of twelve outside scientists, under contract to the FDA and comprising the Select Committee on GRAS Substances of the Federation of American Scientists for Experimental Biology (FASEB), embarked on a study of the use and safety of substances on the GRAS list. One step in the review process was a survey of all scientific studies of GRAS substances conducted and published throughout the world in the last fifty years. The size of the task is indicated by the fact that over sixteen thousand such studies were reviewed on a single ingredient. In addition, the committee reviewed information furnished by the FDA on how the substances are used by the food industry and in what quantities.

Once identified, the material on each item was summarized and then supplemented by any available animal test data. The FASEB then reported its findings to the FDA, categorizing each substance in one of four ways:

1. affirmed as generally regarded as safe and maintained on the GRAS list
2. placed on a new GRAS list, but with various restrictions
3. converted to a regulated food additive status with strict controls over its use
4. banned from use in food

GRAS Review Update—1978

By February 1, 1978, the scientific group had reached the halfway mark. It had submitted scientific evaluation documents on more than 250 of the ingredients it had selected for study and, when safety questions had arisen, had presented recommendations as to how consumer health might best be protected.

The committee reported at this time that it had so far found that most of the substances "present no hazard to health from current uses or as they might be used in the future." The scientists expressed some reservations or concern, however, regarding about 6 percent of GRAS substances. They included: caffeine; monosodium glutamate (MSG); protein hydrolysates; licorice, licorice extracts, and ammoniated glycyrrhizin; sucrose; nutmeg, mace, and their essential oils used as flavors; caramel used as color.

Caffeine—Naturally occuring caffeine (tea, coffee) was not considered, only the use of caffeine as an additive (as in cola beverages). The committee could not agree in their evaluation of the potential harmfulness of caffeine as an additive. Some felt it might be a hazard for those, especially children, who consumed excessive amounts. Others felt in the absence of studies showing harmful effects, an adverse judgment could not be made. The final recommendation was that long-term studies, checking for birth defects or behavioral problems especially, should be undertaken.

Monosodium glutamate (MSG)—The committee, in a tentative report, found no evidence of hazard to adults at present levels of use (though "Chinese restaurant syndrome" is caused in some consumers who ingest it) but were concerned about possible hazards to infants from MSG in baby food and recommended it not be eaten by infants under twelve months of age. Mothers took this very much to heart, and U.S. baby food manufacturers withdrew the additive from their product.

Protein hydrolysates—Are used as protein supplements (made from casein) and flavor enhancers (HVP from vegetables). The committee tentatively found no evidence of hazard but recommended further study and that they no longer be added to commercial infant formulas, strained baby food, or junior food.

Licorice, licorice extracts, and ammoniated glycyrrhizin—Are used as flavors. The committee felt that normal use was not hazardous but that overindulgence can cause a temporary elevation in blood pressure.

Sucrose products—From cane and beet sugar, and dextrose products from corn, were found harmful only in the same way as all sugars—as a cause of tooth decay. The committee suggested additional studies because of the excessive consumption of sweeteners.

Nutmeg, mace, and their essential oils—Used as flavors were not found hazardous, although the committee said further studies were required.

Caramel color—In itself was found safe but the committee recommended that limits be set on certain trace compounds produced in caramels by some types of processing.

Additives—Benefits Versus Risk

The value of additives depends on who is doing the talking. The manufacturers of additives and of processed and fabricated foods wax poetic when describing all the wonderful things additives do for the consumer. Upon looking into the matter, consumers often find that most additives are there for the convenience or increased profits of the manufacturer, or are useful to advertising copywriters. These are not consumer benefits and not worth a risk to the consumer.

Vitamins and Minerals

Additives such as vitamins and minerals are supposedly added to foods to make the consumer healthy. Now that nutrients (even added ones) may be listed on the package, some foods even furnish "100% of the RDA" for several vitamins and some minerals. The question arises whether it is desirable, or even wise, to get all one's RDA requirements in one item of one meal. What about an overdose caused by eating, in addition, a presumably balanced diet the rest of the meal and the rest of the day? After all, vitamin additives are merely vitamin supplements, and we all know that you can take too much of a vitamin supplement. All that "100%" may do is cause us to ingest a megadose without our knowing it. In a world where all your foods provided 100 percent of the RDAs, you might run into trouble rather quickly. Come to think of it, some experts say you don't need supplements at all if you "eat right." If they are correct, we should get our nutrient needs the way they occur in foods, not from fortified or enriched foods (which have either been denatured first or were never meant to contain those nutrients in the first place).

Another point is that nutrients can really cause problems if they are not in balance and if they are not ingested with other nutrients that complement them. Can we trust the fortified and enriched foods to be supplemented that scientifically? Even multivitamin supplements contain various combinations of nutrients. How can you tell the right one to take in view of all the supplements you are getting in your diet?

True, the government makes the food manufacturers put in some nutrients—such as vitamin D in milk—but that's a smidgin compared to what's dumped into some foods, many of which wouldn't be able to claim much in the way of food value without them. Isn't it conceivable that oatmeal, which contains no additives or any other ingredient besides the rolled oats—which apparently help prevent colon cancer—is healthier than a cereal that is almost half sugar, with much of the good processed out of the grain, and a spoonful of nutrients added for bragging purposes?

U.S. Recommended Daily Allowances (U.S. RDAs)

(for adults and children over 4 years)

Protein	
Protein quality equal to or greater than casein	45 g
Protein quality less than casein	65 g
Vitamin A	5000 IU
Vitamin C (ascorbic acid)	60 mg
Vitamin B_1 (thiamin)	1.5 mg
Vitamin B_2 (riboflavin)	1.7 mg
Niacin	20 mg
Calcium	1000 mg
Iron	18 mg
Vitamin D	400 IU
Vitamin E	30 IU
Vitamin B_6	2 mg
Folic acid	0.4 mg
Vitamin B_{12}	6 mcg
Phosphorus	1000 mg
Iodine	150 mcg
Magnesium	400 mg
Zinc	15 mg
Copper	2 mg
Biotin	0.3 mg
Pantothenic acid	10 mg

Artificial Colors and Flavors

Since these have been gone into thoroughly in their own sections, suffice it to say that the industry says they are used because the consumer wants them. Red coloring is pretty; yellow coloring makes margarine look more like butter and baked goods look rich in eggs. In other words, artificial colors and flavors disguise processed and fabricated foods, making them look something like the real thing. The danger is that generations of children will grow into adults without knowing what real food looks and tastes like and will be unable to recognize and protect themselves against non-nutritive imposters. If this early exposure to processed and fabricated foods leads to a lower consumption of real food and to ingestion of hazardous substances, the health of the nation may be endangered. On the other hand, children brought up on real food will more easily reject any other kind.

Phyllis Lehmann of the FDA describes the typical lunch as follows: "Take a typical lunch, for example: sandwich, instant soup, gelatin dessert, and a cola drink. The bread has been fortified with vitamins and also contains an additive to keep it fresh. The margarine has been colored pale yellow—or, if you use salad dressing, it has been made with emulsifiers to keep it from 'separating.' The luncheon meat contains nitrite; the soup an additive to keep it from becoming rancid; the gelatin, red coloring to make it pretty. Finally, the cola to wash it all down—without coloring, flavoring, sweeteners or artificial carbonation, the pause that refreshes is nothing more than plain water!''

Actually, Ms. Lehmann's description is by no means complete—there are many, many more additives in most of the items listed than are mentioned. Just look at the labels the next time you buy gelatin, soup, bread, margarine, or salad dressing. And then consider that if they conform to the government's standard of indentity for that item, there are probably additional additives that are not required to be listed on the label.

Other Additives

Not all additives are known to be harmful; many may truly be harmless and perfectly safe. The additives to avoid are the ones that are used to cover inadequacies in the product, make it look better than it otherwise would, make possible the use of inferior and less expensive ingredients, and add color and flavor that trick the consumer into thinking it is attractive and ''tasty.''

Additives that keep food from going stale (See Chapter 8, Forever Foods—The Food Processor's Dream) or rancid, make it moister or fluffier or crunchier than it would be naturally, are no boon to the consumer. Anything that keeps something ''fresh'' when it is really too old to be good food any longer—the ''Shangri-La'' vegetables that have not been allowed to wither and die—anything that is totally artificial but propped up by modern technology is something you don't really want to eat. And there is always the possibility that more advanced technology may—in the future as it has in the past—disclose that these substances are harmful.

The consumer may be paying a high price in health for ''convenience.'' The instant foods, mixes, and soups that don't even have a can to call their home are all highly processed and exist only by virtue of the possibly unhealthful additives that hold them together, and they are not even your best food dollar buy. And many of them, ironically, take longer to prepare than the same dish made from scratch.

Frozen foods are better and often freer from additives—some of them may actually be higher in nutrition than ''fresh'' produce—but read the label. Some are close to their original condition while some are processed into another substance entirely. You have a choice.

Saccharin, Nitrates and Nitrites—
Clearly Toxic Allowed Food Additives

Saccharin, nitrates, and nitrites are still allowed to be added to foods, although the use of saccharin is restricted and the label on foods containing it must say so, with an accompanying government-mandated warning. The FDA has continued to allow saccharin on the basis that it is important for diabetics, for whom it is thought to be a safer sweetener than sugar (from a blood sugar standpoint). The manufacturer says the public wants saccharin, regardless of how harmful it may be and that may be true.

Sodium nitrate and sodium nitrite, used as food preservatives, have the dubious distinction of being among the few additives that have actually caused deaths among Americans (nitrite is a known carcinogen). The FAO/WHO Expert Committee on Food Additives reported in 1965; "It is impossible to make an estimate of an acceptable dose for babies of six months of age or less on the basis of animal experimentation or clinical experience." (At that time, all of the leading brands of baby foods contained nitrate.)

In 1972 the WHO Committee wrote, in its twenty-third report, "The Committee discussed nitrites with respect to their acute effects such as methaemoglobinaemia and the production of potentially carcinogenic nitrosamines (as a result of reaction between nitrites and various amines). At the present meeting the Committee discussed in detail a recent study showing in rates the occurrence of lymphoma due to nitrates." Committee recommended that further studies be made and said that meanwhile it would be "premature" to change the acceptable daily intake (ADI) levels of 9–0.5

Actually, the good news is that you not only have a choice but that you can see to it the choice of more wholesome and safer food is widened. If you won't buy the fake food, more real food will start appearing in the stores. After all, even a food processor will settle for half a loaf.

Saccharin, Nitrates and Nitrites—
Clearly Toxic Allowed Food Additives (continued)

milligrams per kilogram of body weight and 0.02 milligrams per kilogram of body weight for nitrates and nitrites respectively.

Michael F. Jacobson, director of CSPI, has said of nitrite, "It is one of the most toxic chemicals in our food supply. Dozens of persons have died from nitrite poisoning and countless others have been incapacitated. Nitrite's toxicity is due to its ability to disable hemoglobin, the molecule in the red blood cells that transports life-giving oxygen." In August 1978 the USDA and the FDA announced that a study at the Massachusetts Institute of Technology had clearly shown nitrite to cause cancer.

Nitrates and nitrites are used to kill botulinum spores, but the scientists say both that they are not uniformly effective in doing so and that there are other ways to control botulism. They are also used to make smoked meats the attractive pink color so desirable in ham, bacon, frankfurters, and luncheon meats. The manufacturers say that these products would otherwise be an unattractive gray and that consumers wouldn't buy them. According to Mr. Jacobson, "Nitrite is added to more than seven billion pounds of meat and fish annually."

The FDA, which still has not banned the use of saccharin or nitrites, wrote to me in response to my query on June 15, 1979, without explanation or attempted justification, "At the present time, saccharin and nitrites are the only two marketed food additives that we believe have shown themselves to be clearly toxic."

CHAPTER 32

Watchdog in the Pantry—The FDA

If the FDA had no other mandate than that of keeping our food free from spoilage, unsanitary handling, and contamination—including checking up on food storage, processing conditions, and personal and plant hygiene—it would have its hands full. For not only is the whole United States its province, the FDA is also responsible for all the food items that are manufactured outside this country but imported and sold here. Just a short glimpse of the problems the agency encounters and handles are enough to make a consumer extremely uncomfortable with food; the wonder is that FDA inspectors are able, at the end of the day, to sit down to dinner with any real enjoyment.

Accidents Will Happen

The commonest reason foodstuffs are found unfit for human consumption are often accidents that have occurred during storage. In many cases the manufacturer or wholesaler is not even aware that there has been any contamination of the food, or thinks it is too little to be a hazard. Frequently the company calls in the state health department or an FDA inspector to determine whether a problem exists. Here are some examples from the FDA files.

The Truck That Slid off the Mountain

In March 1980 a forty-five-foot double semitrailer refrigerated truck, running on a highway near Lewistown, Montana, in a heavy rainstorm, slid off the road into floodwaters. It was carrying 300 cases of frozen king crab from Seattle to Chicago, and 74 of the cases were contaminated by the floodwater and by thawing. Under the supervision of the Central Montana Health District, the 226 uncontaminated cases were transferred to another refrigerated truck and sent to their original destination. The contaminated crab parts were placed under embargo and eventually seized and disposed of by the FDA.

Where There Was Smoke

Truck fires are another way food is sometimes spoiled. In the case of Colorado Specialty Foods, one of their carrier trucks caught fire and almost ten thousand pounds of foodstuffs and other contents were damaged. The company asked the Colorado Health Department to help them dispose of the now useless material—approximately $17,000 worth of foods, vitamins, and cosmetics—and the Denver FDA office supervised its voluntary destruction by the Denver company. Out of the entire lot the only salvagable items were the fifty-pound bags of fructose crystals; only two of those bags had been damaged.

Animals and Insects Eat Too

An even more common problem is infestation by rodents or insects, either live or in the form of insect fragments and rodent traces of various sorts. Apartment dwellers constantly battling mice and roaches, and country dwellers coping with the seasonal infestations of carpenter and other ants and an assortment of small animals, can appreciate the scope of the problem. So can any gardener or cook who picks the worms out of the cabbage, the thrips out of the lettuce, and the unidentified insects nestled in the raspberries. The FDA does not expect the impossible—the absolute absence of all such foreign matter—but it does set allowable levels, and any amount over that means the product is liable to seizure. Generally the summary of the action reads like one of the following:

- "In a number of lots of peanuts in a rodent-infested warehouse, some lots of peanuts contained rodent filth, and all lots of peanuts had been held under unsanitary conditions." (Product was released to the dealer for salvaging.)

- A sample of sesame seeds from a General Bonded Warehouse contained "live and dead insect larvae, insect webbing, and beetle-type insects."

(Product was sent to a farm in Texas, where it underwent reconditioning by sifting through four screens of various sizes with air blowers. Even after reconditioning, 125 bags of seeds had to be destroyed, but the rest of the 1,928 fifty-pound bags were released for human consumption.)

Since the confiscated food represents a financial loss to the owner, offenders sometimes go to elaborate lengths to defeat FDA inspectors.

The Case of the Stolen Molé

A particular brand of molé, the spicy chocolate sauce that is used in classic Mexican cuisine, had been banned from entry into the United States because of repeated instances of contamination with "insects and rodent filth." Imagine the surprise of the U.S. Customs agents at the Laredo, Texas, border station when their search of a Mexican tractor trailer revealed a false front behind which were 415 cases of that same molé.

When José de J. Esquada was identified as the owner of the truck, he said the truck had been stolen and, also, that he was not acquainted with the man who had been driving the truck. The FDA investigators found the product in local food stores, to whom it had been sold by Esquada and two other wholesalers. Esquada still denied any knowledge of Donna Maria molé and tried to prove his innocence by insisting he had no food storage facilities. But on being pressed, he seemed to recall having a warehouse in Dallas. The Dallas warehouse contained infested molé, along with other food products, which FDA inspectors seized under a court order. And a retail store employee recognized the truck driver as one of Esquada's.

Esquada, apparently not at all intimidated by these proofs and proceedings, next illegally removed from the Texas warehouse some of the contaminated products, which had been embargoed. This was the last straw. A state court fined him for that specific action, a federal court ordered the $35,000 worth of products destroyed, and customs agents seized the truck and the trailer with the false front.

Repeat offenders are not treated leniently, as the following instances demonstrate.

The Inscrutable Food Products

Jar-Yu King was a food warehouse owner in Kansas specializing in Oriental foods, of which he was the major supplier to restaurants and other users in the Kansas City area. In 1979 his warehouse was discovered to be "accessible to and overrun by rodents." Upon pleading guilty, he was fined $1,000 and given a year's probation, with the understanding that he hire a qualified exterminator to keep his warehouse free of rodents.

Apparently this was not done, however, since barely two years later a return visit by FDA investigators found "an active rodent infestation, with bags of rice contaminated with rodent pellets and urine, and quantities of sweet sauce in plastic bags extensively damaged by gnawing." In view of the previous violations and the continued unsanitary conditions, King was found guilty by a jury and sentenced to a year in prison. The judge said "work in the Leavenworth federal prison kitchen or commissary" might be beneficial, but the reader might think this was cruel and unusual punishment to inflict on the unsuspecting prisoners.

Man-Made Contamination

Not all the contaminants are of insect or rodent origin; pesticides, insecticides, and various chemicals are sometimes the problem. In recent years, as certain pesticides and insecticides have been banned for use in the United States, the FDA has been confronted with an additional problem in the form of imported food that contains "poisonous and deleterious substances" that cannot legally be used in this country.

Another way poisons get into our foods is through the contaminated environment—as is the case, for example, in mercury and PCBs in fish, weed killers, and pesticides in meat and milk and on produce. Unlike spoiled or decomposed foods, these poisons are detectable only through analysis. Since many of these foods, such as fresh produce, must be marketed as quickly as possible, analysis and testing must be done without causing any delay in distribution. Other raw materials are shipped all over the country for processing—grains into flour, corn into meal, potatoes into chips—and testing must be done all along the line in case problems have been created by unsatisfactory shipping and storage conditions. Here is a look at some of the aspects of this enormous job.

Contamination by Association

An unexpected kind of contamination occurred when a Kansas City trucking firm loaded a shipment of flour close to a shipment of paint thinner. It was a long, hot ride to the destination in Denver, and both the manager and the dock supervisor at the Denver terminal remarked a strong odor of paint thinner in the truck. They conscientiously set the flour aside, and a sample of both it and the paint thinner was picked up by the Colorado Department of Health. When analysis confirmed that the flour had been contaminated by the paint thinner odors, the whole load—approximately six thousand pounds of flour—was buried in a local landfill.

Out of the Frying Pan

It often happens that the very steps taken to control one problem end up creating another. Here are two examples.

Squeaky-clean milk is the aim of milk processors, and detergents are used in every step of milk processing. The trick is to use the detergents to clean the milk cans, carrier trucks, pipes, and other equipment without getting any of the cleaning materials into the milk itself. A suspiciously low bacterial count led inspectors in England to detergent-cleaned milk cans that had not been properly rinsed after cleaning. The Department of Agriculture routinely includes warnings in their literature to dairy farmers that detergents that find their way into milk can "seriously hinder the growth of desirable bacteria used in the preparation of cheese and cultured milks." In other words, instead of saying carelessness may make the consumer ill, the USDA wisely equates it with effects that might cost the dairyman money.

In another instance a milling company controlled the more or less inevitable insect problems that plagued their products with the pesticide ethylene dibromide (EDB). EDB is a powerful soil fumigant that had been found effective also for treating stored grains. In the six months prior to January 1984 Birkett Mills Company had used approximately seventy gallons of a mixture containing EDB in one of its mills. In 1984 the U.S. Environmental Protection Agency decided to ban use of EDB for this purpose and to reduce the acceptable level to 900 parts per billion in grain. Even before the ban had been announced, the company stopped using EDB as a fumigant. Unfortunately, it had already gotten into the mill's products, and a routine check by the FDA revealed levels of 13,566 parts per billion in the buckwheat flour in a Philadelphia warehouse. As nearly as could be determined, the contaminated flour was part of 3,500 pounds that had been processed at the mill where the EDB had been used. A second plant, that had never used EDB, had processed about 1,750,000 pounds of light and dark buckwheat flour, hulled grain, and other products. Unfortunately, the grain from the first mill had been shipped to the second mill and the firm had no way of knowing which lot had been shipped to which customer. The result was recall and destruction of all the grain. And the miller was hit with a double whammy when the investigators also had to destroy 500,000 pounds of two-and-a-half-year-old flour that was found to be insect infested.

The eventual happy ending was that subsequently new batches of flour passed all tests with flying colors.

Outright Noncompliance

Many times pesticides and insectides have been allowed to be used in or near plants and animals that will eventually be used as human food. Sometimes the rationale for their use is claimed that they are not harmful to consumers; sometimes it is that they will not get into the food or, if used in the food (as happens, for instance, when some substance is injected into a beef animal), that they will disappear before the food reaches the consumer. When the discovery is made that the substance is harmful or that residues do persist in the food at the retail level, a further determination is made as to whether an "acceptable" level can be established; if so, only foods containing residues above that level are considered illegal.

However, since use of these substances came about in the first place because they made it possible for food to be produced more profitably by the manufacturer (whether farmer, cattleman, dairyman, processor, or anyone else in the food production chain), there were always those who secretly refused to obey the new law that deprived them of some of these profits. The only weapon the FDA has against illegal use of banned substances is the information turned up by the tests and analysis routinely made on all food (except that food under the jurisdiction of the USDA, which performs the same sort of function). The FDA files are crowded with examples of illegal residues; here are just a few.

The DES Smugglers

In the 1940s DES, a synthetic hormone, was popular with pregnant women because it was thought to prevent miscarriage. Even back then it was a known carcinogen, but that, somehow, was not as important as its ability to bring a pregnancy to term. It was discovered, also, that DES had a salutary effect on animals; they grew fatter quicker, on less feed—resulting in a considerable reduction in the cost of raising chickens, cattle, and sheep.

Along the way there had been indications of danger and restrictions on its use, but nothing very serious. Mothers got upset, however, when it developed that teenage girls whose mothers had taken DES seemed to have a much higher incidence of vaginal cancer. In 1947 DES was approved for implantation in live chicken's necks; however, residues were found in the liver and skin fat of the chickens, so this use was banned in 1959. Meanwhile, in 1954 it had been allowed as an additive to cattle feed and in 1957 was used as an oral drug for sheep.

It seemed as if the passage of the Delaney Amendment, which prohibits any substance that causes cancer to be used in food for man or animals, would automatically ban all these uses of DES, a known carcinogen. The situation was complicated, however, because DES-contaminated products that were already on the market were not covered by the law; identical, but new, products were. Distinguishing between the two proved difficult, so Congress exempted DES in cattle feed provided it wouldn't harm the animal and no residue could be found in any edible part of it.

In time, as so often has happened in the history of the FDA, analytical methods became more sophisticated, and residues that had not formerly been detectable began to show up. But it took until 1979 for a complete ban on the use of DES in all livestock to be passed. By that time, possibly, the livestock industry had stopped taking DES bans seriously; in any case, it was firmly convinced of the benefit to it of DES and, as seems to be common with commercial users of any poisonous substance, had developed an attitude that everyone was making a great fuss over nothing. Whatever the reason, in 1980—when no DES should have been in use any longer— FDA investigators found that its continued use was widespread. Over 435,000 heads of cattle were uncovered with DES implants in what the Kansas City *Star* called "the biggest veterinary drug scandal in U.S. history."

By 1982 contraband DES was so profitable that it was actually being smuggled into the country. The FDA, with the help of the Canadian Mounted Police and the Ontario Provincial Police, captured a Canadian resident at the Port of Alexandria Bay in New York State with vials of a milky white substance, a syringe, and other related materials. Tests showed it was indeed DES, mixed with penicillin.

The FDA had information that the DES had been intended for three New York producers, who were injecting it into their veal calves. The producers were carefully watched and were caught when they brought the calves to market and USDA inspectors, with the help of the FDA's veterinary laboratory, found DES in the animals. A fourth producer in the state was also found using the substance, whereupon the state's Department of Agriculture and Markets quarantined 1,184 animals on the four farms, and a restraining order preventing further use of DES was issued.

Although they at first denied any guilt, the producers eventually agreed not to market any treated animals and to stop using DES from then on. They also agreed to pay for the cost of the FDA's monitoring of compliance through regular testing of the calf kidneys and livers. If any DES residues are found in any of the tests, all the animals in that lot may be sold for nonfood use only—animal as well as human.

The Case of the Tainted Wine

Human nature is apparently the same all over; noncompliance with food laws seems to occur in every country. A famous case, which most readers will remember since it occurred in August 1985, involved Austrian wine and at least one brand of German wine that had been contaminated with a poisonous substance used in antifreeze, diethylene glycol.

The German wine was discovered after the Austrian contaminated wine, when the West German authorities informed the United States that it had found that forty-four different labels of German wine—all of them expensive—contained the same chemical. Though the German government assured the Americans that none had been exported to the United States, Norris Alford, chief of product compliance at the Federal Bureau of Alcohol, Tobacco and Firearms, thought it best to check; 1,350 cases of contaminated German wine, thought to be all that were contaminated, were found in random testing of bottles on the shelves of liquor stores around the country. Subsequent investigation revealed that although the Austrian wine had been deliberately doctored to make it resemble sweeter, more expensive varieties, the German wine had apparently inadvertently been contaminated either by passing through the same machinery used by the Austrian wines or, possibly, by being mixed with Austrian wines. The scandal shook up the Austrian wine industry and has resulted in tighter laws and production regulations.

The Ubiquitous Aflatoxin

Not all the FDA's problems are man-made; those that arise from nature can be even more difficult to control. One such substance is aflatoxin, a "poisonous and deleterious substance" that occurs naturally in a number of crops, such as peanuts and corn.

Aflatoxins are natural by-products of two common molds, *Aspergillus favus* and *Aspergillus parasiticus*. Highly complex organic chemicals, they are toxic in high concentrations and are suspected carcinogens. Unlike ergot, a toxic grain fungus that has been known to man for centuries, aflatoxins were discovered only twenty-five years ago and have so far defeated all efforts to cope with them.

It was thought at first that aflatoxins arose when susceptible food products were improperly stored, and early efforts focused on this aspect. Further study revealed that they can also be found on crops growing in the field. Since there is no way to determine visually which crops are infected, the only method of control is through testing. Faced with the problem of setting "acceptable" levels in foods, the FDA has had to adopt the policy that "any product containing identifiable amounts of aflatoxin be considered adulterated and prohibited from entering the marketplace.

The extent of the problem can be illustrated by an incident in 1977, when two-thirds of the corn crop in some Southeastern states was found to be contaminated. The agency prohibited any corn moving across state lines, but as a federal agency, it had no authority to control the movement of corn within a state or to check the aflatoxin content of products made from corn. Some of the states, including Florida, stepped up their own sampling and analysis programs and worked with the FDA to try to identify any contaminated corn that might be being processed within the state. This met with some success, as was seen in the recall of six tons of cornmeal and grits that were removed from two hundred retail stores in southern Florida because they were found to be contaminated.

Study of aflatoxin is continuing, and recently it has been found that peanuts, for example, are often free from aflatoxin but become contaminated by infected shells. This has led to changes in the shelling and processing areas that may reduce the cross-infection. Improved analytical techniques have also allowed the setting of 20 parts per billion as the acceptable level in all susceptible foods.

The best solution would be preventing the formation of aflatoxin-forming molds on the crops; efforts to do this have so far been unsuccessful, so the FDA maintains its vigilant effort to prevent contaminated foods from reaching the marketplace.

In May of 1980, for example, shelled peanuts were destroyed at Salt Lake City, Utah. In 1977 shelled corn found to be contaminated was salvaged by converting 71,000 bushels to gasohol and reconditioning the remaining 25,000 bushels for use in chicken feed; cottonseed found to be contaminated was destroyed, at Yuma, Colorado, in 1978.

The Mercury That Hasn't Gone Away

In 1970 consumers were upset by reports of a toxic substance, mercury, that had been found in high concentrations in freshwater fish. Mercury occurs naturally in earth and rocks, and in fresh and saltwater, sometimes in substantial quantities. Seawater, for example, contains a mean mercury content of 0.15 parts per billion (ppb). Natural mercury does not seem to affect the wholesomeness of food fish, but mercury is also created as a product of industrial pollution in levels so unnaturally high as to contaminate fish. Like PCBs, DDT, dieldrin, endrin, lead, and cadmium, these pollutants are not particularly biodegradable, and their presence persists long after the cause of the contamination has been removed. All these pollutants have gotten into our food chain and are regularly detected by FDA analysis.

As a result of the Canadian scientists' discovery of excessive mercury, both Canada and the United States banned commercial and sport fishing in lakes and rivers found to have a higher concentration. Saltwater fish, including cod, haddock, hake, halibut, herring, mackerel, sardine, shrimp, swordfish, and tuna, were also tested with the result that of all the species, only tuna and swordfish were found to contain amounts in excess of 0.5 parts per billion (the tuna was canned, the swordfish frozen). Further testing showed that most commercial tuna had acceptable levels or less, but 95 percent of the swordfish appeared seriously contaminated.

As a result of these findings, consumers were warned not to eat swordfish, and the eating of any fish taken from many polluted lakes and rivers was totally banned. Today consumer fears about ingesting mercury have been partly blurred by concern over PCBs, DDT, endrin, and other similarly dangerous substances that are turning up in ever-increasing quantities in fish of all sorts. At a time when we are being urged to replace some of our consumption of red meat with the more healthful fish, it is discouraging to know that we may be replacing one danger with another. Unfortunately, all these pollutants have long-term effects on our health, so it is impossible to know how sick they are making us. You can be tested to find out how much mercury is already in your system—if you are an avid eater of canned tuna, you might want to do so—but there must be some better way of protecting your food than turning yourself into a human pincushion. Strengthening the laws the FDA is supposed to enforce would be a giant step in the right direction.

In case you think the pollution problem has been done away with in recent years, here are some recent FDA cases:

- 1981: Swordfish steaks and swordfish fillets—"The articles contained the added poisonous or deleterious substance mercury, in a quantity which might render the article injurious to health." (The swordfish had been imported from Japan.)
- 1982: Swordfish steaks (same description).

- 1982: Salmon eggs (several commingled lots)—The article contained the added poisonous and deleterious substance polychlorinated biphenyls, and the quantity of polychlorinated biphenyls in the article exceed the prescribed 5 ppm tolerance. (Released to the fisheries for salvaging.)
- 1984: Swordfish—"The article contained the added poisonous and deleterious substance, mercury." (Ordered destroyed.)

Although pollution and fish contamination hasn't gone away, awareness counts. Testing for pollutants is now routine, and especially hazardous conditions are usually detected and publicized in the media. The consumer is warned away from Hudson River bass and fish of various kinds from the Great Lakes whenever levels become "excessive." In addition, individual effort to eat as great a variety of fish, both freshwater and salt, in as many forms as possible (fillet, whole, canned, fresh) will help (see also Part Three, Real Food).

PART SIX

Getting
The Facts

CHAPTER 33

The Nutrient Connection

Since ancient times folk healers have believed that many ills could be treated successfully with substances derived from nature. Regard for most natural substances declined in the nineteenth and twentieth centuries, when great strides were made in the development of synthetic drugs and medications. Some natural substances, such as digitalis and curare, were still utilized, but more and more the laboratory was looked to as the source of help. In the United States plant medicine was generally put on the back burner by all but a few health food advocates who persisted in thinking not only that natural remedies were best in treating illnesses, but that illnesses could actually be prevented by proper diet.

Now the tide appears to have turned, and the public is suddenly being inundated with new discoveries about the prevention and cure of diseases through nutrition. Many of the new theories are based on little more than hope, or a slight indication that diet may help reduce the incidence of cancer, heart disease, hypertension—whatever is uppermost in the public's mind at the time.

In spite of all the contradictory pronouncements, studies, recommendations, and advice, some patterns are becoming apparent. For example, there is general agreement that you can't go wrong by cutting back all fats. If you go overboard on this and try to eliminate saturated fat and eat polyunsaturated fat exclusively instead, the next study may tell you you're headed for trouble. Analysis of most of the dietary findings and recommendations seem to indicate that the old advice of eating a "balanced diet" is still sound. The best plan seems to be everything in moderation, including various kinds of fiber, vegetables, dairy foods, fresh fruit, cereals, and whole grains, and, above all, a diet high in real foods and very, very low in fake foods.

In Part Seven, Taking Charge of Your Life and Your Health, you'll find some specific guidelines on following this regimen. In this part you'll get a clearer picture of what is really known about nutrition and what is persistent myth.

CHAPTER 34

Those Elusive Nutrients

Why You May Need Vitamin Supplements

Part and parcel of the argument that goes on about whether or not the average American needs vitamin and mineral supplements is the idea of eating "a balanced diet,"—that is, one that supplies all the essential nutrients. Theoretically, anyone eating such a diet would have no need to supplement it.

There are four problems with the balanced-diet notion.

1. Individual nutrient requirements vary, often considerably, from the "average." One individual may be so genetically constituted as to achieve perfect health following the RDA tables as a guide. Another may need four or five times that amount for the same health level. A third person may require, for instance, twice as much vitamins C and E but only half as much A.
2. The amount of vitamins one person needs can change, influenced by illness and exposure to pollutants, chemicals, or other stresses. Even if it were possible to get enough of the essential nutrients from food sources, the individual would have to constantly adjust certain items in the diet according to changing needs. It is usually easier and more convenient for a person to effect these temporary changes by taking more or less of the nutrient in supplement form; additionally, supplements will not affect the caloric balance already achieved.
3. We unknowingly ingest, under the misconception that it is real food, an untold amount of fake or denatured (edible but not nutritious) food. Specific recommendations for a so-called balanced diet—such as choosing from the four food groups and other guidelines—do not

differentiate between whole fruit and fruit drinks, chicken breast and fast-food chicken nuggets, or canned and fresh vegetables. Instead we are told to eat so much dairy, so much meat, and so much of other generalized food items. Since there are more no- or low-nutrition foods sold, the odds are against the unguided consumer buying the foods that contains the maximum nutrition—yet that is the premise behind the food groups and recommendations.

4. From harvest to food processor to dinner table is a long, arduous journey, and many nutrients are lost along the way. Many foods that start out loaded with good nutrition end up pleasing our jaded palates but accomplishing little else.

Presently many consumers are trying to remedy the deficiencies in the nutritional requirements caused by modern life, by taking supplements. The sensible way to use supplements is just that, as supplements. They do not take the place of real food. It is still important to get as many nutrients as possible from food itself; only in that way can we also get the as yet unknown but essential elements that nature has built in. The value of supplements is limited by our still very limited nutritional knowledge; we are constantly discovering the importance of nutrients of which we were unaware just a few years ago.

Without a tame analytical chemist in the kitchen, it is impossible to know that good still remains in the food you are putting into your mouth, but it helps to know how to choose wisely, what to avoid, and how to handle and prepare food so as to retain whatever good may have survived in it by the time you get it home.

Vitamin C

Vitamin C is the most commonly taken vitamin supplement. Thanks to the work and writings of Dr. Linus Pauling, and in spite of studies by the Mayo Clinic and others to the contrary, the public seems to have decided empirically that vitamin C intake far over the RDA amount helps prevent colds and possibly a number of other ills, such as cancer and high serum cholesterol. Since the worst opponents can say is that taking large quantities is a waste of money and that in some individuals there is a slight chance that massive amounts may cause kidney stone formation, vitamin C supplements are probably here to stay.

Vitamin C is adversely affected by heat (cooking, pasteurization, food processing), and exposure to air, oxygen, water, and light. It is not surprising, therefore, that the best sources are raw freshly picked foods; even oranges with a high vitamin C content will lose more and more the further they are from the tree and the more they have been processed. Some foods, such as liver (the only meat that contains appreciable amounts of this vitamin) are useless as a source because they are never eaten raw. Here are examples of the difficulty the consumer encounters in trying to get the maximum vitamin C from natural sources.

From Oranges

You probably look to oranges and orange juice to fill most of your RDA of vitamin C; let us see how satisfactory this is.

The RDA for "ascorbic acid" is 60 milligrams, the amount supposedly provided by one 6-ounce glass of 100 percent pure orange juice. The USDA's Composition of Foods table provides the following information:

Food and Description (100 grams)	Ascorbic acid (mg)
oranges, raw,	
peeled fruit, all	
commercial varieties	50
California:	
navels (winter oranges)	61
valencias (summer oranges)	49
Florida:	
all commercial varieties	45

In other words, the amount of vitamin C varies according to season (winter oranges contain more than summer), variety of orange, and what state the oranges are grown in. And according to the following table, the same vitamin C content is found in the fresh-squeezed orange juice from the raw fruit as in the whole fruit itself, except that in the juice table we have the Florida listing broken down in more detail, as follows:

(Florida juice)	Ascorbic Acid (mg)
early and midseason oranges	
(Hamlin, Parson Brown, Pineapple)	51
late-season valencias	37
temple	50

Since these nutrient values are given for fresh-squeezed juice, let us see what happens to vitamin C with processed juice.

Canned	Ascorbic Acid (mg)
unsweetened	40
concentrate, unsweetened	
undiluted	229
diluted, 5 parts water	47
Frozen concentrate, unsweetened	
undiluted	158
diluted, 3 parts water	45

As you would expect, juice from the whole orange comes out best, frozen concentrate next, and canned last. Generally, even canned or frozen fruits appear to retain vitamin C fairly well. Let us see what the vitamin C situation is when the consumer buys it at the store.

There are no regulations that stipulate how much vitamin C 100 percent pure orange juice must contain; seasonal and varietal variations are understood. About 90 percent of the juice produced in the United States comes from Florida (California produces primarily eating oranges), and more and more of it is sold in the form of concentrate that has been mixed with water, pasteurized, bottled, and sold chilled in the refrigerated section of the market. Only a few brands sell whole orange juice that has been pasteurized but has not been made from concentrate.

The Connecticut Agricultural Experiment Station (a similar station exists in every state) analyzed twenty-four different brands of reconstituted chilled orange juice packed in plastic-coated cardboard containers. Although all the products were dated, indicating when the juice should be removed from sale, there was no way of telling from the carton how much time had elapsed since "bottling."

Unlike riboflavin, vitamin C is retained better if stored in the refrigerator in glass containers rather than cardboard. This is due to the fact that vitamin C can be decreased by exposure to oxygen and the glass containers exclude oxygen more successfully. Some manufacturers contributed this information (the length of time from bottling to code date), revealing a range from 16 to 49 days, with an average of 27 days. The study found "The effective vitamin C contents . . . decreased at an average rate of about 2 percent per day during an average period of 16.5 days when stored unopened at 40° F." But loss of effective vitamin C in some brands differed greatly from the average; the range was "from none to 76.5 percent." And, of course, there is further loss as the carton is opened and during home storage.

So in estimating whether you are getting your RDA of vitamin C from that 6-ounce glass of 100 percent pure orange juice, you have to allow considerable leeway. Fortunately, most consumers deliberately consume much more than the RDA amount of C, so the amount in a single glass of juice is not critical.

Juice Drinks

Generally speaking, juice drinks are not a good source of vitamin C; most of them don't even pretend to be. The categories are self-limiting, since only the 100 percent pure citrus drinks are high in vitamin C, and juice drinks, by definition, are low in their content of pure juice. Unless vitamin C has been added, the amount they contain is bound to be negligible. A juice drink must by law contain at least 30 percent juice; ades (except lemon and lime) must contain at least 15% juice (lemon- and lime-ades at least 12.3 percent juice); drinks and punches (except lemon and lime) at least 10 percent (lemon and lime at least 6 percent); flavored drinks may contain less than 10 percent; artificially flavored products need not contain any juice.

Drinks in these categories may be sold in the form of water and juice, juice concentrate, instant mixes, or powders. They may contain either (or both) artificial and natural flavors, but frequently the flavor is due mostly to high sugar content (note the second ingredient—after water—listed on the label). Colors are added to give the appearance of the type of juice they imitate (the consumer expects orange drinks to be orange-colored even though no orange juice is included in the list of ingredients). Although comparatively little juice is required to be in these drinks by law, the Connecticut Experiment Station analysis of seventy different brands of juice drinks found that about a fifth of them had less than the legal amount; of the ten that claimed they were fortified with vitamin C (according to the labels), four had none and one had less than claimed. Considering the loss of vitamin C from 100 percent pure orange juice, the amount of the vitamin still to be found in the highly processed juice drinks does not constitute incentive for purchasing them.

Tomato Juice

Tomatoes and canned tomato juice are generally thought of as good and comparatively inexpensive source of vitamin C, but consumers often worry that a large can of juice, stored in the refrigerator after opening, may lose its C rapidly. The Food Research Institute of Canada's Department of Agriculture reported on a study in 1983 of the variation of vitamin C concentration in canned tomato juice under various conditions. An encouraging finding was that "short-term refrigerated storage of opened cans had little effect on the total vitamin C levels." The scientists expressed concern, however, "regarding the validity of data in nutrient composition tables," because of the possible effect on the vitamin C content due to changes in the different tomato varieties used, new processing techniques, and more elaborate marketing systems.

As expected, a study of twenty-six different brands of canned juice, made during three consecutive crop years, showed a good but variable vitamin C content. According to the report by L. Faye Russell and W. John Mullin of the institute, not one of the brand samples contained the amount of vitamin C—16 milligrams per 100 grams—claimed in the USDA Composition of Foods table on their labels. The table given in the report, giving the L-ascorbic acid content of commercially canned tomato juice, showed a range from a low of 6.5 to a high of 15.1 milligrams per 100 grams of juice, with most of the samples falling well below the high. The study concluded: "Overall, the vitamin C content of canned tomato juice appears to be extremely variable and is generally overestimated in tables of nutrient composition. Brand names provide no aid to the consumer in predicting vitamin C levels."

From the consumer's standpoint, an encouraging comment from the study, is, "However, the total vitamin C content of tomato juice appears to be maintained during short-term storage in the home after the can has been opened." In spite of this information, canned tomato juice is still considered a good source of vitamin C; it just isn't quite so good a source as you may be led to believe, and allowances must be made for both natural and man-induced variations in the amount to be found in any given can.

Produce

Fresh raw vegetables, such as cabbage, green leafy vegetables, and potatoes, are a good source of vitamin C—when they truly are fresh. Dousing them with sulfites to make them look fresh, removing wilted outer leaves, wetting them down, and other similar marketing practices make it difficult for the consumer to make an informed choice. This is serious because bruised or old vegetables, subjected to these practices and stored for several days in the store at room temperature, have substantially reduced amounts of vitamins A and C. The USDA reports, for example, that "fresh" raw green beans may lose up to 50 percent of their vitamin C when left unrefrigerated for twenty-four hours.

It is frequently claimed that one of the reasons our diet is so much "better" than it used to be is because we have year-round availability of a much wider variety of fresh foods and that we are no longer limited to the short seasons of, for example, many garden vegetables. A simple and startling example of the lack of validity in this argument is what happens to spinach under these new conditions. We undoubtedly eat more spinach than ever before, not only because it is always available but also because new varieties have been developed with less of the bitter taste that made it undesirable to many adults and almost all children. It has been rediscovered as a salad green—it has even acquired a certain cachet as such—and now that it comes all nicely washed and bagged in plastic, the cook doesn't even have to put it in the washing machine (set to cold water) to get rid of the sand.

According to the USDA Composition of Foods table, raw spinach contains 51 milligrams per 100 grams of vitamin C, and cooked spinach, boiled and drained, 28 milligrams per 100 grams, making raw spinach an easily available and good source, and even cooked spinach a reasonably good source, especially since frozen cooked spinach apparently retains the same level as the fresh cooked. (Although it is noteworthy that this applies only to the frozen whole leaf spinach; for frozen chopped spinach, the vitamin C content in the cooked product drops to 19 milligrams per 100 grams. If you prefer chopped, pureed, or creamed spinach, take an extra minute and do it yourself from the fresh or frozen whole leaf.)

The catch is that the USDA tables do not distinguish between the vitamin C in spinach at "field level," when it is being harvested, and the vitamin C remaining after being subjected to commercial marketing conditions, and studies have shown that the loss in the second instance can run as high as 90 percent. According to the Canadian Food Research Institute, the USDA tables are usually "composites of analytical data from samples assayed at or near harvest." Since the consumer rarely gets to eat spinach this fresh, it is clear that the tables are not a good guide to the vitamin C content to be expected in the spinach served up in the average American home.

A 1983 report from the institute on the vitamin C content of fresh spinach said, "Out-of-season fresh spinach is four to thirteen days post harvest when it reaches consumers in the northern United States and Canada. Previous work has indicated that enzymatic destruction of vitamin C begins as soon as vegetables are picked and continues through transport and handling (e.g., washing, packaging) due to bruising and wilting. Consequently the data provided by the tables of nutrient composition, such as USDA Handbook No. 8, are in need of updating." This is a polite way of stating a devastating fact about those widely used tables that serve as the key source for much menu planning and for nutrition guidance.

Actual vitamin C levels in fresh spinach are described as "extremely variable, as well as unpredictable." Neither is there much the consumer can do about it. As the report states further: "Unfortunately, the consumer has no way of judging the vitamin content when selecting fresh spinach, beyond a cursory visual examination." What the consumer *can* do is encourage more local farming so that the spinach can be bought nearer to the time it is harvested, or even, when possible, grow it in a home garden. It is an easy crop; the season is short but spinach can be grown at least twice—in the spring and fall—even in northern states, and it takes comparatively little room.

Dehydration also saps vitamin C and other vitamins as well. When you bring vegetables of this sort home, store them in the vegetable bin of your refrigerator or in plastic bags to avoid dehydration. (This is not necessary for potatoes if you can keep them in a cool, dark, dry place.)

The interior of your refrigerator, especially if it is frost free, is quite dry. To see the destructive effect of dehydration experiment with two heads of fresh lettuce—iceberg is especially dramatic. Store one in the vegetable bin and the other, unwrapped, on the refrigerator shelf. In a short time the shelf-stored head of lettuce will be not so much wilted as dried out and obviously inedible. Doing this to even a far tougher vegetable like cabbage will produce the same result, though it will take a little longer. On the other hand, too much moisture is detrimental, too, and washed vegetables should be shaken as dry as possible and wrapped loosely in paper toweling before storage in the bin. (Do not forget about them or they will rot . . . and the whole point of fresh vegetables is to eat them fresh.)

How Packaging Can Retain—Or Lose—Nutrients

Riboflavin Retention

Milk is far and away the best source of riboflavin (vitamin B_2), and in this regard, one of the few good things that has happened to milk in recent times is the switch from packaging it in glass bottles to plastic or wax-coated cardboard cartons. The old-fashioned method of leaving a bottle of milk at the back door was destructive to its riboflavin content; riboflavin is sensitive to ultraviolet rays and strong light, regardless of whether it is sunlight or artificial light. If you leave milk in a glass in the sun for three and a half hours, it can lose as much as three-quarters of its riboflavin content.

Although many consumers prefer the taste of milk stored in glass bottles—some even take it out of the carton and store it in glass when they get it home—they should be aware of the potential for nutrient loss and not count on the riboflavin content of milk so stored as an important addition to their diet. If you leave milk in the refrigerator for your children to drink when they come home from school, use mugs and cover them with foil caps.

Fortunately, riboflavin is stable under heat, so hot milk is a good source, as are canned and dried milk. About 10 to 20 percent is lost in pasteurization or other milk processing techniques, but that is considered an acceptable tradeoff for the sake of safety. Whole, raw milk, properly stored, has the highest riboflavin content, but unless it is produced under ideal conditions, it may be unhealthful due to bacterial contamination.

Freezing does not seem to destroy appreciable amounts of riboflavin, so frozen meats and vegetables may be good sources, providing the drip water (as the foods are thawed) is used in cooking rather than discarded. The drip water, which most people throw away without thinking twice about it, is rich in nutrients (see table, p. 312), and as much as 4.15 percent of the riboflavin in a frozen pork roast can be lost during defrosting.

The old, generally discarded custom of adding sodium bicarbonate to the cooking water of some vegetables in order to retain their green color was very destructive of the vitamin C. Steaming vegetables briefly, without raising the cover until they are done, is a more healthful way of getting the same effect.

Olive Oil

You may not think of olive oil as a particularly perishable product, yet how olive oil is packaged affects its nutrient content. Since the USDA Composition of Food tables do not list olive oil separately from salad oils, and since salad oils are not listed as having any food value other than their fat—and therefore energy—content, the consumer might wonder what difference it makes how it is packaged. The answer is that although the oil will eventually deteriorate, consumers assume that a reliable brand of oil purchased in a reliable store will be in good condition. In addition, we are learning more every day about the value of olive oil in our diet.

When it became possible to classify oils as saturated or unsaturated, it was discovered that oilive oil fell into a neutral category. Much more recently it has been discovered that olive oil is not merely neutral but actually has a positive and beneficial effect on the body's handling of cholesterol. Much more work will have to be done now that food scientists have broken this much new ground, and packaging may prove to be just as critical in retaining the beneficial qualities of olive oil as it has been for retaining the value of other foods.

A study that was completed in 1985 by two food scientists, A. K. Kiritsakis, of the Department of Food Science, Higher Technical Educational School in Salonika, Greece, and L. R. Dugan, of the Department of Food Science and Human Nutrition at Michigan State University in Lansing, compared virgin olive oil stored in bottles made of two different kinds of materials, transparent glass and polyethylene plastic. Half of the containers of both kinds of bottles were stored in rooms where they were exposed to sunlight for four hours a day and diffused light for the remainder of the day. Half of the containers were completely covered with aluminum foil, creating total darkness. The study showed that "the presence of any light was unfavorable," and the more light exposure, the more damage was done to the olive oil.

Oxidation, for example, occurred slowly in darkness, faster in diffused light, and fastest in direct sunlight. This would seem to indicate that clear glass bottles would be less desirable than plastic ones, but as it turned out, the matter was much more complicated. Glass packaging gave better protection against oxidation than the polyethylene, due to the high permeability of the plastic, which allowed air to enter and therefore oxidation to take place, with significant deterioration in the color of the oil even in diffused light. After three months of storage, even in diffused light, in polyethylene bottles, the olive oil had developed an off taste and had lost most of its original color. The oil stored in the transparent glass bottles in the presence of sunlight quickly lost all its color and about 70 percent of its carotene.

The study concluded that bottling in transparent plastic containers would be the least desirable packaging, since the oil would be easily oxidized even in the diffused light of a supermarket. The ideal container would appear to be "bottles that are not transparent and that are not permeable to oxygen, in order for oxidative deterioration to be minimized during storage."

How This Helps the Consumer   The consumer can apply the results of this study to home storage by keeping unopened olive oil in a dark cupboard and, if purchased in a large quantity, storing only a small part of it in a handier small, opaque container in a dark place. It is not advisable to keep open olive oil on a table or counter in the popular and decorative glass cruets that are commonly used. The cruets should be kept for serving oil at the table and returned to the dark after use.

Pasta Packaging

The effect of packaging on an entirely different type of product from any we have mentioned so far was the object of a study reported in the September–October 1984 issue of *Cereal Chemistry*. Conducted by E. M. Furnya and J. J. Wathesen of the Department of Food Science and Nutrition at the University of Minnesota at St. Paul, it analyzed twenty enriched pasta products, purchased from retail stores, for their riboflavin content.

Riboflavin was chosen because the niacin and iron with which most pasta products are enriched are considered stable in this type of product, and the stability of enriched thiamin is dependent on temperature variations and water activity. Riboflavin, on the other hand, as we have seen, is light sensitive and more liable to be affected by packaging not designed with that sensitivity in mind.

The light sensitivity of riboflavin was first discovered in 1944, when it was found that it decomposed rapidly in milk exposed to light. Studies of pasta revealed that this characteristic was not peculiar to milk. In fact, a single layer of macaroni, exposed to moderate intensities of light, lost more than half its riboflavin content the first day. After thirty-five days a further 10 percent had been lost. Pasta protected from light retained its riboflavin content. Unlike milk, however, the rate of loss of riboflavin in pasta was not increased with an increase in the intensity of the light.

Pasta products are usually packaged in one of three types of containers: transparent bags, solid paperboard cartons, or paperboard cartons with transparent windows. The study was conducted with eight brands of enriched elbow macaroni and spaghetti taken from the front of the store shelves and then stored in the dark until they were analyzed. Ten packages were of the transparent bag variety, five were solid paperboard cartons, and five were paperboard cartons with transparent windows.

As might be expected from what we now know, all but one of the paperboard cartons (with and without transparent windows) were within or above the standards of identity riboflavin requirement (which is expressed as a range rather than as a single amount) for enriched pasta. Of the ten packaged in transparent bags, 50 percent had a riboflavin content below the standards of identity requirement. Knowing this, the informed consumer will probably choose to forgo the attractive transparent bags of pasta in favor of the more nutrition-preserving paperboard cartons.

Once again the USDA Composition of Foods table could not be counted on in planning one's nutrient intake. It gives riboflavin values for enriched and not enriched spaghetti, but since it does not take into account differences in packaging, these values as given may be off by as much as 50 percent.

The Perfect Package

Even these few instances of the effects of packaging on the retention of nutrients show there should be support for packaging that does more than just contain the item and protect it from casual contamination. It is clear that scientists are learning much more about packaging with each study, especially about the vulnerability of nutrients in food and about the difficulty in retaining them from the time of harvest to the consumer's kitchen. It is the job of the manufacturer, not the consumer, to ensure packaging that will provide maximum nutrient retention, but, from the examples already given, it is obvious this is not being done. Most of the studies that compare various types of packaging show sharp differences among them in nutrient retention, depending on packaging materials used or on the design of the package (as with the cardboard pasta box with a window), but even years after these studies have reported their findings, poor packaging (from a nutrient-retention viewpoint) continues to be used.

The reasons for this are many. Food packaging has become an extremely complex industry. Not only are the available materials numerous but new ones are being invented faster than the manufacturer can keep up with them. It is not enough for a manufacturer to decide to use a "plastic" container. If the plastic is cellophane, there are over a hundred types of cellophane-containing films and laminates, and each type has its own particular property of moisture or gas permeability, burst strength, stretch ability, and flexibility—to name just a few of the properties that must be considered in protecting a given food product. If a plastic bottle is ruled out because it allows more oxygen penetration than a glass container, the plastics industry promptly gets to work to try to develop a plastic with the impermeability of glass. Years ago, when clear glass was found unsuitable for certain products, dark brown glass was developed. The old adage, Necessity is the mother of invention, could almost be the motto of the packaging industry. A symbiotic relationship exists between the food packager and the food scientist, the latter discovering the kind of protection his newly "invented" food requires, the packager trying to provide it—even, if necessary, creating a new material—and all at a competitive price.

Some products require two containers: a primary one that comes in direct contact with the contents and a secondary one that does not touch the contents. The requirements for the two containers are entirely different. In the case of saltines, for example, the inner containers protect the product from moisture and help keep it fresh and allow uniform packing so that the individual crackers are less liable to crumble or break in shipping, the outside box displays the labeling information, stores easily on the supermar-

Nutrient Stability and Light and Oxygen Exposure

Some nutrients are stable when exposed to light and oxygen; some are not. This list will help the consumer purchase and handle food so as to obtain the greatest amount of a given nutrient.

Light-stable Nutrients

choline
inositol
niacin
pantothenic acid
thiamine

Light-sensitive Nutrients

vitamin A
vitamin C (ascorbic acid)
carotenes (pro-A)
vitamin B_{12}
vitamin D
essential fatty acids
folic acid
vitamin K
vitamin B_6
riboflavin
vitamin E

Oxygen-stable Nutrients

biotin
inositol
vitamin K
niacin
pantothenic acid
vitamin B_6
riboflavin

Oxygen-sensitive Nutrients

vitamin A
vitamin C (ascorbic acid)
carotene (pro-A)
vitamin B_{12}
vitamin D
essential fatty acids
folic acid
thiamine
vitamin E

ket shelf, is recognizable for the type of product, and is strong enough to stand up under normal marketing conditions. Two containers are bound to be more expensive than one, so they must be able to be advertised as a consumer benefit (worth a higher price), and the primary container must make it possible to create a less expensive secondary container than would otherwise be necessary.

Each food has its own requirements. In one case a moisture-proof material is needed to keep moisture out; in another instance the problem is to keep

Nutrient Stability and Heat

Those nutrients that are heat sensitive tend to be decreased by cooking. The consumer can decide which foods to serve raw and which cooked, when preparing food in the home kitchen, if the degree of loss is known. This table does not differentiate among the various methods of cooking—steaming, boiling, broiling, or baking—but rather gives a range. The cook can often retrieve lost nutrients by, for instance, using the water in which foods have been boiled, or skimming the fat off baked and roasted foods and using the natural gravy that remains.

Nutrient	Heat Stable (S) or Unstable (U)	% Cooking loss
vitamin A	U	0–40
vitamin C	U	0–100
biotin	U	0–60
carotenes (pro-A)	U	0–30
choline	S	0–5
vitamin B_{12}	S	0–10
vitamin D	U	0–40
essential fatty acids	S	0–10
folic acid	U	0–100
inositol	U	0–95
vitamin K	S	0–5
niacin	S	0–75
pantothenic acid	U	0–50
vitamin B_6	U	0–40
riboflavin	U	0–75
thiamine	U	0–80
vitamin E	U	0–55

moisture in. And it may be that different materials work best in these two different situations, even though both must be moisture-resistant.

All of which is offered simply as an indication of the complexity of packaging and to show how impossible it is to expect the consumer to know which package to buy. Even the transparent plastic window in the cardboard pasta box may be made eventually from a plastic with a fair to good range of resistance to sunlight. A plastic rated "Good" in this respect would retain more light-sensitive nutrients than one rated "Fair," but the consumer would have no way of judging which plastic has been used.

Price of the item, which could be a guide, is not, as the cost of the item may have more to do with the manufacturer's desired profit margin than with manufacturing costs. Now that food is simply another product, like underwear, increased profits are liable to receive more consideration than is consumer benefit. As we see in another section, expensive chocolates and inexpensive chocolates both can be found using vanillin, even though the few cents' savings gained through using this artificial flavoring instead of the much more delicious vanilla bean is a fractional percentage of the cost of the expensive candy.

Aside from the cost, the manufacturer's perception of what constitutes a package with the greatest consumer appeal affects his decision as to what materials to use. When Pringles went to tube-shaped cans instead of the traditional potato chip bag, it made a virtue of the uniform shape of the chips (derived from their processing technique), as compared to natural chips whose shape cannot be controlled, and they did this partly by creating a can with the familiar shape of tennis ball containers, which had a certain cachet. The untraditional container also drew attention away from the amount it contained. Without comparing label information, it was harder for the consumer to know whether the bag or the can contained more chips—and, therefore, to make any real price comparison. (It was not impossible, but it was harder, and the hurried consumer often gives up on price comparisons of optional "fun" items, like snack foods.)

"Edible" Packaging

The consumer may hardly even be aware of some "packaging," such as the waxes used on fresh produce (see also Chapter 19, Tracking Down Real Fruit, for a discussion of the dangers of waxed foods), and there seem to be more every day. One of the newest is spray coating, which is increasing the use of edible packaging. Before the invention of spray coating, edible packaging was more or less confined to such things as sausage casings, cheese rinds, and similar more-or-less natural "containers." With spray drying, gelatins, gum arabic, and similar materials can be combined with artificial flavorings, preservatives, and similar additives to form a coating that goes completely unnoticed.

Of course, not all coatings are undesirable. Raisins, for instance, are coated with starch to prevent them from moistening the rest of the commercial breakfast cereal, much as a home baker dredges them with flour before adding them to the batter so that they will not sink to the bottom of the baked muffin. If labeling were so complete that the consumer knew all the

Handling Frozen Food

While most people are careful to cook frozen vegetables in little or no water, many do not give any special thought to handling frozen meat. As the following figures show, the value of the high vitamin B complex content of pork can be considerably reduced by not utilizing the drip water that develops during defrosting. Save it and add to gravy, sauce, or roasting pan.

Nutrient	*Percentage Lost (in drip water from thawing)*
niacin	10.7
thiamine	9.02
vitamin B_6	8.71
tryptophan	7.15
pantothenic acid	6.95
vitamin B_{12}	5.06
riboflavin	4.15

ingredients in the package, spray-dried ingredients would also be revealed, either as harmless or as undesirable. The problem with them now is that their presence may go undetected and so cannot be avoided.

As you can see, there are many aspects to consider in packaging. The consumer is right to feel that the first priority should be given to the preservation of the highest proportion of the maximum number of nutrients, but this is unlikely to be the case, since this aim does not take priority in any other aspect of food processing and distribution.

The Consumer's Role in Nutrient Retention

The consumer is the one who suffers if edibles are eaten under the misapprehension that they are nourishing when they are not. Even when the consumer is well informed about diet and makes wise choices, creating a diet that is varied and well balanced in theory, the actual result may be nutritionally disappointing.

As we have seen, many things will have happened to food—even fresh produce—from the time it is harvested to the time we eat it. Additionally, its nutrient content will vary, even at the time of harvest, according to

---

Nutrients Down the Drain

Many rice recipes call for washing the rice before cooking. If you do, this is the percentage of various nutrients that three washings will send down the drain.

Nutrient	Percentage Lost
iron	21.3
riboflavin	16.9
calcium	10.1
niacin	9.1
phosphorus	4.7
thiamine	4.6
nitrogen	2.3

---

season, soil, degree of maturity, weather during various periods of growth, method of harvesting, and the specific variety that was grown. Washing, trimming, storing, packing, transporting, and packaging will all take their toll. The more a food is processed, the greater the possibility of nutrient loss. For instance, if a food is blanched before freezing, then cooked in boiling water (which is later discarded) and allowed to stand on a steam table—all before being served—there will be nutrient losses every step of the way. The industry estimates that no more than 25 percent of nutrients are generally lost in processing, but that is an industry estimate and may be somewhat optimistic. Considering the large diversity of processes, it is not a particularly meaningful figure, but even a 25 percent loss may mean a great deal to the consumer trying to plan a high-density diet.

So-called TV dinners, where many of the foods are not only prepared for freezing but often are actually precooked and then cooked again in the reheating process, usually combine a number of foods with varying degrees of sensitivity. Canned foods, with their obvious changes in texture and flavor, usually heavily bolstered with salt to make them palatable, are claimed to be fairly nutritious. It may well be that they are, compared not to garden-fresh produce but to the green beans or tired carrots that have traveled several thousand miles to get to your store's produce department. But this is a compared-to-what-equation; a canned green bean and a green bean just picked from your garden and eaten raw in a salad or briefly steamed are almost different vegetables. They certainly look different and taste different, and it would be hard to imagine that the same percentage of nutrients survives in both foods.

The more the consumer eats prepared foods, take-out foods, highly processed foods, and out-of-season foods, the less likely it is that the necessary amount of essential nutrients can be gotten from diet alone. Our entire food manufacturing (including raising of food), processing, and distribution systems may be unwittingly undermining our health. Perhaps it is time to consider some of the creative new approaches to decentralizing the production of our food and putting it back in the hands of smaller, more local producers. Since producing enough food to feed us all is no problem—a fact to which our bulging warehouses testify—perhaps what should concern us in the future is improving quality.

Making the Most of Vitamin C

Vitamin C is the most popular of all vitamin supplements and is frequently taken in quantities far above the RDA suggested amount as insurance against an inadequate intake. While that is controversial, no one disputes that nutrients ingested as part of one's food are generally better utilized by the body and are more desirable than in supplement form.

As we have seen, vitamin C is both light- and heat-sensitive and begins to be lost as soon as a fruit or vegetable is harvested. But here are some facts that will help you get the maximum nutrition from your vegetables.

• Locally grown produce will have more vitamin C than produce from other areas. It will have lost fewer nutrients, including C, because it has had to travel the shorter distance to your kitchen.

• Vegetables picked in the afternoon have more C than those harvested in the morning, after a night of darkness. Sunlight is detrimental to vitamin C *in* picked fruits and vegetables but sunlight *on* growing produce increases its vitamin C content. For instance, tomatoes are highest in vitamin C when grown in full sun, not shaded by their own leaves, and picked on a sunny afternoon. (Of course, as gardeners know, an unshaded tomato is liable to get "sunburned," so if you grow your own, don't take too much foliage off your plants.) Peas grown up netting will be richer in C because more of the pods are exposed to the sun.

• Vegetables and fruits picked when they are mature, but not old, will be more nutritious. This is especially true of green beans, peas, peppers, and tomatoes; it is not so important for root vegetables, such as beets and potatoes.

• Refrigeration will slow the loss of vitamin C. For instance, kale will lose up to 70 percent of its vitamin C if left in a 70-degree temperature for 48 hours. If kept at the 40 degrees of the refrigerator, it will lose only about 5 percent in the same period.

CHAPTER 35

Friends and Foes— Nutrient Interactions

Although nutrients are often discussed as if all that were needed was to get enough of them into our bodies, we are learning now that how well we utilize the nutrients we ingest is affected by a number of factors. Certain illnesses, other nutrients, drugs, pollutants, and even differences in lifestyle, age, and genes affect not only how much we need but how much our bodies will absorb at a given time. Here are just a few examples of food and drug interactions that can minimize or enhance nutrient utilization.

Alcohol

Alcohol should not be combined with antibiotics, anticoagulants, antidiabetic drugs (including insulin), narcotic analgesics, antihistamines, tranquilizers and sedatives, or antidepressants. With drugs that have a tendency to cause drowsiness, alcohol can strongly enhance that effect. In addition, alcohol lowers the threshold for allergic reactions and may trigger an adverse reaction even in cases when you were not aware of an allergy. A nondrug example is the case of numerous people who first discovered they were allergic to peanuts when they consistently had an allergic reaction when spending an evening in a bar. The combination of alcohol and peanuts (served as a free snack) lowered the overall allergy level and allowed a mild peanut allergy to become more serious. Certain vitamins and minerals, especially B_1, B_6, B_{12}, folacin, iron, magnesium, and zinc, may be depleted by excessive alcohol consumption.

Anticoagulants

See *Vitamin K* entry if taking coumarin or other anticoagulants.

Antacids

Although the directions on many antacid packages suggest they should be taken an hour after meals, it is also recommended that they should not be taken within two hours of eating milk and milk products. (See also *Over-the-Counter Drugs.*)

B Vitamins

See individual B vitamins. See also *Alcohol, Colchicine, Hydralazine, INH, Lactose, Mineral Oil, Neomycin, Oral Antidiabetic Agents, Oral Contraceptives, Sulfites.*

B-complex Vitamins

B-complex vitamins are an example of how important it is to get as many nutrients as possible in their natural combination in the foods in which they occur, and how important it is to take supplements with caution. Nature requires a balance of these vitamins in the body, and too much of one may actually create a deficiency in another. When you take individual B vitamins you may upset the body's balance so that you benefit less, rather than more, by taking the additional supplement. As a general rule, all the B vitamins represented in a B-complex formula should be taken together at the same time; whether the amount contained in a particular brand is sufficient, even according to the RDA amounts, is something you should check by reading the label.

Ascorbic Acid (Vitamin C)

Foods and beverages high in ascorbic acid, such as fruits, fruit juices, and many soda beverages (see labels), can cause some drugs—for example, antidepressants—to dissolve too quickly. (See also *Iron, Oral Contraceptives.*)

Caffeine

See *Iron.*

Calcium

Rhubarb, spinach, and other foods high in oxalates can decrease the bioavailability of calcium. This effect can be offset by eating increased vitamin D and milk products that contain lactose and calcium. (See also *Lactose.*)

Colchicine

This drug, prescribed for gout, inhibits intestinal nutrient absorption, especially of vitamin B_{12}; it is not usually a problem unless taken over a prolonged period.

Vitamin D

Vitamin D increases absorption and utilization of calcium and phosphorus. When used as an additive for foods lacking it, such as milk, it is usually in the form of irradiated ergosterol from yeast.

Diuretics

Since diuretics flush water out of the system, they inevitably deplete the body of nutrients at the same time. Attention has focused on potassium depletion because diuretics are commonly given for heart conditions, such as congestive heart failure, to control edema. Since heart patients may also be taking digitalis, potassium depletion is especially serious; it may make the heart more sensitive to the effects of digitalis, and a normal dose may become an excessive one. For this reason people taking diuretics should make a point of eating a potassium-rich diet.

Vitamin E (Alpha-tocopherol)

Polyunsatured fats naturally contain vitamin E, which is an antioxidant and essential to counter their strong oxidative effects on the human body.

Manufacturers, however, sometimes process out the vitamin for separate sale, leaving the consumer without the protection nature provided. Vitamin E also favors iron absorption and protects carotene and vitamin A with its antioxidant ability.

Fats and Oils

Eating fatty foods before taking griseofulvin (for fungus infections) can cause an increase of the drug's level in the blood.

Thiamine (Vitamin B_1)

Thiamine functions as an enzyme to help the body utilize carbohydrates, oxidizing glucose to supply energy. (See also *Sulfites*.)

Hydralazine

This is another drug prescribed for high blood pressure, and it can deplete the body's supply of vitamin B_6. Taking extra amounts of the vitamin, either in supplements or in food rich in B_6, may not solve the problem, since hydralazine acts by inhibiting production of the enzyme that converts the vitamin into a form the body can use, or sometimes by combining with the vitamin to form a compound that is not metabolized but excreted.

INH

The antituberculosis drug INH acts like hydralazine to deplete vitamin B_6 by inhibiting the enzyme necessary for the human body to make use of B_6. Equally, it may instead combine with the vitamin to create a compound that the body excretes rather than utilizes.

Iron

Vitamins C and E aid iron absorption, but large quantities of chocolate, cola drinks, coffee, and diet powders may inhibit it because of their caffeine content. Soy products also interfere with iron absorption, an important point to remember when feeding young children who may have a lactase deficiency and have substituted soy milk for cow's milk. Soy products fortified with iron may mislead the consumer into assuming a higher quality of bioavailability than is actually the case. Citrus products, on the other hand, enhance iron absorption.

Isotretinoin

Prescribed for some skin diseases, this drug is not compatible with vitamin A supplements inasmuch as it is a vitamin A derivative and the combination could lead to an overdose.

Lactose

There is some evidence that lactose (milk sugar) increases calcium retention in children. It also enhances the growth of microorganisms that synthesize several of the B vitamins.

Vitamin K

One of the beneficial effects of vitamin K, enhanced clotting of the blood, can be a disadvantage if anticoagulants, to prevent or reduce clotting, have been prescribed. If such a drug is being taken, it might be wise to reduce the intake of leafy green vegetables temporarily.

Licorice

Since licorice contains a substance that can cause an elevation in blood pressure, it should not be eaten in excessive amounts. In addition, it could counteract the effect of medication taken to lower blood pressure. Licorice has long been a popular flavor for medications, but because of this, most American manufacturers now use a synthetic flavoring agent. Many imported products still contain nautral licorice and should be eaten only in limited quantities by those with problems with blood pressure levels.

MAO (Monoamine Oxidase) Inhibitors

These drugs, which are often prescribed for high blood pressure and for depression, should never be taken with foods that contain tyramine. Foods in this category include aged or fermented foods but also many that don't fall in either of those categories. Specific foods to avoid include sharp or aged cheese, Chianti and sherry wines (or any wines in excess), pickled herring, certain fermented sausages (salami, pepperoni), yogurt, sour cream, and other fermented milk products, beef and chicken livers, canned figs, fava or broad beans, avocados, soy sauce, and any active yeast preparations.

The interaction between the tyramine in these foods and MAO inhibitors can raise blood pressure to life-threatening levels, sometimes causing brain hemorrhage or even death; at the least, this combination may result in severe headaches. There is also a possibility that all the foods reacting with MAO inhibitors have not yet been identified; for instance, cola drinks, coffee, chocolate, and raisins are suspect but not proved. Anyone experiencing headaches when taking MAO should check promptly with the doctor and be prepared with a list of foods eaten within the past forty-eight hours.

Milk and Milk Products

Tetracycline prescriptions will usually contain a warning not to be taken with milk and milk products. This is because their calcium content impairs the absorption of tetracycline and, in effect, reduces the size of the dose prescribed. Not only would this affect the immediate condition for which the drug had been prescribed, but also might reduce the pescribed dose to a subclinical dose; if antibiotics are taken in subclinical doses (less than certain minimum amounts), they may create resistance to them on your part, as well as resistant bacteria and, in the long run, will be harmful rather than beneficial. (See also *Antacids.*)

Mineral Oil

Using mineral oil as a laxative may not be advisable because it depletes the body of B vitamins and also inhibits nutrient absorption by the intestine. Vitamin D absorption can be affected by as little as four teaspoons of mineral oil taken twice a day. Older people, who frequently experience constipation, are liable to use mineral oil as a "natural" laxative, and they are often also less likely to get sufficient exposure to the sun to replenish their vitamin D supply in that way. Absorption of vitamin K and carotene (a precursor of vitamin A) is also interfered with by mineral oil ingestion.

Always check laxative ingredients on the label to see if mineral oil is a primary ingredient, and ask your doctor whether it might be wiser to switch to a bulk laxative.

Neomycin

An antibiotic that acts on vitamin B_{12} in the same way as colchicine.

Oral Antidiabetic Agents

All tend to impair absorption of B_{12}, a problem if the agents are taken over a long period of time.

Oral Contraceptives

Oral contraceptives deplete folic acid and vitamin B_6, as well as increasing the need for C, B_1, B_2, B_{12}, and folacin. They may also increase blood levels of vitamin A and iron. Ideally anyone taking them should eat an especially well balanced diet in order to avoid subclinical deficiencies.

Over-the-Counter Drugs (OTC Drugs)

Since a doctor's prescription is not needed for OTC drugs, they are often taken in excessive quantities, creating nutrient deficiencies. Antacids are commonly overused and can lead to phosphate depletion. If you take an antacid regularly, you may notice muscle weakness and the symptoms of vitamin D deficiency. In any case, it would be better to eliminate the cause of the stomach upset and to discontinue eating the foods and/or beverages that are causing it.

Smoking

Tobacco smoking reduces the level of vitamin C in the blood.

Sulfites

The adverse effect of sulfites on thiamine is so well known that they have long been banned for use in meats and other foods that are particularly rich sources of thiamine.

Thyroid Medications

When taking thyroid medication, it is advisable to limit the intake of soybeans, rutabagas, brussels sprouts, turnips, cabbage, and kale. All these vegetables contain goitrogens, which inhibit production of thyroid in the body and could possibly cause goiter.

Chapter 36

Fats Under Fire— When Scientists Disagree

Using the example of the disputed role of cholesterol and fats in heart disease (HD), this chapter will deal with differences of opinion that exist among top experts in the field, as revealed in published reports over the past few years.

The 198? RDAs—A Standoff

On October 12, 1985, *The New York Times* ran an editorial headed "Standing Fast on Diet." The first paragraph read, "After intense debate, the National Academy of Sciences has made a sound decision: not to change its nutritional guidelines for Americans." The story behind the academy's decision, of critical interest to every American, follows.

Approximately every five years the RDAs are reevaluated in light of recent advances in knowledge of human nutrition, changes in the average American's life-style, disease statistics, and other factors. This is done by the Food and Nutrition Board of the National Research Council, part of the National Academy of Sciences. The board consists of fifteen scientists who meet to discuss and establish the recommended dietary allowances (RDAs).

In May 1980 the board published its dietary recommendations in a twenty-page report titled "Toward Healthful Diets." Among its findings were that there was no reason for the average healthy American to restrict consumption

---

The 1980 Food and Nutrition Board

The distinguished scientists who made up the 1980 board were as follows:

Chairman: Alfred E. Harper, department of biochemistry, University of Wisconsin, Madison

Vice Chairman: Henry Kamin, department of biochemistry, Duke University Medical Center, Durham, N.C.

Roslyn B. Alfin-Slater, division of environmental and nutritional science, University of California School of Public Health, Los Angeles

Sol H. Chafkin, Ford Foundation, New York, N.Y.

George K. Davis, nutrition laboratory, University of Florida, Gainesville

Richard L. Hall, science and technology, McCormick and Company Inc., Hunt Valley, Md.

Gail G. Harrison, department of family and community medicine, University of Arizona, Tucson

Victor Herbert, Veterans Administration Medical Center, Bronx, N.Y.

Ogden C. Johnson, scientific affairs, Hershey Foods Corporation, Hershey, Penna.

David Kritchevsky, the Wistar Institute, Philadelphia, Penna.

Robert A. Neal, department of biochemistry, Vanderbilt University School of Medicine, Nashville, Tenn.

Robert E. Olson, department of biochemistry, St. Louis University School of Medicine, St. Louis, Mo.

George M. Owen, School of Public Health, University of Michigan, Ann Arbor

William B. Robinson, Institute of Food Science, Cornell University, Geneva, N.Y.

Irwin H. Rosenberg, section of gastroenterology, University of Chicago, Chicago, Ill.

---

of cholesterol or fat intake (except to maintain normal body weight). Their basis for such a recommendation was that no clearcut evidence had been produced that reducing serum cholesterol by means of low-cholesterol diets could prevent coronary heart disease and, in addition, that the recommendations of some groups to modify saturated fats and cholesterol had not been shown to be entirely free of risk.

These recommendations burst upon the scientific community like a bombshell and reaction was strong, immediate, and vocal. The American Medical Association expressed strong approval. The American Heart Association expressed equally strong disapproval. During the news conference at which the report was presented to the press, Dr. Robert E. Olson, the board member who wrote the report, indicated that the board had been influenced by the fact that most of the evidence of adverse effects of high saturated-fat diets were based on studies of populations, and he said that such studies did not provide an adequate basis for recommending dietary modifications. Until such evidence had been provided by clinical and animal studies, he said, the board would retain its recommendations. In the text of the report the board also spoke of "concern about promising tangible benefits from controversial recommendations that could alter people's lives and habits." It further stated, "Sound nutrition is not a panacea, good food that provides appropriate proportions of nutrients should not be regarded as a poison, a medicine or a talisman. It should be eaten and enjoyed."

The recommendations were that the American diet should consist of a wide variety of foods, including "appropriate servings of dairy products, meats or legumes, vegetables and fruits, and cereal and breads"—the usual food groups that have been the basis of official diet recommendations for many years. It did, however, suggest reduction of salt intake and maintenance of normal weight.

Those of the press who disagreed with these findings made a lot of the fact that the National Dairy Council, the United Egg Producers, and the National Livestock and Meat Board were pleased with these findings, although they had never commented on the favorable attitudes of the makers of polyunsaturated oils and products, such as margarine, when previous studies that had seemed to indicate that polyunsaturates were better than saturates had been reported.

The New York Times seemed somewhat disturbed by the panel's report and recommendations but, in reporting on it, did say, "For human beings . . . the link between cholesterol and fat in the diet and heart disease is largely circumstantial." Adding, "In virtually every society yet studied, researchers have found that the more fat and cholesterol in the diet, the higher the average blood cholesterol level in the people and the higher the death rate from coronary heart disease." In other words it did not say that any connection between high serum cholesterol and heart disease had been proved, but it tacitly indicated that such a connection exists. This, of course, is exactly the "studies of population" that the board had specifically rejected as satisfactory evidence.

In spite of the *Times*'s reporters' obvious effort to objectively report on a subject on which they felt strongly, an editorial (June 3, 1980) was less tactfully worded. The Food and Nutrition Board was upset by the editorial and responded to it in a Letter to the Editor (*New York Times*, June 16,

1980) by Professor Alfred E. Harper, chairman of the Food and Nutrition Board. Dr. Harper wrote:

> The vehement and emotional reaction of the editorial staff of *The New York Times* to the publication "Toward Healthful Diets," which was released last week by the Food and Nutrition Board . . . verges on the hysterical.
>
> The board had the termerity to conclude, that, because the scientific evidence was inadequate, it could not propose a general recommendation concerning consumption of cholesterol for the U.S. population as a whole. Both the American Medical Association and the Canadian Health Protection Branch reached this conclusion three years ago. The board also concluded that it was inappropriate to make a general recommendation concerning fat consumption for the public at large. It suggested instead that recommendations with regard to fat consumption should be made specifically for different age and population groups.
>
> A June 3 editorial condemned the board for not endorsing the view that a recommendation to reduce consumption of cholesterol and fat is an appropriate public policy action for lowering the incidence of chronic degenerative diseases. Has the board been subjected to this coercive attack because it has had the effrontery to disagree with the established opinions of the editors? Are we to assume that *The Times* does not condone differences of scientific opinion? . . .

The Times certainly made whatever amends might have been called for by its editorial by publishing Dr. Harper's letter in full, under the fair heading "Fat, Cholesterol and Free Scientific Inquiry."

By the April 1981 issue of *The Harvard Medical School Health Letter,* further commentary had appeared. As the letter summed it up under the heading "The Cholesterol Controversy" (not apparently in any reference to Dr. Pinckney's book of the same name):

> The question of whether cholesterol is bad for us has been very much in the news since the National Research Council last summer suggested that there was insufficient evidence to recommend dietary changes. This year began with a renewal of the controversy when the January 8 issue of *The New England Journal of Medicine* printed a report supporting the theory that increased cholesterol and fat in the diet do increase the risk for heart disease. However, just one week later, the January 16 issue of the *Journal of the American Medical Association* carried a report from the Framingham Heart Study suggesting that low levels of blood

cholesterol in men correlate with an increased risk of cancer. Obviously, all of this becomes confusing for the person trying to decide whether to reduce cholesterol and fat in his or her diet. Dr. Donald Berwick, a pediatrician, is a health practice analyst for the Harvard School of Public Health and co-author of a book from that institution entitled *Cholesterol, Children and Heart Disease*. We have asked him to sort out this controversy and to address the ultimate question, "What should we do about our diet?"

Dr. Berwick agreed that the evidence was circumstantial but felt it sufficient to implicate serum cholesterol in heart disease. His recommendations were the usual ones: reduce the amount of fat in the diet, substitute polyunsaturated fats for saturated fats. He agreed that the Framingham Heart Study and other studies have "suggested that people with low cholesterol levels and people who take cholesterol-lowering drugs may increase their risk of having cancer," but dismissed it with the comment, "The meaning of this result is still unclear." Of course, given the lack of consensus in the scientific community, the letter could probably just as easily have come up with an expert who would have agreed with the board's recommendations. Another opinion, one way or the other, did not really resolve the consumer's dilemma.

Three years later the matter still had not been sorted out, nor had a consensus been reached, but the tide seemed to be turning for cholesterol. *The New York Times* (November 21, 1984), in discussing margarine, wrote, ". . . confusion regarding margarine's health benefits is still widespread, fostered by contentions in some scientific quarters that the role of fats and cholesterol . . . in heart disease has been overemphasized and that the methods used to make margarine negate some of its potential benefits to the heart create possible cancer hazards. . . . there is no ironclad evidence to support one view or another . . ." And instead of recommending replacing saturated with unsaturated fats, the article reflected more recent scientific opinion in stating, "Heart experts generally suggest that a third [of dietary fats] come from saturates, a third from monounsaturates and the rest from polyunsaturates." Since statistics indicate that the average American consumes two-thirds of his or her fats as saturates, this still amounts to a recommendation that the amount of the saturated fat ingested be reduced, but it does give it an equal place in the diet with polyunsaturates, and it does refer to the newest thinking that for health reasons all fats, regardless of what kind, should be reduced to the point that they comprise no more than 30 percent or less of the total calories consumed.

The article also takes note of the possible carcinogenic effects of margarine consumption due to the creation of trans fatty acids by the process of hydrogenation. Trans fatty acids are unnatural substances that have not only been linked to increased risk of cancer but may also negate the supposed cholesterol-lowering benefits of polyunsaturates. In addition, they may interefere with the formation of essential body chemicals, prostaglandins. When to these adverse effects of substituting butter for margarine is added the dangers referred to in the previous chapter of cooking with polyunsaturated fats (through the creation of toxic, cancer-causing substances), the unproved possibility that the cholesterol and saturated fat in butter may be unhealthful seems like a small risk. And there is no question that butter still tastes better and is a more natural product.

Unfortunately, the *Times* article closes with the recommendation, contrary to the thrust of the article as a whole, that after you reduce overall consumption of fat, you "consider replacing whatever saturated fats remain in the diet with unsaturated ones." This seems to ignore what the article has just said about reducing all fats in a one-third to one-third to one-third ratio, and about the possible dangers of margarine and of hydrogenated fats in general.

By December 13, 1984, a panel convened by the prestigious National Institutes of Health was back to recommending that Americans reduce dietary cholesterol—only this time the recommendation was tempered slightly by the phrase "especially those [Americans] considered to have a high cholesterol level," and by less extreme dietary restrictions, such as, "eat less butter, margarine, oil and other fats over all, and replace some or all animal fats with margarine and oil.""Less butter" and "some animal fats," represented a considerable advance over "no butter" and "all animal fats" in earlier recommendations.

The panel did, however, take the position in their report that elevated blood cholesterol is a direct cause of heart disease and not just an associated risk factor. Their conclusions were based on a wide range of evidence, presumably gathered from both sides of the cholesterol fence. This included the recently completed NIH study called the Lipid Research Clinics Coronary Primary Prevention Trial (CPPT), sponsored by the National Heart, Lung and Blood Institute.

The CPPT study showed that reducing high serum cholesterol could reduce the incidence of heart attacks. It was conducted among 3800 middle-aged men with serum cholesterol levels of at least 265 milligrams per deciliter of blood (in the top 5 percent of adult Americans' serum-cholesterol levels). It was hoped that this study would at last persuade the majority of physicians to encourage their patients to crack down on thier cholesterol intake. (A 1984 study by the National Heart, Lung and Blood Institute had revealed that of sixteen hundred physicians, only 39 percent subscribed to the choles-

The 1984 National Institutes of Health Panel

The distinguished scientists who made up the NIH panel and arrived at findings the opposite of the Food and Nutrition Board:

Dr. Daniel Steinberg, chairman and professor of medicine, University of California, San Diego

Dr. Sidney Blumenthal, former senior consultant in health sciences, Columbia University, New York, N.Y.

Dr. Richard Carleton, chief of cardiology, Memorial Hospital, Providence, R.I.

Nancy Chasen, public interest attorney, Bethesda, Md.

Dr. James Dalen, physician-in-chief, University of Massachusetts Medical Center, Worcester, Ma.

John T. Fitzpatrick, attorney, Fairfield, Ct.

Dr. Stephen B. Hulley, professor of epidemiology and medicine, University of California, San Francisco, Ca.

Dr. Gregory O'Keefe III, Island Community Medical Center, Vinalhaven, Maine.

Dr. Elijah Saunders, head of division of hypertension, University of Maryland School of Medicine, Baltimore, Md.

Dr. Robert E. Shank, professor of preventive medicine, Washington University School of Medicine, St. Louis, Mo.

Dr. Arthur A. Spector, professor of biochemistry, University of Iowa, Iowa City, Iowa.

Dr. Robert W. Wissler, professor of pathology, University of Chicago, Chicago, Ill.

Dr. Richard D. Remington, vice president for academic affairs, University of Iowa, Iowa, City, Iowa.

---

terol-equals-heart-disease theory.) Unfortunately the study didn't include any women; it included only the middle-aged, those with high cholesterol, and those who took cholestyramine (a cholesterol-lowering drug) daily. The control group received a placebo so as not to give the plan away. The results showed 155 heart attacks in the group on the drug; 187 for those taking the placebo.

Though the panel had no problem indicting cholesterol as the villain, other experts did not always agree. One who disagreed was Dr. Edward H. Ahrens, Jr., head of the cholesterol metabolism laboratory at Rockefeller University, who felt cholestyramine played an important part in the results. Other critics thought it questionable that the results of a study among such a specialized group should be applied to healthy adults of other ages. No studies seem to have been done to date among those with normal cholesterol levels, and whether lowering their cholesterol would be healthful or harmful is completely unknown. (See also Chapter 30, The RDAs—What They Really Mean.)

Where Does This Lack of Consensus Leave the Consumer?

The 1980 Food and Nutrition Board and the 1984 National Institutes of Health Panel consist of distinguished experts, whose credentials are impressive—at least to a layman—yet they cannot agree on whether high serum cholesterol has been shown to cause heart disease and whether it is advisable to eat as little saturated fat and as much polyunsaturated fat as possible. On the other hand, studies have been reported to the public that heart disease may be caused by many factors, of which cholesterol may be only one, and that polyunsaturates may have some definitely undesirable effects.

The lesson to be learned from this lack of consensus is that nutrition is a science apparently still in its infancy, and no guidelines, no matter how impeccable their source, should be considered cast in concrete. Avoiding dietary extremes will save the consumer from making any serious mistakes as well as permitting a life-style that is much easier to follow. As is shown throughout this book, the conclusions of preliminary reports are sometimes presented as established fact, longheld nutrition "truths" are discovered to be myths, and we constantly must question our premises in light of new knowledge.

In addition, even if we wish to take heed of current guidelines, we need to be sure they are being accurately represented. To use fats as an example once again, the American Heart Association's current recommendations suggest approximately equal intake of the three kinds of fats—saturated, polyunsaturated, and monounsaturated—yet you will frequently see this presented only as "The ideal diet should consist of no more than 30 percent fat, of which only 10 percent should be saturated." I find that most consumers interpret this statement to mean the ratio should be 10 percent saturated to 20 percent unsaturated fat, which is not at all what the American Heart Association is recommending.

PART SEVEN

Taking Charge of Your Life and Your Health

Chapter 37

How to Cope with the Changing American Diet

Americans are not eating the way their grandparents did; they couldn't even if they wanted to. Changing life-styles, urbanization of the population, growth of agribusiness, increased food transportation and processing, information and misinformation about good nutrition, changing patterns of health and disease—all have had their effect on what America eats.

Changing Life-styles

Two-family incomes are becoming the norm, and as the number of full-time housewives decreases, so does the amount of home cooking in American households. Today it is estimated that forty cents of every dollar spent on food goes for restaurant or take-out food, and that figure is rising steadily. When both partners work, both are liable to be too tired, too busy, and too disinclined to cook at home. Singles are even less likely to prepare a meal for themselves (and the number of singles in the population is also growing). This change in life-style affects not only what Americans are eating but often means a loss in nutrition through further processing and handling of food. It also means less control over the content of one's food and makes it harder to detect nonfood, the fake food that physically fills the stomach without nourishing the body.

Diet and nutrition books are full of tips on how to stay on your diet when eating out; it isn't easy. Hamburgers, pizza, french fries, sweet rolls, and those cute little loaves of bread that come on their own bread boards with a little bread knife are not the best foods for a steady healthful diet.

In addition, most restaurant food is different from home-cooked food, even if you eat what you would have made at home. Broiling a steak at home can easily be accomplished without additional fat, but the restaurant often pampers you by tossing on butter or brushing with oil. And since labor costs are greater than food costs for restaurants, methods of cooking are usually chosen on the basis of how expeditious they are. That butter is often used because it makes it easier to broil something rather than because the dish requires it. Without the extra fat, greater care must be taken if foods are not to dry out, stick, and become messy to clean up—which explains why you often get your broiled restaurant-prepared fish (ordered for its cholesterol-lowering properties) literally—and unappetizingly—swimming in butter.

In addition to problems of preparation, there is the difficulty of knowing whether restaurant food is real or fake. In the supermarket it is up to the consumer to read and decipher the information on the label; in a restaurant you may not know about the imitation cheese on your pizza, the imitation whipped cream on your imitation ice cream, and the imitation hard-boiled eggs in your egg sandwich.

Urbanization of the Population

Small local farms have almost disappeared. State after state is now passing laws allowing farmland to be appraised on a different, lower basis if the heirs agree to use it only as farmland; before those laws were passed, or where they still do not exist, the inheritance appraisal of farmland is the price it would bring if sold to developers. The children of farmers could not afford the tax burdens of this new appraisal and potential farmers were being lost to the nation as the sons and daughters were forced to sell the land to pay the taxes.

Appearances can be misleading. Connecticut, for example, looks rural because it has more forestland today than it did in colonial times, but most of the local farms are gone. Twenty years ago residents of Westport, Wilton, and other Fairfield County towns an hour or so from New York City could buy rich, creamy milk, cheese, ice cream, and heavy cream (not ultrapasteurized) from local dairies. You could even get milk that was not homogenized. Farmers in every town sold their own fresh-killed turkeys and chickens, eggs, and every kind of fresh vegetable in season. The apple orchards telegraphed their presence in the fall by the scent of ripe, fresh apples as soon as you came within two or three miles of the cider mill, and the cider was tangy and sweet, without a hint of preservative or pasteurization.

In just two decades most of these sources of fresh food have disappeared; housing developments have risen on the farmland, and people drive for miles to shop at the few farmers' markets that remain. Our fresh produce now comes from thousands of miles away—often from other countries. We gain, to some extent, in variety but lose in nutrition, freshness, and flavor, and in the intangible benefits to the human spirit that come from being in contact with food that has been freshly gathered.

Growth of Agribusiness

One of the reasons for the decline of the small farmer is the growth of large farming businesses that are run by businessmen, trained in profit-and-loss, cost-benefit, bottom-line practices. The product, instead of being automobiles or refrigerators, just happens to be food, but as little concession as possible is made to that fact; the emphasis is on how to increase the profit margin, not on the taste, nutrition, or intergrity of a crop. The infamous plastic tomato of winter supermarkets, picked unripe before the flavor components can develop, ripened by gas to look like a tomato, bred to be as hardy as a tennis ball so as to withstand the rigors of harvesting, sorting, packing, and shipping, designed through selective breeding to be uniform in size and shape so that it can be processed by machines instead of people, is the ideal "food" crop. It is bought almost exclusively to add a touch of color to salads and garnishes; it is certainly not bought for its flavor or texture.

There are other disadvantages to mega-agriculture besides the quality of the food it produces. Chemical fertilizers are more "efficient" than natural fertilizers, but continued use of chemical fertilizers creates dead soil. Soil bacteria, which are essential to the creation of topsoil (the only natural material plants can grown in), and which make soil nutrients available to plants, cannot feed on chemical fertilizers; they must have organic material. Without organic material, their soil factories shut down, and instead of being a living source of nutrients, the soil becomes a holding medium for chemicals. Chemical fertilizers will grow crops, but these crops will contain only a few limited nutrients and usually none of the trace elements, which more and more we are discovering to be essential to healthy human growth. For years there were some soil scientists who insisted that plants would contain the same nutrients regardless of the fertility of the soil in which they were grown; somehow these scientists were never called upon to explain why we then had to add iodine to food raised on soil away from our sea coasts but not to crops grown on soil near the sea. We now know that food grown in depleted soil will be depleted in nutrition, and we are being confronted with actual nationwide subclinical deficiences of elements such as zinc. And one of the ways in which a zinc deficiency in food plants may be created is overfertilization with phosphorus—one of the three chief nutrients provided by chemical fertilizers.

Another disadvantage to agribusiness is the tendency to grow single crops. From a planting, raising, and harvesting standpoint, it is more efficient and profitable to grow large areas of a single crop. This crop has usually been developed into a single hybrid bred genetically for qualities that are desirable from a manufacturing and distribution standpoint. Growing a single strain of a single food—whether potatoes, wheat, corn, or other plant— creates a wonderfully easy opportunity for the insects, bacteria, and diseases compatible to that crop to destroy it. Efforts have been made, especially in Canada, to maintain a seed bank of discarded strains so that, in the event of a worldwide catastrophe—brought about because we have spread this one-strain, one-crop system throught the globe—we will be able to grow plants resistant to the organisms that have destroyed the one hybrid strain everyone was growing. Rice and wheat, both of which have been very heavily hybridized, are considered especially vulnerable to destruction.

Increased Food Processing and Distant Transportation

When food is big business, it makes sense to centralize and mechanize its production as much as possible. And since agribusiness often involves the food processor as well as the grower, it is natural that plants should be bred both to produce as much as possible in a given space and to produce food with the characteristics best suited to its processing.

Inevitably, centralization means most consumers live far from the point of origin of their food, and since nutrients are lost with every minute that passes after the moment of picking, even fresh produce has probably lost nutrients by the time it reaches the consumer. And since the fresh appearance of the food is compromised by too long an interval between harvesting and selling (appearance is highly regarded for its sales appeal), methods have had to be devised to create at least the appearance of freshness (see Chapter 9, Forever Fresh—The Sulfite Story). The waxing of fruits and vegetables is an example of the ingenuity that has been applied to this problem (see Chapter 19, Tracking Down Real Fruit).

Never has there been a time when so many Americans have been so conscious of nutrition. Unfortunately, there has also never been a time when the consumer has been bombarded with so much fragmented information and misinformation. The RDAs are a weak reed to lean on (see Chapter 30, The RDAs—What They Really Mean), and in an increasingly competitive marketplace, advertising is growing more and more misleading. Television provides snippets of information in one-minute segments, and the print media jump on every bandwagon ("The Danger of a Calcium-Deficiency to American Womanhood"), with a weather eye kept on possible advertisers. The growth of such consumer organizations as the Center for Science in the Pulbic Interest, with their serious and informative publications, shows how hungry the public is for basic facts clearly presented, yet confusion is rampant.

Changing Patterns of Health and Diseases

All this might not be so serious if it were not undermining our health. Although we brag about having eliminated many of the infectious diseases, others, such as heart disease, cancer, birth defects, hospital-related infections, and new diseases, such as Legionnaire's Disease and AIDS, have more than taken their place. Many of these diseases have long, or even unknown, periods of incubation; the state of the nation's health twenty or thirty years from now cannot even be guessed at.

How Americans Have Changed Their Diet

American sugar consumption is now at its highest in history—an average of 850 calories per person per day. Eighty-two percent of it comes from processed foods: from breakfast cereals, vegetable juices, bread, salad dressings, canned vegetables, candy, ice cream, pastry, soup, and sauces—every time the American consumer markets, loads of hidden sugar come home along with the groceries.

In an effort to cut down on voluntary sugar intake—the ten teaspoons of sugar in a can of Coca-Cola, for example—Americans have turned to a dubious alternative. Artificial sweeteners have not generally proved to be a safe substitute for sugar, however, and whether aspartame, the newest candidate, will prove as undesirable as cyclamates and saccharin remains to be seen.

At the present time Americans are still consuming between 40 and 50 percent of their calories in fats—52.6 pounds per person per year. To be sure, many have switched to a larger proportion of unsaturated fats (which, as we have seen, may be an unhealthful thing to do), in an effort to lower their cholesterol. Many authorities recommend lowering this intake to 30 percent or less, but it isn't that easy, because here again, hidden fats account for much of the total. There is a growing use of liquid oils by food processors, and fast-food outlets have been criticized for their excessive use of beef fat, tallow, and palm oil (even higher in saturated fat than beef fat) in the preparation of their fish and chicken dishes and their french fries. Both these food sources are heavily utilized by the working consumer. It is the processed foods, not the pat of butter we add to our baked potato, that are the major source of our dietary fat, and their hidden calories (a fast-food baked potato with topping may hide more than 1½ grams of fat in its "deluxe" depths) that make it difficult to keep track of fat intake.

Consumption of whole grains and whole grain products has decreased markedly. White bread and wheat bread (brown, but not made with whole wheat) have replaced whole-grain baked products. Hot cereals, such as oatmeal, are eaten much less than formerly, and their sugary cold-cereal replacements, even when fortified to the hilt, are no substitute.

Salt is still eaten in excessive amounts—15 grams per person per day. But many manufacturers rely solely on salt to supply the "flavor" of their products, and consumers respond by buying those products instead of more wholesome—but less salty—items. Now that high blood pressure is in the news and low-salt diets are recommended to alleviate it, Americans are trying to cut down on their salt intake. Yet even if you throw out the family salt shaker, you still have to contend with salt in almost every processed food you buy; a snack of potato chips or salted peanuts is enough to put you over your ideal daily ration. It is an uphill battle at best, and some of the strategies, such as overuse of potassium salt substitutes, may create more problems than they solve.

At the turn of the century the American diet derived about 30 percent of its protein from animal foods. Today the figure is up to 70 percent. In recent years red meat has been indicted as a source of cholesterol; and recently we have been told to cut down on protein intake in favor of carbohydrates. The beef industry is unhappily trying to grow leaner, more pesticide- and antibiotic-residue-free meat, but Americans may never go back to the consumption of steaks and beef roasts in the amounts of just a few years ago. On the other hand, in spite of the proliferation of salad bars and pasta salads, the year-round distribution of fresh produce is not being fully utilized. Consumption of fresh fruit, of which Americans once ate 134.7 pounds per person per year, has dropped to 83.2 pounds per person per year. Fresh vegetables have mostly given way to processed vegetables, which, although consumed in greater quantities (62.5 pounds on the average today, compared to 14.5 pounds in 1910), do not contain the nutrients of garden-fresh vegetables, and, if canned, often contain considerable added salt. We are consuming great quantities of potatoes, but mostly in the form of french fries, both frozen and fast food (the industry uses more than 75 percent of the total amount of frozen french fries packed each year). Potatoes are a good food, normally low in fat, but french fries have more than eight times as much fat as a baked potato (you could even add that pat of butter and still come out ahead).

The Silver Lining

Although the average woman spends less time in the kitchen than she used to, the average man spends more—barely, but more. A much larger proportion of consumers are asking questions about nutrition and are concerned about additives, pesticides, and artificial ingredients. The consumer is becoming more sophisticated about nutrition advice and more skeptical if it comes from industry sources. Beef producers are responding to the drop in sales by trying to persuade the consumers that they are growing leaner beef and using few antibiotics in its preparation; the pork producers are responding to the concern over fatty meats by developing pork that is much leaner than it has ever been. Low-salt foods are now available in supermarkets instead of only in a small corner of one shelf in a health-food store, and low-fat foods are being promoted, although it will take better labeling to reveal whether they are really as low in fat as the consumer thinks they are. Low-calorie frozen dinners are being exposed by consumer groups when their labels are not quite accurate as to the number of calories contained within.

These examples show that people power can change the ways of food manufacturers: if you won't buy it, they will try to make it better. Sales speak louder than words.

USDA Extension Service branches throughout the country are monitoring food products within their states and producing clear, readable, informative material, analyzing various types of food items, and these are available to the public. Nutrition information is no longer relegated to the "women's pages" (which no longer exist as such) of newspapers but appears in high-circulation publications such as *Reader's Digest* and *Family Circle,* and in many unexpected publications.

Rich French cooking has been lightened up, thanks to nouvelle cuisine, which has been replaced by even simpler, more sensible food, which is even presented as food, not as an art form. Heavy sauces and cream soups

Dietary Guidelines to Lower Cancer Risk

Recommendations from the American Institute for Cancer Research

1. Reduce the intake of dietary fat, both saturated and unsaturated, from the current average of approximately 40 percent to a level of 30 percent of total kilocalories.
2. Increase the consumption of fruits, vegetables, and whole-grain cereals.
3. Minimize the consumption of salt-cured, smoked, or charcoal-broiled foods.
4. Drink alcoholic beverages only in moderation.

Liberal consumption of dark green and deep yellow fruits and vegetables; vitamin C–rich fruits and vegetables; other fruits and vegetables; dried beans and peas; whole grains and whole-grain cereals is recommended. Enriched or refined grains are omitted, as the institute carefully explains, "not because foods made from these products are harmful, but because they have a lower density of some important nutrients . . . [they] do not have to be omitted from the diet, but cannot be substituted for whole grains. . . ."

Moderate consumption of low-fat milk, yogurt, and cheese; lean meat, fish, and poultry is recommended.

Very moderate consumption is recommended for whole milk, high-fat cheese; nuts and seeds; eggs; fatty meats; salt-cured, smoked, and charcoal-broiled foods; sausage and game. Part of the difference between the moderate and very moderate consumption groups is that while both provide protein, the very moderate group is high in fat.

Sparse consumption is recommended for the "empty calorie group," including rich desserts, sweets, fats and oils, and alcohol.

are offered less often, though rich desserts are more popular than ever.

The public has increasingly embraced foods that were once eaten only by health freaks—yogurt, tofu, sunflower and pumpkin seeds, tropical fruits (besides pineapple and bananas), and vegetables like snow peas, avocados, and salad greens other than the ubiquitous and not particularly nutritious iceberg lettuce.

Scientists are discovering that scurvy and beri-beri are not the only deficiency diseases. As evidence is mounting that diet may contribute to, if not actually cause, illness. It is also being recognized that it is sometimes possible to cure illness through diet.

We are beginning to discover that consumers are not homogeneous, and that we need to know ourselves and what our needs are. Slide-rule nutrition that says everyone should eat this much of this and that much of that doesn't work, because of our individual needs and differences. It's more work to have to listen to your body, but it's rewarding.

It's almost never too late to help yourself to better health. If you stop smoking, your lungs will immediately begin to recover from their damaged state. If you start eating right, your body will gratefully try to get back on course. If you exercise sensibly, your cholesterol may go down, the flab may firm up, and your eyes may start to sparkle. We're not only living longer, we are often given second—and third and fourth—chances to correct our earlier mistakes and improve the quality of the life ahead of us.

Some Americans are not living as well as they used to and some Americans are living better than they used to; which way you choose is up to you.

Chapter 38

Making the Most of Real Food

You know by now that eating well isn't going to be easy. On the other hand, I hope you also realize that it isn't impossible. What you need are guidelines to help you make wise choices. Menus are all very well, but no compilation of menus can take care of all occasions—or the rest of your life. You need the ability to determine for yourself what the best foods are, how and where to compromise, and what are the hard, what the easy choices. Real food is out there, and consumer demand for it will increase the supply.

Here is an annotated checklist to guide you.

Your Real Food Checklist

1. Eat a balanced diet.

   A balanced diet means eating the range of nutrients the human body requires for optimum health. It used to be thought this was necessary every day, but averaging food intake every three days is now considered by many experts a satisfactory procedure. It used to be thought, for instance, that we needed to eat a complete protein at one sitting to get the full protein benefit. If we ate rice at breakfast and beans at lunch (a complete protein combination), it was thought to be less desirable than a lunch of both rice and beans. The latest thinking seems to be that the different kinds of protein can be eaten at different times of the day and that they will still be utilized as complete.

Aim at a balanced diet by choosing from the old reliable Basic Four Food Groups—milk, meat, vegetables and fruit, and bread and cereal.

Milk includes all milk products. Meat includes fish, eggs, legumes, and cheese as well as meat. Vegetables and fruit are best fresh, next best frozen. Eat some raw and some steamed or lightly cooked. Bread and cereal should come only from whole-grain products. Corn is good food but should not be eaten to the exclusion of whole grains. Rice should preferably be brown, or converted if you want white.

Servings need not be large. Three ounces of meat or fish is an adequate day's supply. If you tolerate milk products, they can be eaten in greater quantity. A quart of milk a day may not be too much if you are limited in other foods.

It's unlikely you will eat too much of either vegetables or fruit; enjoy them fully. Whole-grain products can be an easy source of valuable dietary fibers and can make quick, easy, wholesome meals—think of the wide variety of open and closed sandwiches, the range of pastas, the good-for-you hot and cold breakfast cereals. If you choose carefully what you eat them with, bread and cereal products are not fattening and are an excellent source of good-quality carbohydrates. If you are cutting down on your fat intake, they will fill you up, keep you from getting hungry between meals, make a good snack (whole rye crackers with a dab of cottage cheese or some mashed sliced banana), and contribute valuable nutrients.

2. Eat a variety of food.

One of the dangers of following suggested menus is that you will get into a rut. Even when substitutes are offered, you may be too busy or too tired to juggle them and end up eating the same old thing week after week.

There's a whole wonderful world of foods out there. Eating should be an adventure, not a chore. By eating a variety of foods, you almost guarantee yourself a more rounded diet, and you are bound to minimize intake of any one group of chemicals. Next to avoiding chemical additives entirely, the best thing is to eat a little of a lot of different kinds. If you vary your diet, you will automatically do this.

You may not realize that it's easier to eat a wider variety of foods if you cook from scratch. Take something as basic as an egg. You can eat it scrambled, fried, boiled, poached, coddled, curried on toast, in an eggnog, Benedict, in a custard, in a cake, as meringue (egg white only), in a potato salad—the list is endless. And the same is true of every food you can think of. A can of soup is just a can of that kind of soup. A stockpot of chicken broth is zucchini soup, cream of broccoli, pot au feu, rice pilaf (try it with parsley and pine nuts), chicken pot pie, sautéed cucumbers, and a better cold remedy than almost anything in your medicine chest. (And I haven't scratched the surface of the possibilities.)

Once you get over the idea that cooking is boring and discover the relaxation of preparing your own delicious *real* food, you'll have a lot of fun. It's a great way to make friends or entertain; letting people loose in the kitchen is a guaranteed ice-breaker. Start with easy things and work up. Broiling a free-range chicken with a dash of garlic powder and a sprinkle of lemon juice, and tossing a mixed green and vegetable salad with your own vinaigrette dressing (olive oil, vinegar or more lemon juice, paprika, dry mustard, a dash of hot pepper) takes all of twenty minutes and is a gourmet meal.

The next night you can mix the left-over salad (dressing and all) in the blender, and heat slightly while you cook spaghetti. The salad becomes the vegetable and the sauce, the spaghetti is good carbohydrate, and the real Parmesan cheese you sprinkle on freely is the protein. The whole meal is quick, delicious, cheap, and fit for company. Fruit for dessert, of course.

3. Eat moderately.

If you enjoy your food, you will savor it. It's surprising how much easier it is to eat smaller portions when what you're eating is worth tasting and stopping to enjoy. Fast food is prepared and served— and eaten—like fast food. You deserve more pleasure out of your food than that.

Real food is easier to enjoy than fake food because it has more subtleties of taste and texture. Once your palate has become used to real food, you will be amazed at how much alike most fake food tastes, partly because it usually contains too much salt and sugar and too little actual flavor.

Eating moderately will lead you to focus on quality rather than quantity. Your figure, your health, and your life-style will all benefit. It's fun to discover you can tell the difference between good food and poor food. You don't have to be able to tell what wine it is from a single sip, but it's interesting to recognize the various spices and have some notion of how a sauce has been put together. You'll never be lonely again when you become interested in quality food— and you'll make interesting friends.

4. Be relaxed.

Some people get so uptight about nutrition that they forget that eating is one of life's natural pleasures. Think of a kitten lapping up a bowl of cream with closed eyes, a puppy gnawing away at a bone (and later burying it for future enjoyment). When you see scenes of African lions tearing away at their lunch, they don't look tense and starving—they look happy.

Our world is full of schoolchildren tossing unopened or half-eaten sandwiches in the school trash, dieting women picking with resignation and distaste at lettuce leaves, men enduring their tasteless (because salt-free) chicken. It needn't be that way. Real food and variety and moderation will restore these jaded appetites. If you don't have the build you may not be as thin as you like, but if you eat right, you certainly won't be fat and you'll be bursting with vitality and the joie de vivre that is much more attractive than skinny nervousness. Women are told they cannot be too rich or too thin so they lose the fun of inexpensive pleasures (sunsets are free and good food doesn't have to be costly) and normal meals. Comfort people with good food simply prepared; they will bless you, and you will never lack for friends.

5. Avoid processed foods.

The more somebody else has done to your food, the less nutritious and real it is. If you are making rice, don't buy it with all sorts of flavors or vegetables or other ingredients. Make brown or converted rice and add your own nuts, vegetables, herbs, or spices. It takes only a minute, for heaven's sake, and eliminates all the unnecessary additives and artificial flavors, and you can stretch one pot of rice to several different dishes on different nights. You food budget will shrink, and your health and well-being will bloom.

Don't settle for instant. Quick Quaker Oats take five minutes; you'll never convince me you can't get up five minutes earlier to eat a tasty, hearty, cancer-preventing hot cereal instead of the instant that you make by pouring hot water in a bowl. If you need any more convincing, compare the ingredients in instant products and the real thing.

If you absolutely, positively need that extra five minutes of sleep, eat cold cereal, but eat real cold cereal, like Grape Nuts, not a candy bar cut up in small pieces with fruit flakes. Candy bars are not fit for breakfast, and the heavily sugared cereals TV tells kids they like are just that. You wouldn't send your children off to school with a chocolate bar, but if you let them eat a bowl of cereal whose only real value is the milk that wets it down, the effect is the same. One well-known professor of nutrition at Rutgers University was once asked by a group of food technologists to whom he was lecturing what he thought of cold cereal. It was a daring question, and the audience was hushed, waiting for his answer. The professor waited a moment, then grinned and said, "I think cold cereal is great . . . It gives texture to milk."

Why eat instant mashed potatoes? Read the label. Real potatoes are good food and not fattening. Serve them with yogurt instead of butter and milk or sour cream, if you need to. Chances are you could use the small amount of butter and milk that is needed to make superlative mashed potatoes and simply omit a fast-food lunch or some other processed food you eat almost automatically without thinking of its fat content.

Consider eating good wholesome butter instead of margarine. Here again, what are you avoiding, and at what price to nutrition? And wouldn't you be better off cutting down on the fancy TV dinners or "buttered" popcorn at the movies?

Speaking of popcorn, it's good food and satisfactorily filling. Just leave out the butter and salt; you may be really surprised at how good it tastes. Ask at the movies to have the "butter" (it isn't really, of course) and salt left off, and enjoy your movie and your snack that much more.

Why buy peanut butter with "less sugar"? Peanut butter is good food, but it doesn't need *any* sugar and you can buy peanut butter made with nothing but peanuts. Why settle for less than the real thing?

6. Buy fresh foods fresh.

By now you are probably getting the idea. Buy fresh fruits and vegetables. Don't try to buy too far ahead. If you must buy ahead, handle it carefully at home so that as few nutrients are lost as possible. All through the book are lots of tips; you'll gradually learn smart storage as well as smart shopping.

If lettuce or cabbage has been "trimmed," buy heads that haven't. The outer leaves are a giveaway if vegetables are tired; that's why they are removed.

If fruit or vegetables are heavily waxed, ask your produce manager whether he can get any that aren't. Maybe you can buy more produce in season and learn to make more use of true winter vegetables when the others have to travel from Brazil or Mexico to get to your table. Save your money and get more nutrition for it by not rushing the season—the first strawberry, the first peach, the first grapefruit are the most expensive, the poorest quality, and the least nutritious. Why not wait and get your money's worth?

Frozen foods may have more nutrition than tired, out-of-season fresh. Just avoid those that are combined, sauced, or otherwise added to. If it's something you can do in your own kitchen, you'll be better off doing it there. And you'll save enough to get some timesaving appliances if cutting and chopping is a chore.

7. Be adventurous.

Try different combinations. The first person to think of chopping cranberries with raw oranges broke new ground and scored a hit. Nouvelle cuisine involves mostly lighter sauces and unusual combinations, often introducing fruits to dishes that never had them before.

You don't have to have a winner every time. How often have you read a review of an expensive new restaurant only to find the reviewing commenting, "The duck à la kiwi, however, didn't quite make it and at $20 a portion was especially disappointing." If you strike out, grin and add some cheese and yogurt to the scrambled eggs and sprinkle with parsley before serving as a substitute. (It helps to have some blueberry muffins in the freezer that you can warm up.)

Better Bacon

Bacon is used not only as a breakfast treat or a garnish to a mixed grill, but also crumbled in salads and to enhance grilled cheese sandwiches, burgers, and many other foods. Aside from the question of its nitrite content (which vitamin C is said to counteract to some extent), the problem with bacon has always been how to get rid of the fat.

A quick and easy solution is to microwave the bacon strips for 4 or 5 minutes at high power, then let them "rest" for another 4 or 5 minutes. The trick is to use a baking dish with a grill or gravy channels. All the fat will drip down out of the way and only crisp, perfectly cooked strips of meat will be left. Just be sure to cover the bacon with a sheet of paper toweling before turning on the power so the fat doesn't splatter.

You can make all sorts of dips, butters, and cheese spreads just by looking at the selection at the store and duplicating them at home. Instead of paying $3 for a small carton of cucumber spread, take a few minutes to peel and quarter a cucumber and an onion and blend them with cottage or cream cheese. Violà. And think of the money you've saved. Just be brave and try it. What can you lose?

Men are great cooks and very inventive. If you're a man and you've never cooked, discover your hidden talent and do yourself good at the same time. I never knew a man who couldn't cook once he really gave it a try.

8. Avoid the artificial.

Artificial colors, artificial flavors, and chemical additives are not in your best interests. You needn't try to eliminate them totally if that is difficult, but make an effort to avoid them as much as possible. Read the labels; compare brands.

Some of your aches and pains may be due to sensitivities to some of these additives, or you may be allergic to them. Try to eat additive-free and see how your health improves.

Extralean Hamburger—Is It Better?

While consumers are cutting back on overall beef consumption, hamburgers remain popular because they are quick to prepare and tasty. In an effort to cut down on fat and cholesterol intake, some consumers are paying premium prices for chopped meat labeled lean or extralean; the question is whether it is any better than the regular ground beef.

A number of studies have been done recently and all have come to much the same conclusion: you're better off with the regular hamburger than with the fancier, and more expensive, versions. For instance, a recent study by nutritionists Kenneth Prusa, Ph.D., and Karla Hughes, Ph.D., of the University of Missouri–Columbia, found that the act of broiling the burgers got rid of most of the extra fat but left a tasty burger. Lean and extralean lost not only fat but also moisture and came out dryer and tougher.

On Your Own

Well—you're on your own, but you're not unarmed. And best of all, you can take charge of your own life and health if you want to. It may be a little work—but so is jogging or aerobics or job hunting or dressing for success or taking a trip or raising a family or anything worth doing. And like all those things, taking charge of your own life brings a wonderful sense of accomplishment and satisfaction.

Appendix

Where to Get Information About Specific Products

Here are the names and addresses of some of the major food and beverage corporations. In addition, some companies now feature toll-free "800" telephone numbers on their packages. If the company you want to call is not listed below, check the product package or call the 800 Directory Assistance operator. If there is no 800 number, you can obtain the regular phone number of any corporation from your local library.

Do not hesitate to ask the company for a list of ingredients or for nutrition information about its food or beverage product. Your request will show the manufacturer that you care about your health, and may result in product improvements.

Anheuser Busch, Inc.
One Busch Pl.
St. Louis, Mo. 63118
Manager, Consumer Relations
314-577-3093

A&P Supermarkets
Great Atlantic and Pacific Tea Co.
2 Paragon Drive
Montvale, N.J. 07645
Consumer Relations Manager
201-573-9700

Armour Food Products
15101 N. Scottsdale Rd.
Scottsdale, Ariz. 85260
Consumer Representative
602-998-6184 or 998-6347

Baskin Robbins 31 Ice Creams
Glendale, Calif. 92101
Manager, Publicity and Public Relations
818-956-0031

Beatrice Foods Co.
2 N. LaSalle St.
Chicago, Ill. 60602
Corporate Relations
312-558-4199

Borden, Inc.
180 E. Broad St.
Columbus, Ohio 43215
Manager, Consumer Response Dept.
614-225-4511

Campbell Soup Co.
Campbell Pl.
Camden, N.J. 08101
Director, Consumer Relations
609-342-4800

Carnation Co.
5045 Wilshire Blvd.
Los Angeles, Calif. 90036
Manager, Corporate Relations
213-932-6000

351

Dannon Company, Inc.
22-11 38th Ave.
Long Island City, N.Y. 11101
Director, Consumer Relations
718-361-2240

Del Monte Corp.
P.O. Box 3575
San Francisco, Calif. 94119
Supervisor, Consumer Affairs
415-442-4803

R. T. French Co.
One Mustard St.
P.O. Box 23450
Rochester, N.Y. 14692
Consumer Representative
716-482-8000

General Foods Corp.
250 North St.
White Plains, N.Y. 10625
Manager, Consumer Service
914-335-2500

Gerber Products Co.
445 State St.
Fremont, Mich. 49412
Supervisor, Consumer Relations
616-928-2000

H. J. Heinz Co.
1062 Progress St.
Pittsburgh, Pa. 15212
Manager, Consumer Relations
412-237-5740

Hershey Foods Corp.
14 E. Chocolate Ave.
P.O. Box 815
Hershey, Pa. 17033
Manager, Customer Relations
717-534-7500

Hunt-Wesson Foods, Inc.
1645 W. Valencia Dr.
Fullerton, Calif. 92634
Manager, Consumer Relations
714-680-1430

ITT Continental Baking Co.
Box 731
Halstead Avenue
Rye, N.Y. 10580
Director of Nutrition and Consumer Affairs
914-899-0225

Kellogg Co.
235 Porter St.
P.O. Box 3423
Battle Creek, Mich. 49016
Manager, Consumer Services Dept.
616-966-2268

Kentucky Fried Chicken
P.O. Box 32070
Louisville, Ky. 40232
Group Manager, Consumer Affairs
502-456-8300

Kraft Consumer Service
Retail Food Group, Kraft, Inc.
Glenview, Ill. 60025
Manager, Consumer Service
800-942-0481 (in Ill.); 800-323-0768
   (outside Ill.)

Land O'Lakes, Inc.
P.O. Box 116
Minneapolis, Minn. 55440
Director, Consumer Affairs
800-328-4155

Nabisco Brands, Inc.
Parsippany, N.J. 07054
Senior Manager, Consumer Information
201-898-7460

Nestle Foods Corp.
100 Bloomingdale Rd.
White Plains, N.Y. 10605
Manager, Consumer Affairs
914-682-6037

Ore-Ida Foods, Inc.
P.O. Box 10
Boise, Idaho 83707
Manager, Consumer Relations
208-383-6237

Pepperidge Farm, Inc.
Westport Ave.
Norwalk, Conn. 06856
Manager, Consumer Services
203-846-7276

Perdue Farms, Inc.
P.O. Box 1537
Salisbury, Md. 21801
Consumer Relations Coordinator
301-543-3000

Progresso Foods Corp.
365 W. Passaic St.
Rochelle Park, N.J. 07662
Consumer Relations Representative
201-368-9450

Swift & Co.
1919 Swift Dr.
Oak Brook, Ill. 60521
Manager, Consumer Communication
312-850-5966

Quaker Oats Co.
Merchandise Mart Plaza
Chicago, Ill. 60654
Consumer Response
312-222-7111

Welch Foods, Inc.
2 South Portage
Westfield, N.Y. 14787
Director, Corporate Communications
716-326-3131

Stouffer Foods
5750 Harper Rd.
Solon, Ohio 44139
Manager, Consumer Affairs
216-248-3600, ext. 2109

Wendy's International, Inc.
P.O. Box 256
Dublin, Ohio 43017
Community Affairs Manager
614-764-3100

Federal Agencies that Will Help

Federal agencies are constantly compiling statistics, analyzing facts and trends, and funding studies in areas related to consumer health and nutrition. This information is available to you, but it is sometimes difficult to obtain unless you know where to call or write. Here is a list of some of the most helpful agencies. If the person you reach cannot answer your question or send you the material you are seeking, you will often be referred to someone who can.

Agricultural Marketing Service
Dept. of Agriculture
Washington, D.C. 20250
202-447-8998

Bureau of Alcohol, Tobacco and Firearms
 (listed under *U.S. Government*)
Dept. of the Treasury
1200 Pennsylvania Ave., N. W.
Room 6211
Washington, D.C. 20226
202-535-6245

This bureau does for alcoholic beverages what the FDA does for most foods.

Consumer Information Center
Pueblo, Colo. 81009

There are a number of consumer publications on a wide variety of subjects constantly being prepared. Write for a free catalog. Some of the booklets are free; others cost only pennies.

Cooperative Extension Service
Dept. of Agriculture

This service has a number of branches in every state. Consult your local library for the one nearest you. Each branch is serviced by a nutritionist who will answer your nutrition questions and send you all sorts of helpful material, such as a list of foods rich in oat bran, the current U.S. RDA guidelines, and so on.

Food and Drug Administration
Consumer Affairs and Small Business Staff
   (HFO-22)
Dept. of Health and Human Services
5600 Fishers La., Room 13-55
Rockville, Md. 20857
301-443-4166

The FDA is supposed to be watchdog over most of the nation's food to determine the safety of additives such as artificial colors, flavors, etc., and to insure that your food is pure and wholesome and properly labeled (according to the regulations) regarding contents and ingredients. Questions in these areas should be directed to the Maryland staff. If, however, you think a food or beverage you have bought has something wrong with it—a bulging can of tomatoes, strange material in a soft drink container, frozen fish that doesn't seem to be what it says on the label—the place to call is your local FDA branch. You may find the number in your phone book under the U.S. Government listing for Health and Human Services, Food and Drug Administration. If you cannot find it, your local library can get the nearest branch number for you.

Food and Nutrition Service
Dept. of Agriculture
3101 Park Office Center Dr., Room 512
Alexandria, Va. 22302
703-756-3276

Human Nutrition Information Service
Dept. of Agriculture
Federal Bldg., Rooms 360 and 364
6605 Belcrest Rd.
Hyattsville, Md. 20782
301-436-8617

Meat and Poultry Hotline
Food Safety and Inspection Service
South Bldg., Room 1163
Dept. of Agriculture
Washington, D.C. 20250
800-535-4555

Use this number to report any untoward experience you may have with meat or poultry, or to ask any urgent question you may have about meat or poultry you have eaten.

Office of the Consumer Advisor
Dept. of Agriculture
Administration Bldg.
Washington, D.C. 20250
202-382-9681

Note: *If you have a problem but do not know which agency to contact, you can call the Federal Information Center (FIC) for advice and referral. There is at least one FIC in every state and your local library can give you the number.*

Bibliography

Action Levels for Poisonous or Deleterious Substances in Human Food and Animal Feed. Food and Drug Administration, Center for Food Safety and Applied Nutrition, Industry Programs Branch, Washington, D.C. 1985.

Agricultural Information Clearing House, Information Office of Public Affairs. Phone communications, various. USDA. Washington, D.C. 1985–86.

Alter, Stewart. "Nutrition: What's the Recommended Allowance in Food Advertising?" *Magazine Age*. December 1980.

Alternative Sweeteners. The Calorie Council, Atlanta, GA.

American Heart Association. "Statement About Results of Coronary Primary Prevention Trial. (CPPT)." NR 84–3362. Washington, D.C. Jan. 10, 1984.

Anderson R. "Chromium Intake, Absorption and Excretion of Subjects Consuming Self-Selected Diets." *American Journal of Clinical Nutrition*. Vol. 41. 1985.

"A Shoppers' Guide to Margarines." Health & Nutrition Newsletter, Columbia University School of Public Health & Institute of Human Nutrition, March 1986.

Barbour, Beverly Anderson. "Pros and Cons of Whole Grain Breads." *School Foodservice Journal*. July/August 1978.

Berg, Eric N. "The Sugar Industry Turns Up Its Sales Pitch." *The New York Times*. Nov. 17, 1985.

Boffey, Philip M. "Panel Suggests Role of Cyclamate in Cancer May Be an Indirect One." *The New York Times*. June 11, 1985.

Brody, Jane E. "Heart Disease: Big Study Produces New Data." *The New York Times*. Jan. 6, 1985.

Brown, J. J. et al. "Salt and Hypertension." *The Lancet*. Vol. 2. Aug. 25, 1984.

Brown, Dr. Virgil. "Some Ounces of Prevention That Lower Heart Risk." *The New York Times*. Aug. 31, 1986.

Brunton, Jerry. Animal Health Institute. Phone communication. Washington, D.C. 1985.

355

Burkett, Dennis P. "Dietary Fiber and Disease." *Journal of the American Medical Association*. Aug. 19, 1974.

Burros, Marion. "Diet Guidelines Revised by Heart Association." *The New York Times*. Aug. 27, 1986.

_____. "Those Old Saws About Food." *The New York Times*. July 19, 1986.

Code of Federal Regulation. Food Labeling. Title 21, Section 100–199. Current.

Cohen, J. D. "Role of Nutrition in the Management of Hypertension." *Clinical Nutrition*. Vol. 3. July/August 1984.

Cristol, Richard E., Deputy Director, Food Additives Council. Phone communication. Atlanta, GA. 1985.

Corn and Hog Farming. Office of Governmental and Public Affairs, U.S. Department of Agriculture. Washington, D.C. 1977.

Cronin, Frances. Diet Appraisal Research Branch, USDA. Phone communication. Beltsville, MD. 1985.

David, J. A. et al. "Glycemic index of foods: a physiological basis for carbohydrate exchange." *American Journal of Clinical Nutrition*. Vol. 34, no. 3. March 1981.

Denny, Cleve, Director of Research, National Food Processors Association. Phone communication. Washington, D.C. 1985.

Diet, Nutrition and Cancer Prevention. U.S. Department of Health and Human Services, Public Health Service and National Institutes of Health. 1985.

Dietary Guidelines for Americans. 2nd Ed. U.S. Department of Agriculture and U.S. Department of Health and Human Services. 1985.

"Dietary Guidelines Committee Stalls on Key Cholesterol Question." *Nutrition Action*. Center for Science in the Public Interest. July/August 1984.

Dignan, Dennis M., Food technologist, Plant and Protein Technology, FDA. Phone communication. Washington, D.C. 1985.

"Dyes in Your Food." Public Citizen Health Research Group Health Letter. March/April 1985.

Eater's Digest, Q&A. "Butter Buds and Egg Beaters." *Nutrition Action Health Letter*. Vol. 12, no. 6. July/August 1985.

Economic Effects of a Prohibition on the Use of Selected Animal Drugs. U.S. Department of Agriculture, Economics, Statistics and Cooperative Service. Agricultural Economic Report No. 414. Washington, D.C. November 1978.

Elsas, Louis, Director of Division of Medical Genetics, Emory University. Phone communication. Atlanta, GA. 1985.

Enig, Mary G. et al. "Dietary Fat and Cancer Trends—a Critique." *Federation Proceedings*. Vol. 37, no. 9. July 1978.

Environmental Nutrition. "Diet/Hypertension Research Update." Vol. 8, no. 5. May 1985.

Erwteman, T. M. et al. "Beta Blockade, Diuretics, and Salt Restriction for the Management of Mild Hypertension." *British Medical Journal*. Vol. 289. Aug. 4, 1984.

Fabricant, Florence. "On Display, 'Fresh' Food in Packages." *The New York Times*. Apr. 18, 1984.

"Fast Fries Fried in What?" Editorial. *The New York Times*. June 27, 1986.

FDA Enforcement Report. Dec. 19, 1979.

FDA Enforcement Report. Mar. 19, 1980.

FDA Enforcement Report. May 21, 1980.

FDA Enforcement Report. July 9, 1980.

"FDA Monitoring Programs for Pesticide and Industrial Chemical Residues in Food." 106 pages. Study Group on FDA Residue Programs, Department of Health, Education and Welfare, Public Health Service, FDA. Rockville, MD. 1979.

Fenner, Louise. "That Lite Stuff." *FDA Consumer*. June 1982.

"Fish, Fatty Acids, and Human Health." Editorial, *New England Journal of Medicine*. Vol. 312, no. 19. May 9, 1985.

Food Additives. International Food Additives Council. Atlanta, GA.

Food Defect Action Levels. Current Levels for Natural or Unavoidable Defects in Food for Human Use That Present No Health Hazard. U.S. Department of Health and Human Services, Public Health Service, Food and Drug Administration, Center for Food Safety and Applied Nutrition. Washington, D.C. Current through April 1984.

Friedwald, William T. Heart, Lung and Blood Institute, National Institutes of Health. Phone communications. Bethesda, MD. 1985.

"Fruit, Fish and Gamma Rays." Editorial. *The New York Times*. Sept. 24, 1986.

Furuya, E. M. et al. "Packaging Effects on Riboflavin Content of Pasta Products in Retail Markets." *Cereal Chemistry*, Vol. 61. September/October 1984.

Giddings, George. Isomedix, Inc. Correspondence and phone communications. Whippany, NJ. 1985.

Gillin, Francis D. University of California Medical Center. Phone communications. San Diego, CA. 1985–86.

Gofman, John. University of California at Berkeley. Phone communication. Berkeley, CA. 1985.

Goodman-Malamuth, Leslie. "McHeartbread. Cardiologists Underscore Dangers of a High-Fat Diet at Fast-Food Restaurants." *Nutrition Action Health Letter*. January 1986.

Greenberg, Richard. American Council on Science and Health. Washington, D.C. 1985.

"Growing Oranges." U.S. Department of Agriculture, Office of Governmental and Public Affairs. Washington, D.C. July 1978.

Hankin, Lester. "Quality of Tomato Paste, Sauce, Purée, and Catsup." A report of a cooperative study by the Connecticut Agricultural Experiment Station, New Haven, and the Food Division of the Connecticut Department of Consumer Protection. New Haven, CT. January 1986.

Hankin, Lester et al. "Comparison of Code Data Reliability for Freshly Bottled Whole, Lowfat and Nonfat Fluid Milk." *Journal of Food Protection*. Vol. 43, no. 3. March 1980.

———. "Keeping Quality of Pasteurized Milk for Retail Sale Related to Code Date, Storage Temperature, and Microbial Counts." *Journal of Food Protection*. Vol. 40, no. 12. December 1977.

_____. "Relation of Codes Dates to Quality of Milk Sold in Retail Markets." *Journal of Food Protection.* Vol. 43. New Haven, CT. February 1977.

_____. "Quality of Tofu and Other Soy Products." A cooperative study by the Connecticut Agricultural Experiment Station and the Connecticut Department of Consumer Protection. Bulletin No. 810. New Haven, CT. March 1983.

_____. "Quality of Butter and Blends of Butter with Oleomargarine." Bulletin No. 813. Connecticut Agricultural Experiment Station. New Haven, CT. July 1983.

Harper, Harold A. "Concerning Vitamins." *Western Journal of Medicine.* December 1978.

Hart, Ronald W. et al. *Report of the Color Additive Scientific Review Panel.* September 1985.

Havighorst, C. R. "Alaskan Pollock Builds New Seafood Industry." *Food Engineering.* Vol. 56. February 1984.

HHS News Release: P80–22. Food and Drug Administration. May 30, 1980.

Holmberg, S. D. et al. "Drug-resistant Salmonella from Animals Fed Antimicrobials." *New England Journal of Medicine.* Vol. 311. Sept. 6, 1984.

Holmberg, Scott. Phone communication. Center for Disease Control. Atlanta, GA. 1985.

Hopkins, Harold. "The Color Additive Scoreboard." *FDA Consumer.* Vol. 14, no. 2. March 1980.

Hulley, S. B. et al. "Alcohol Intake, Blood Lipids, and Mortality from Coronary Heart Disease." *Clinical Nutrition.* Vol. 3. July/August 1984.

Industry Programs Branch, Center for Food Safety and Applied Nutrition, FDA. Phone communication, various. Washington, D.C. 1985.

Interim Dietary Guidelines. Committee on Diet, Nutrition and Cancer of the National Research Council. March 1984.

"Is Irradiated Food Safe or Necessary?" Public Citizen Health Research Group Health Letter. March/April 1986.

Jacobson, Michael F. "Food Technology." *New England Journal of Medicine.* Vol. 313, no. 7. Aug. 15, 1985.

_____. "Undoing Delaney." Nutrition Action Health Letter. Vol. 12, no. 7. September/October 1985.

Jelinek, C. "Occurrence and Methods of Control of Chemical Contaminants in Foods." *Environmental Health Perspectives.* Vol. 39. 1981.

Keys to Quality. Food Buying Guides from USDA. U.S. Department of Agriculture, Agricultural Marketing Service. Slightly revised, July 1973.

Kornhauser, A. et al. "Effect of Dietary Beta-Carotene on Psoralen-Induced Phototoxicity." *Annals of the New York Academy of Science.* 1985:453:91–104.

Kromer, George. "Current Status and Future Market Potential for Cottonseed." Economic Research Service, U.S. Department of Agriculture. Dec. 13, 1977.

_____. "Market Situation for Oils and Fats and the Fatty Acid Industry." Pulp Chemicals Association Annual Meeting. San Diego, CA. Mar. 30, 1978.

_____. "U.S. Food Fat Consumption Trends." *The Fats and Oils Situation.* Economic Research Service, U.S. Department of Agriculture. April 1974.

_____. "World Fats and Oils Situation and U.S. Tallow Prospects." Economics, Statistics and Cooperative Services, U.S. Department of Agriculture. Oct. 31, 1978.

Kromer, George et al. *Fats and Oils Situations.* Economics, Statistics, and Cooperatives Services, U.S. Department of Agriculture. February 1979.

Kromhout, Daan, et al. "The Inverse Relation Between Fish Consumption and 20-year Mortality from Coronary Heart Disease." *New England Journal of Medicine.* Vol. 312, no. 19. May 9, 1985.

Kulkarni, K. "Advice from the Dietitians: Sweeteners: Past, Present and Future." *Diabetes Educator.* Vol. 9. Winter 1984.

La Vecchia, C. et al. "Dietary Vitamin A and the Risk of Invasive Cervical Cancer." *Int. J. Cancer.* 1984:34:319–322.

Lecos, Chris. "Fructose: Questionable Diet Aid." *FDA Consumer.* Vol. 14, no. 2. March 1980.

Lenfant, Claude et al. Science Press Briefing on the Lipid Research Clinics Coronary Primary Prevention Trial (LRC-CPPT). Lister Hill Auditorium, National Institutes of Health. Bethesda, MD. Jan. 12, 1984.

Le Riche, W. Harding. *A Chemical Feast.* Facts on File Publications. New York. 1982.

Leverton, Ruth M. *Fats in Food and Diet.* Agriculture Information Bulletin No. 361. U.S. Department of Agriculture. Washington, D.C. November 1974.

Levinson, S. et al. "Supplemental Vitamin A Prevents the Acute Radiation-Induced Defects in Wound Healing." *Annals of Surgery.* 1984:200:494–5121.

Levy, Stuart B. Tufts University School of Medicine, New England Medical Center. Phone communication. Boston, MA. 1985.

Liebman, Bonnie F. "Light Foods You Can Lean On." Nutrition Action Health Letter. Vol. 13, no. 8. September 1986.

Lukaski, Henry C. Agricultural Research Service, Human Nutrition Research Center. Phone communications. USDA. Grand Forks, ND. 1985.

Lukaski, Henry C. et al. "Influence of type and amount of dietary lipid on plasma lipid concentrations in endurance athletes." *American Journal of Clinical Nutrition.* January 1984.

McMichael, John. "Fats and Atheroma: An Inquest." *British Medical Journal.* Jan. 20, 1979.

McNiel, Douglas W. "Impact of Mechanically Boning Red Meats." *National Food Review.* April 1978.

"Magazine Nutrition Tips Often Have the Wrong Ingredients." *Magazine Age.* December 1984.

"Margarine, the Better Butter?" *Consumer Reports.* February 1979.

Maserei, I., L. Rouse. "Effects of a Lacto-ovo Vegetarian Diet on Serum Concentrations of Cholesterol, Triglyceride, HDL-C, HDL2-C, HDL3-C, Apoprotein-B and Lip(a)." *American Journal of Clinical Nutrition.* Vol. 40. September 1984.

Meat and Poultry Inspection. The Scientific Basis of the Nation's Program. Prepared by the Committee on the Scientific Basis of the Nation's Meat and Poultry Inspection Program, Food and Nutrition Board, Commission on Life Sciences, National Research Council. 209 pages. National Academy Press. Washington, D.C. 1985.

Meggos, H. N. "Colors—Key Food Ingredients." *Food Technology*. Vol. 39: January 1984.

Meister, Kathleen A. et al. *Antibiotics in Animal Feed: A Threat to Human Health?* American Council on Science and Health. Summit, NJ.

Muller, H. G. and Tobin, G. *Nutrition and Food Processing*. Avi Publishing Co. Westport, CT. 1980.

"Nitrite Levels in Bacon." Food Safety and Inspection Service, USDA. Rules and Regulations, Federal Register. Vol. 51, no. 115. June 16, 1986.

"No Need to Cry Over Spoiled Milk." *Environmental Nutrition*. Vol. 8, no. 3. March 1985.

"Nutrition and Diet Exchange Information: Lean Cuisine." Stouffer Foods Corporation. Solon, OH. 1981.

"Nutrition in Your Garden." Press Service Sheet. National Garden Bureau, Inc. Willowbrook, IL. August 1984.

"Nutrition Labeling—Terms You Should Know." FDA Consumer Memo. Rockville, MD. March 1974.

"Oat Bran's Cholesterol-Lowering Effect Reviewed." *Nutrition Report*. April 1986.

Oliver, Thomas. *The Real Coke, The Real Story*. Random House, NY. 1986.

Ono, K. et al. "Nutrient Composition of Lamb of Two Age Groups." *Journal of Food Science*. Vol. 49. September/October 1984.

Pardridge, William. University of California at Los Angeles. Phone communication. 1985.

Pear, Robert. "Labeling for Food to Be Broadened." *The New York Times*. Aug. 18, 1985.

Pennington, Jean A. Thompson. *Dietary Nutrient Guide*. Avi Publishing Co. Westport, CT. 1983.

Phillipson, Beverly E. et al. "Reduction of Plasma Lipids, Lipoproteins, and Apoproteins by Dietary Fish Oils in Patients with Hypertriglyceridemia." *New England Journal of Medicine*. Vol. 312, no. 19. May 9, 1985.

Pinckney, Edward R. "The Biological Toxicity of Polyunsaturated Fats." Paper presented at 22nd annual Minnesota Academy of Family Physician's Refresher. Minneapolis, MN. Apr. 5, 1972.

_____. "The Potential Toxicity of Excessive Polyunsaturates." *American Heart Journal*. Vol. 85, no. 6. June 1973.

_____. "Is Commercialism Controlling the Controversy Over Cholesterol?" *Medical Counterpoint*. Vol. 3, no. 5. May 1971.

Pinckney, Edward R. et al. "Vitamin E: Some Negative Observations on Alleged Positive Actions and Some Potential Adverse Reactions." Research Foundation for Plastic Surgery, Beverly Hills, CA. 1975.

Pollack, Earl S. et al. "Prospective Study of Alcohol Consumption and Cancer." *New England Journal of Medicine*. Vol. 310, no. 10. March 8, 1984.

Potter, Norman N. *Food Science*. 4th ed. Avi Publishing Co. Westport, CN. 1986.

Prince, Jeffrey, Director, National Association of Restaurants. Phone communication. Washington, D.C. 1985.

Russell, L. F. et al. "Vitamin C Content of Fresh Spinach." Food Research Institute, Agriculture Canada. Ontario, Can. November 1983.

Schmeck, Harold M., Jr. "Hunger for Salt Found to Be Powerful Instinct." *The New York Times:* Aug. 9, 1983.

Schroeder, Henry A. "Losses of vitamins and trace minerals resulting from processing and preservation of foods." *American Journal of Clinical Nutrition.* May 1971.

Schweigert, B. S. "The Food Ingredients Dilemma in the Modern Marketplace." *Food Technology.* Vol. 38. January 1984.

Shepherd, James et al. "Effects of Dietary Polyunsaturated and Saturated Fat on the Properties of High Density Lipoproteins and the Metabolism of Apolipoprotein A-1." *Journal for Clinical Investigation.* American Society for Clinical Investigation. August 1977.

Snyder, P. O. et al. "Effect of Hot-Holding on Nutritional Quality of Food." *School Food Service Research Review.* Vol. 8. Spring 1984.

Somers, Ira I. *Food Labeling. Some Questions Answered.* National Canners Association. Washington, D.C. 1971.

"Sweet Talk About Sweetened Cereals." *Consumer Reports.* March 1978.

"Sweeteners: Are Any of Them Safe?" *Consumer Reports.* November 1985.

"Tainted Cheeses: How Dangerous?" *The New York Times.* Aug. 27, 1986.

"Termite's Delight. These Breads Get Their Fiber from Wood Pulp." *Nutrition Action Health Letter.* Vol. 12, no. 7. September/October 1985.

Tritsch, George L. "Irradiated Food." Letters to the Editor. *The New York Times."* June 30, 1986.

Tucker, Kitty, President, Health and Energy Institute. Interview. Washington, D.C. 1985.

Underwood, E. J. *Trace Elements in Human and Animal Nutrition.* Academic Press. New York. 1977.

Urbain, Walter. Michigan State University. Phone communications. East Lansing, MI. 1985–86.

U.S. Fats and Oils Statistics, 1961–1976. Economic Research Service, U.S. Department of Agriculture. Washington, D.C. June 1977.

Valberg, L. S. et al. "Effects of Iron, Tin and Copper on Zinc Absorption in Humans." *American Journal of Clinical Nutrition.* Vol. 40. September 1984.

Vetter, J. L. "Fiber as a Food Ingredient." *Food Technology.* Vol. 38. January 1984.

"Vitamin Nutrition and the American Consumer. A Position Paper for Industry." Food Department, Roche Chemical Division, Hoffman–La Roche, Inc.

Vuolo, L. et al. "Review: Putative Mutagens and Carcinogens in Foods." *Environmental Mutagen.* 1985:7:577–598.

Wahl, P. W. et al. "Distribution of Lipoprotein Tryglyceride and Lipoprotein Cholesterol in an Adult Population by Age, Sex and Hormone Use." Pacific Northwest Bell Telephone Co. Health survey reported in *Atherosclerosis.* Vol. 39. 1981.

Wang, Chi-Sun. Oklahoma Medical Research Center. Phone communications. Oklahoma City, OK. 1985.

Weimer, Jon. "Nutrition Labeling: The Unresolved Issues." *National Food Review.* U.S. Department of Agriculture, Economics, Statistics and Cooperatives Service. Washington, D.C. Summer 1980.

"What Is Food to One . . ." Editorial, *New England Journal of Medicine.* Vol. 311, no. 6. Aug. 9, 1984.

Wholesomeness of Irradiated Food. Joint FAO/IAEA/WHO Expert Committee Report. Technical Report Series 659. World Health Organization. Geneva, Switzerland. 1981.

Wilkins, Tracy. Virginia Polytechnic Institute and State University. Phone communications. Blacksburg, VA. 1985.

Willett, Walter C. et al. "Diet and Cancer—an Overview." *New England Journal of Medicine.* Vol. 310, no. 10. Mar. 8, 1984.

Williams, Roger J. et al. *A Physician's Handbook on Orthomolecular Medicine.* Keats Publishing. New Canaan, CT. 1979.

Yale Medical Library, Computer Search Service, New Haven, CT. Various citations.

Yogogoshi, H. et al. "Effects of Aspartame and Glucose Administration on Brain and Plasma Levels of Large Neutral Amino Acids and Brain 5-Hydroxyindoles." *American Journal of Clinical Nutrition.* Vol. 40. July 1984.

Index